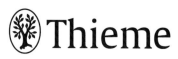

# Skull Base Cancer Imaging

## The Practical Approach to Diagnosis and Treatment Planning

**Eugene Yu, MD, FRCPC**
Associate Professor of Radiology and Otolaryngology–Head and Neck Surgery
University of Toronto
Toronto Joint Department of Medical Imaging
University Health Network
Princess Margaret Cancer Centre
Mount Sinai Hospital and Women's College Hospital
Toronto, Ontario, Canada

**Reza Forghani, MD, PhD, FRCPC**
Associate Chief
Department of Radiology
Jewish General Hospital
Assistant Professor of Radiology
McGill University
Clinical Investigator
Segal Cancer Centre and Lady Davis Institute for Medical Research
Jewish General Hospital and McGill University
Montreal, Québec, Canada

813 illustrations

Thieme
New York • Stuttgart • Delhi • Rio de Janeiro

Executive Editor: William Lamsback
Managing Editor: J. Owen Zurhellen IV
Director, Editorial Services: Mary Jo Casey
Production Editor: Naamah Schwartz
International Production Director: Andreas Schabert
Editorial Director: Sue Hodgson
International Marketing Director: Fiona Henderson
International Sales Director: Louisa Turrell
Director of Institutional Sales: Adam Bernacki
Senior Vice President and Chief Operating Officer: Sarah Vanderbilt
President: Brian D. Scanlan

**Library of Congress Cataloging-in-Publication Data**

Names: Yu, Eugene, editor. | Forghani, Reza, editor.
Title: Skull base cancer imaging : the practical approach to
   diagnosis and treatment planning / [edited by] Eugene Yu,
   Reza Forghani.
Description: First edition. | New York : Thieme, [2018]
   | Includes index.
Identifiers: LCCN 2017018194 (print) | LCCN 2017019519 (ebook)
   | ISBN 9781626232976 (E-book) | ISBN 9781626232969
   (hardcover : alk. paper)
Subjects:  | MESH: Skull Base Neoplasms–diagnostic imaging
Classification: LCC RD529 (ebook) | LCC RD529 (print) |
   NLM WE 707 | DDC  617.514–dc23
LC record available at https://lccn.loc.gov/2017018194

**Important note:** Medicine is an ever-changing science undergoing continual development. Research and clinical experience are continually expanding our knowledge, in particular our knowledge of proper treatment and drug therapy. Insofar as this book mentions any dosage or application, readers may rest assured that the authors, editors, and publishers have made every effort to ensure that such references are in accordance with **the state of knowledge at the time of production of the book.**

Nevertheless, this does not involve, imply, or express any guarantee or responsibility on the part of the publishers in respect to any dosage instructions and forms of applications stated in the book. **Every user is requested to examine carefully** the manufacturers' leaflets accompanying each drug and to check, if necessary in consultation with a physician or specialist, whether the dosage schedules mentioned therein or the contraindications stated by the manufacturers differ from the statements made in the present book. Such examination is particularly important with drugs that are either rarely used or have been newly released on the market. Every dosage schedule or every form of application used is entirely at the user's own risk and responsibility. The authors and publishers request every user to report to the publishers any discrepancies or inaccuracies noticed. If errors in this work are found after publication, errata will be posted at www.thieme.com on the product description page.

Some of the product names, patents, and registered designs referred to in this book are in fact registered trademarks or proprietary names even though specific reference to this fact is not always made in the text. Therefore, the appearance of a name without designation as proprietary is not to be construed as a representation by the publisher that it is in the public domain.

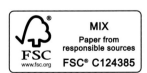

For Grace, Ryan, Charlotte, and my parents

*– Eugene Yu*

To my beautiful wife Veronika, my children Olivia and Alexander, and my parents

*– Reza Forghani*

# Contents

# Foreword

It is a distinct honor to have been invited to write the Foreword for this timely book that highlights and summarizes the current knowledge of imaging as it pertains to the expanding and complex field of skull base cancer. The editors of this text are very well known to me and have made valuable contributions to the field of head and neck diagnostic imaging that have helped to advance knowledge and improve patient diagnosis and care.

The list of contributors that Dr. Yu and Dr. Forghani have recruited for this book reads like a "Who's Who" from the field of skull base cancer imaging, surgery, and radiation therapy. They have selected a most balanced and outstanding group of experts who in each chapter have thoughtfully and skillfully presented a very comprehensive review of the current state of knowledge of skull base imaging and therapy. The textbook includes a very detailed analysis of the various anatomical sites, an understanding of the pathways of tumor spread, and the role of clinical imaging in the diagnosis and treatment of skull base cancer. The material is presented in a clear and concise fashion that includes both critical and contrasting viewpoints for the reader. The book chronicles the current knowledge of understanding that optimizes the best diagnostic radiologic investigations in disease diagnosis and treatment. This text is a most valuable contribution to head and neck oncology and should be considered as compulsory reading for trainees across the disciplines involved in caring for our patients.

Armed with the knowledge contained in this book, clinicians should feel confident that the information provides the best known imaging techniques to help in the diagnosis and treatment planning for our specialties at this time. My congratulations therefore to the editors and authors for their impressive contributions which have culminated in a most comprehensive book.

*Patrick Gullane*
*CM, OOnt, MB, FRCSC, FACS, Hon FRACS, Hon FRCS, Hon FRCSI*
*Wharton Chair in Head and Neck Surgery*
*Past Chair of Otolaryngology–Head and Neck Surgery*
*Professor of Otolaryngology–Head and Neck Surgery*
*Professor of Surgery*
*University of Toronto*
*Toronto, Ontario, Canada*

# Preface

It seems appropriate that the genesis of *Skull Base Cancer Imaging* was during the 25th Annual North American Skull Base Society (NASBS) meeting in Tampa, Florida. Dr. Reza Forghani and I were attending the meeting and had wandered over to the Thieme display booth and ran into Timothy Hiscock. I know Mr. Hiscock very well as he was my editor on another textbook a few years prior. While we were commenting on how beautiful the books were, Tim casually mentioned that the "one thing missing was an up-to-date textbook on skull base imaging." Then came that silent moment with Tim just looking at me as if to say "now this is where you come in." While apprehensive about diving into another textbook endeavor, the opportunity to develop, write, and edit a textbook on a topic that I finding truly fascinating was just too tempting to pass up. This is especially true when that opportunity allowed me to work with a very close friend and colleague such as Reza.

The NASBS meeting is a true multidisciplinary event that brings together the full spectrum of professionals—surgeons, radiation and medical oncologists, pathologists, speech pathologists and radiologists, etc. Experts from each of these specialties are needed to properly treat patients with skull base cancer. Both Reza and I, as radiologists, realize that we are only a small piece of the multidisciplinary team that needs to work together for our patients. As such, when creating the template for this textbook, which is first and foremost an imaging textbook, we realized that it was of utmost importance to have the active input and participation of our colleagues. As head and neck radiologists, our job is to detect and accurately map out the extent of disease. The recognition of certain critical imaging features can have a profound influence on staging and prognosis and can guide and alter treatment options and protocols. This was something that we wanted to highlight in each of the chapters. The individuals who are most knowledgeable about such features are our clinician colleagues. We realized that in order for this imaging textbook to have the best chance to succeed and to have the greatest possible value for the reader, we needed the active input of our clinical colleagues as co-authors and collaborators. We also realized that in any field of medicine, there are always many and, at times, contrasting viewpoints. Thus we made it a point to involve and recruit colleagues from some of the largest, most experienced academic institutions in North America and beyond that, who treat skull base disease. The result is a multidisciplinary as well as a multicenter volume of work.

This book comprehensively covers the various neoplastic diseases that affect the skull base. We have done this by taking an anatomic approach—by dividing the skull base into various anatomic compartments. An overview of the anatomy of each region is first presented, followed by a discussion of the neoplasms that can arise in those locations. Not only are the key differentiating imaging features presented, but the pathophysiology, prognosis, and treatment options are also discussed.

We hope that our book will be of value not just to radiologists, but also to any of our clinical colleagues who are involved in the care of patients with skull base cancer.

*Eugene Yu, MD, FRCPC*

# Acknowledgments

We would like to sincerely thank J. Owen Zurhellen, William Lamsback, and Timothy Hiscock from Thieme Publishers for their support. We also wish to sincerely thank and acknowledge the incredible work and support of our colleagues who participated in this endeavor. And finally we would like to thank our respective families—Grace, Ryan, Charlotte, Veronika, Alexander, and little Olivia—for putting up with us while we spent many hours sequestered away writing and editing.

# Contributors

**Laila S. Alshafai, MBBS, FRCPC**
Assistant Professor
Diagnostic Neuroradiologist, Head and Neck Imaging
Mount Sinai Hospital and University Health Network
Division of Neuroradiology
University of Toronto
Toronto, Ontario, Canada

**Nabeel S. Alshafai, MD, FRCSC, EBNS**
Assistant Professor
Consultant Neurosurgeon and Spine Surgeon
University of Antwerp
Antwerp, Belgium

**Gregory J. Basura, MD, PhD**
Assistant Professor
Department of Otolaryngology–Head and Neck Surgery
Division of Otology/Neurotology-Skull Base Surgery
University of Michigan
Ann Arbor, Michigan

**Aditya Bharatha, MD, FRCPC**
Diagnostic and Interventional Neuroradiology
Division Head, Neuroradiology
Department of Medical Imaging
St. Michael's Hospital
Assistant Professor
University of Toronto
Toronto, Ontario, Canada

**Scott V. Bratman, MD, PhD, FRCPC**
Assistant Professor
Clinician-Scientist, Radiation Medicine Program
Princess Margaret Cancer Centre
Department of Radiation Oncology
University of Toronto
Toronto, Ontario, Canada

**Christopher J. Chin, MD, FRCSC**
Head and Neck Oncology, Anterior Skull Base, and
  Rhinology
Department of Otolaryngology–Head and Neck Surgery
University of Toronto
Toronto, Ontario, Canada

**Hugh D. Curtin, MD**
Professor of Radiology
Chief of Radiology
Massachusetts Eye and Ear Infirmary
Harvard Medical School
Boston, Massachusetts

**Michael D. Cusimano, MD, MHPE, FRCSC, DABNS, PhD, FACS**
Professor of Surgery
Department of Surgery
Division of Neurosurgery
St. Michael's Hospital
University of Toronto
Toronto, Ontario, Canada

**John R. de Almeida, MD, MSc, FRCSC**
Head and Neck Surgeon
University Health Network, Mount Sinai Hospital
Assistant Professor
Department of Otolaryngology–Head and Neck Surgery
University of Toronto
Toronto, Ontario, Canada

**Sheldon D.S. Derkatch, MD, BSc, FRCPC**
Clinical Neuroradiology Fellow
Department of Medical Imaging
University of Toronto
Toronto, Ontario, Canada

**Adam A. Dmytriw, MD, MSc**
University Health Network, Princess Margaret Cancer
  Centre
Department of Medical Imaging
Faculty of Medicine
University of Toronto
Toronto, Ontario, Canada

**Reza Forghani, MD, PhD, FRCPC**
Associate Chief
Department of Radiology
Jewish General Hospital
Assistant Professor of Radiology
McGill University
Clinical Investigator
Segal Cancer Centre and Lady Davis Institute for Medical
  Research
Jewish General Hospital and McGill University
Montreal, Québec, Canada

**Ehab Y. Hanna, MD, FACS**
Professor and Vice Chairman
Director of Skull Base Surgery
Department of Head and Neck Surgery
Medical Director, Head and Neck Center
University of Texas MD Anderson Cancer Center
Houston, Texas

**Chris Heyn, MD, PhD, FRCP(C)**
Assistant Professor
Department of Medical Imaging
University of Toronto
Associate Scientist
Sunnybrook Research Institute
Staff Neuroradiologist
Sunnybrook Health Sciences Centre
Toronto, Ontario, Canada

**Walter Kucharczyk, MD, FRCPC**
Professor
Departments of Medical Imaging and Surgery
  (Neurosurgery)
University of Toronto
Neuroradiologist
Toronto Joint Department of Medical Imaging
Toronto, Ontario, Canada

**Amy W. Lin, MD, FRCPC**
Lecturer
St. Michael's Hospital
Department of Medical Imaging
University of Toronto
Toronto, Ontario, Canada

**Vincent Lin, MD, FRCSC**
Associate Professor, Associate Scientist
Department of Otolaryngology–Head and Neck Surgery
Sunnybrook Research Institute
Sunnybrook Health Sciences Centre
Institute of Medical Sciences
Faculty of Medicine
University of Toronto
Toronto, Ontario, Canada

**Nidal Muhanna, MD, PhD**
Head and Neck Surgical Oncology and Reconstructive
  Microsurgery
Department of Otolaryngology–Head and Neck Surgery
University Health Network
University of Toronto
Toronto, Ontario, Canada

**Brian O'Sullivan, MD, FRCPC, FRCPI, FFRRCSI (Hon),
  FASTRO (Editor-in-Chief)**
Professor, Department of Radiation Oncology
Bartley-Smith/Wharton Chair in Radiation Oncology
Princess Margaret Cancer Centre
University of Toronto
Toronto, Ontario, Canada

**Almudena Perez-Lara, MD, PhD**
Head and Neck Radiology Fellow
Department of Radiology
Jewish General Hospital and McGill University
Montreal, Québec, Canada

**John A. Rutka, MD, FRCSC**
Professor of Otolaryngology–Head and Neck Surgery
University of Toronto
Staff Otologist/Neurotologist
University Health Network
Toronto, Ontario, Canada

**Arjun Sahgal, MD, FRCPC**
Associate Professor of Radiation Oncology and Surgery
Deputy Chief, Department of Radiation Oncology
Site Group Leader, CNS Oncology
Clinician Scientist, Sunnybrook Research Institute
Affiliate Scientist, Toronto Western Research Institute
Director of the Cancer Ablation Therapy/MR Linac Program
Department of Radiation Oncology
University of Toronto
Sunnybrook Health Sciences Centre
Toronto, Ontario, Canada

**Rickin Shah, MD**
Assistant Professor
Department of Radiology
University of Michigan Health System
Ann Arbor, Michigan

**Peter Som, MD, FACR**
Professor of Radiology, Otolaryngology–Head and Neck
  Surgery and Radiation Oncology
Mount Sinai School of Medicine of New York University
Chief of Head and Neck Imaging Section
Mount Sinai Medical Center
New York, New York

**Ashok Srinivasan, MD**
Professor of Radiology
Director of Neuroradiology
Department of Radiology
University of Michigan Health System
Ann Arbor, Michigan

**Sean Symons, BASc, MPH, MD, FRCPC, MBA**
Deputy Radiologist-In-Chief and Head
  Division of Neuroradiology
Department of Medical Imaging
Sunnybrook Health Sciences Centre
Associate Professor
Departments of Medical Imaging and Otolaryngology–
  Head and Neck Surgery
University of Toronto
Toronto, Ontario, Canada

**Allan D. Vescan, MD, MSc, FRCSC**
Assistant Professor
Director of Undergraduate Medical Education
Department of Otolaryngology–Head and Neck Surgery
Faculty of Medicine, University of Toronto
Mount Sinai Hospital
Toronto, Ontario, Canada

**Ian J. Witterick, MD, MSc, FRCSC**
Professor and Chair
Otolaryngologist-in-Chief
Mount Sinai Hospital
Department of Otolaryngology–Head and Neck Surgery
Faculty of Medicine
University of Toronto
Toronto, Ontario, Canada

**Eugene Yu, MD, FRCPC**
Associate Professor of Radiology and Otolaryngology–Head
  and Neck Surgery
University of Toronto
Toronto Joint Department of Medical Imaging
University Health Network
Princess Margaret Cancer Centre
Mount Sinai Hospital and Women's College Hospital
Toronto, Ontario, Canada

# 1 Anterior Cranial Fossa, Nasal Cavity, and Paranasal Sinuses

*Sheldon D.S. Derkatch, Ian J. Witterick, Scott V. Bratman, Almudena Perez-Lara, Hugh D. Curtin, and Reza Forghani*

## 1.1 Introduction

The anterior skull base, nasal cavity, and paranasal sinuses can be affected by a diverse group of neoplastic and nonneoplastic pathology that may transgress the boundaries between these or other adjacent spaces. Understanding the close relationship, patterns of disease spread, and potential complications is essential for optimal diagnostic evaluation of this area. In the case of malignant disease, accurate identification of tumor extent is essential for appropriate staging and preoperative planning and to ensure an optimal resection margin and the best possible outcome for the patient. In this chapter, we will provide an overview of the imaging characteristics of the large array of common and uncommon pathology affecting these regions. However, beyond the morphologic imaging characteristics, we will emphasize clinically important features or patterns of spread, supplemented by commonly used current treatment paradigms. In doing so, it is our hope not to be limited by imaging findings alone but rather focus and emphasize those findings that have the greatest clinical relevance and impact on patient care. In order to help better understand the anatomic pathways of disease spread and anatomic variants that can predispose to complications and are of importance for surgical planning, this chapter will begin with a brief overview of embryologic development, followed by a clinically oriented review of imaging anatomy.

## 1.2 Embryological Development

The formation of the structures constituting the face, paranasal sinuses, and skull base is achieved through an elaborate, highly orchestrated series of cell migration, proliferation, and differentiation controlled by complex cascades of cell signaling systems. A detailed discussion of the embryological development of the anterior skull base and paranasal sinuses is beyond the scope of this chapter and covered in detail elsewhere.[1,2] The purpose of this section is to provide a brief and broad overview of the development of these structures to highlight some key milestones and structures that may help the reader understand important anatomic landmarks, functional units, and basis for variations that may be encountered in clinical practice.

### 1.2.1 Development of the Anterior Skull Base

The cartilaginous neurocranium or chondrocranium forms the base of the developing skull through fusion of adjacent cartilages. The skull base is formed mainly by endochondral ossification, whereas the calvarial vault is mainly formed by membranous ossification.[2,3] Numerous ossification centers are involved in the development of the skull base, but the major ossification centers present at birth are the basioccipital center, the basisphenoidal center, and the presphenoidal center giving rise to the basiocciput, basisphenoid (postsphenoid), and presphenoid, respectively. The orbitosphenoid cartilage, alisphenoid cartilage center, and condensed mesenchyme (intramembranous bone) give rise to the more lateral parts of the sphenoid/sphenoid wings.[4] At birth, there is very limited ossification of the anterior skull base.[5] Ossification of the skull base occurs in an orderly fashion in the first 2 years of life from posterior to anterior and lateral to medial, and by 24 months of age, the anterior skull base is nearly completely ossified. However, small gaps may persist in the nasal roof until 3 years of age and the foramen cecum may ossify as late as 5 years of age.[3]

### 1.2.2 Development of the Nasal Cavity and Paranasal Sinuses

Nasal cavity and subsequent paranasal sinus development begins at the frontonasal prominence with the formation of bilateral oval thickenings of the surface ectoderm, referred to as nasal placodes, that are present by the end of the fourth week.[1,2] Subsequently, these recede into flat depressions called nasal pits (the primordia of anterior nares or future nostrils). From the fifth week of gestation, the nasal pits deepen toward the oral cavity, eventually resulting in an open communication between the oral and nasal cavities. An elaborate cascade of growth and fusion then leads to the downward growth of the nasal septum, formation of the definitive secondary palate, and other structures constituting the nasal cavity. Ectodermal epithelium at the roof of the nasal cavity differentiates into the olfactory epithelium, with the development of olfactory receptor cells having axons that lead into the developing olfactory bulbs.

All paranasal sinuses begin as evaginations or diverticula located along the walls of the nasal cavities that evolve into air-filled cavities in the adjacent bones.[6] As such, they are lined by a pseudostratified columnar-ciliated epithelium similar to that lining the nasal cavity. In adults, the diverticular origins persist as the sinus orifices. The maxillary sinus is the first paranasal sinus to form during fetal life. At birth, the maxillary sinuses are rudimentary and grow slowly until puberty. Full development of the maxillary sinuses occurs after eruption of permanent maxillary dentition at approximately 20 years of age.[7] The ethmoid air cells are the first sinuses to fully develop. At birth, the ethmoid air cells are fully developed in number but not in size. Thereafter, there is progressive development and growth of the ethmoid air cells, and by approximately 12 years of age, the ethmoid air cells have reached their adult size.[6]

The frontal sinus first begins with the appearance of the frontal recess in the lateral nasal cavity wall.[6] A series of pits or furrows then develop in the frontal recess that represent rudimentary ethmoid air cells, each of which has the potential to form the frontal sinus. Occasionally, the frontal sinus may also develop from an ethmoid air cell that has migrated from the ethmoid infundibulum rather than the frontal recess. The main development of the frontal sinus occurs in the postnatal period, with the sinus slowly enlarging to reach maximal adult size near the end of the second decade of life.[6]

At birth, the sphenoid sinus is devoid of air, containing red marrow. Conversion of red to fatty marrow occurs between 7 and 24 months of age and is believed to first start in the presphenoid.[8,9] Marrow conversion then extends more posteriorly into the basisphenoid. The sphenoid sinus starts its major growth in the third to fifth year of life, typically reaching adult configuration by the age of 12 years.[6] The process of pneumatization is typically preceded by fatty marrow conversion. In rare cases, premature arrest of sinus development is proposed as a potential etiology for alterations in the appearance of the skull base that can mimic pathology, referred to as arrested pneumatization of the skull base.[10] These are typically located in the basisphenoid or adjacent skull base. They appear nonexpansile with sclerotic borders, internal fat, and internal curvilinear calcifications and should be recognized as a developmental variant and not misinterpreted as a pathologic process (▶ Fig. 1.1).

# 1.3 Anatomy Overview: Applied Anatomy and Clinically Relevant Variants

## 1.3.1 Anterior Skull Base

The anterior skull base can be broadly described as constituting the floor of the anterior cranial fossa and the roof of the nose, ethmoid air cells, and orbits.[3,11] Posteriorly, the anterior skull base is formed by the lesser wings and anterior body of the sphenoid bone, including the planum sphenoidale, tuberculum sella, and anterior clinoid processes. The bones forming the anterior skull base are the ethmoid (cribriform plate) centrally and the horizontal portion (orbital plate) of the frontal bone more laterally, the latter forming the greater part of the anterior cranial fossa (▶ Fig. 1.2, ▶ Fig. 1.3). More posteriorly, the anterior skull base is formed by part of the body (planum sphenoidale) and lesser wing of the sphenoid bone (▶ Fig. 1.2, ▶ Fig. 1.3). The planum sphenoidale, also sometimes referred to as the jugum sphenoidale, refers to the central plane of the intracranial surface of the sphenoid bone that is anterior to the sella turcica and in between the lesser wings of the sphenoid

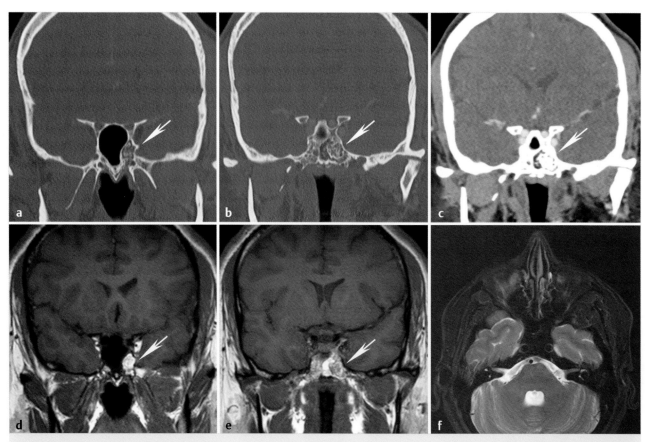

**Fig. 1.1** Arrested pneumatization of the sphenoid sinus. Coronal reformatted images from a high-resolution contrast-enhanced CT displayed in bone (**a,b**) and soft-tissue windows (**c**) demonstrate a nonexpansile, nonaggressive lesion in the basisphenoid with sclerotic borders and internal curvilinear densities/calcifications (*arrow*). The lesion is broader on the left side. A fatty component is clearly seen medially in the lesion on CT (**c**) and high-signal fatty content of the lesion is even better seen on the coronal T1-weighted MR images (**d,e**), with suppression of fat signal resulting in low signal on the axial fat-suppressed T2-weighted image (**f**).

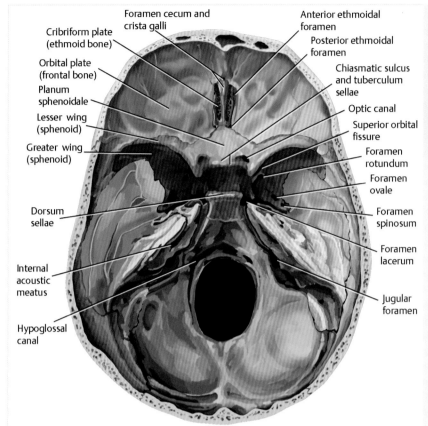

Foramen cecum and crista galli

Cribriform plate (ethmoid bone)

Orbital plate (frontal bone)

Planum sphenoidale

Lesser wing (sphenoid)

Greater wing (sphenoid)

Dorsum sellae

Internal acoustic meatus

Hypoglossal canal

Anterior ethmoidal foramen

Posterior ethmoidal foramen

Chiasmatic sulcus and tuberculum sellae

Optic canal

Superior orbital fissure

Foramen rotundum

Foramen ovale

Foramen spinosum

Foramen lacerum

Jugular foramen

**Fig. 1.2** Anatomy of the skull base, intracranial view. Illustration of the intracranial aspect of the skull base. The anterior skull base can be broadly described as constituting the floor of the anterior cranial fossa, roof of the nose, ethmoid air cells, and orbits anteriorly and the lesser wings and anterior body of the sphenoid bone (planum sphenoidale) posteriorly. Cribriform plate/ethmoid bone (*purple*), frontal bones (*tan*), occipital bone (*green*), parietal bones (*pink*), sphenoid bone (*red*), temporal bones (*grey*).

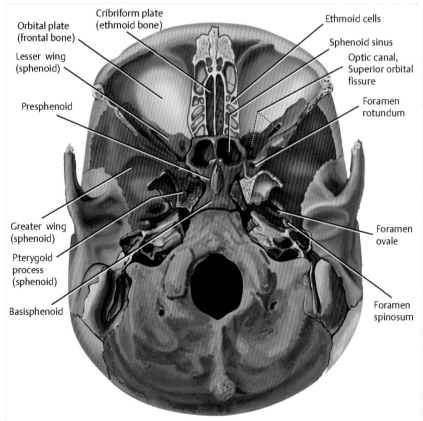

Orbital plate (frontal bone)

Lesser wing (sphenoid)

Presphenoid

Greater wing (sphenoid)

Pterygoid process (sphenoid)

Basisphenoid

Cribriform plate (ethmoid bone)

Ethmoid cells

Sphenoid sinus

Optic canal, Superior orbital fissure

Foramen rotundum

Foramen ovale

Foramen spinosum

**Fig. 1.3** Anatomy of the skull base, extracranial view. Illustration of the extracranial aspect of the skull base, with the orbital roofs, ethmoid air cells, and sphenoid sinus exposed. The anterior skull base can be broadly described as constituting the floor of the anterior cranial fossa, roof of the nose, ethmoid air cells, and orbits anteriorly and the lesser wings and anterior body of the sphenoid bone posteriorly. Cribriform plate/ethmoid bone (*purple*), frontal bones (*tan*), occipital bone (*green*), parietal bones (*pink*), sphenoid bone (*red*), temporal bones (*grey*).

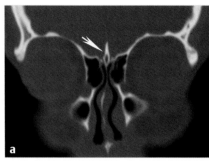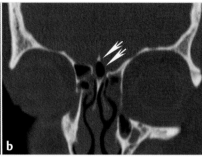

**Fig. 1.4** Coronal reformats from high-resolution sinus CT of two different patients demonstrating examples of (**a**) non-pneumatized crista galli (*arrow*) and (**b**) the less common pneumatized variant (*double arrows*).

on either side (▶ Fig. 1.2). The anterior clinoid processes are formed by the medial part of the lesser wings of the sphenoid and serve as sites of attachment for the anterior part of the tentorium cerebelli anteriorly. The anterolateral boundary of the anterior skull base is formed by the frontal bones. The posterior margin of planum sphenoidale (tuberculum sellae, medially) and the lesser wing of the sphenoid forming the sphenoid ridge (laterally) separate the anterior skull base from the central skull base posteriorly (▶ Fig. 1.2).

Other bony landmarks of the anterior skull base include the frontal crest and crista galli. The frontal crest is a midline ridge between the frontal bones anteriorly and serves as a site of attachment for the falx cerebri (▶ Fig. 1.2). The crista galli is a midline triangular process arising from the ethmoid, also a site of attachment for the falx cerebri (▶ Fig. 1.2, ▶ Fig. 1.4). The crista galli can be pneumatized in approximately 2 to 14% of cases in different studies[12,13,14] (▶ Fig. 1.4). Although pneumatization of this structure represents an anatomic variant, there can be inflammation of the pneumatized crista galli similar to paranasal sinuses and there are even case reports of mucocele formation in this area.[15,16] It has been suggested that the primary origin of the pneumatization of the crista galli is from the frontal sinus.[13]

The foramina of the anterior skull base include those in the cribriform plate, the foramen cecum, and the anterior and posterior ethmoidal foramina (▶ Fig. 1.2, ▶ Fig. 1.3). The cribriform plate contains multiple small perforations that transmit afferent fibers from the nasal mucosa to the olfactory bulbs. At the junction of the ethmoid (cribriform plate) and the adjacent frontal bone, the frontoethmoidal suture contains the foramen cecum, corresponding to a small midline pit anterior to the crista galli. The data on the development, patency, and presence of a functional vein through the foramen cecum is sparse. However, although absent in the majority of the population, there can be rare instances of a patent small emissary vein in children and rarely in adults that interconnects the venous system of the nasal cavity and the superior sagittal sinus.[17,18] When patent, this may represent a potential route for spread of infection/inflammation or rarely be associated with cerebrospinal fluid (CSF) leaks.[17,18,19]

The anterior ethmoidal neurovascular bundles (artery, vein, and nerve) enter the cranial cavity at the junction of the cribriform plate and the orbital plates of the frontal bone anteriorly on each side. Similarly, the posterior ethmoidal canals and attendant neurovascular contents are transmitted through the skull base at the junction of the posterolateral corners of the cribriform plate and the sphenoid. The anatomic variations in the trajectory of these structures, well seen on high-resolution

sinus computed tomography (CT), can be important for surgical planning during endoscopic surgery and will be discussed in more detail in the section on paranasal sinuses.

The anterior skull base has important relations to critical adjacent structures and spaces that need to be taken into account when evaluating different pathology as well as for treatment planning. Superiorly, these are the structures of the anterior cranial fossa, including the frontal lobes as well as the olfactory bulb and tract (olfactory nerve or cranial nerve 1). Inferiorly, these are the nasal cavity and ethmoid air cells medially and the orbits laterally. The applied anatomy of the nasal cavity and paranasal sinuses will be discussed in the next section.

## 1.3.2 Nasal Cavity and Paranasal Sinuses

### Nasal Cavity

The nasal cavity is a triangular area divided on each side by the nasal septum (▶ Fig. 1.5). The horizontal central part of the roof of the nasal cavity is formed by the cribriform plate of the ethmoid bone (▶ Fig. 1.5), separating the nasal cavity from the anterior cranial fossa. Posteriorly, the nasal cavity roof is formed by the anterior aspect of the body of the sphenoid and the superior turbinates, with bilateral interruptions for the sphenoid sinus ostia. Anteriorly, the nasal cavity roof slopes down along the inner aspect of the nasal bones and nasal spine of the frontal bone.

The olfactory fossa is formed by the cribriform plate, separated at the midline by the crista galli. The cribriform plate has a medial lamella inferiorly and medially and a lateral lamella that is vertical or slanted (▶ Fig. 1.5).[20] The lateral lamella of the cribriform plate is the thinnest structure in the skull base and as such represents a site of potential breach or injury, vulnerable to surgical trauma during exenteration of disease from the anterior ethmoid air cells in the area of the superior attachment of the middle turbinate.[21,22,23] It connects to the fovea ethmoidalis, the roof of the ethmoid labyrinth that is formed by the orbital plate of the frontal bone. In a classic study in 1962, Keros classified the depth of the olfactory fossa, as defined by the height of the lateral lamina of the cribriform plate, into three categories. Type 1 corresponds to a depth of 1 to 3 mm, type 2 to a depth of 4 to 7 mm (most common), and type 3 to a depth of 8 to 16 mm (▶ Fig. 1.6). The height of the lateral lamella and corresponding depth of the olfactory fossa is directly related to the surgical risk of intracranial entry[24] and iatrogenic CSF leak following endoscopic endonasal surgery for benign and malignant disease. Therefore, the greater the height or depth, the greater the risk.

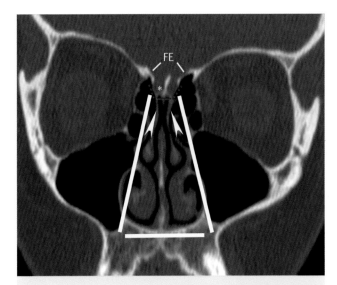

**Fig. 1.5** Coronal reformat from a high-resolution sinus CT demonstrates basic anatomy of the cribriform plate and triangular-shaped nasal cavity (*solid white lines*). The cribriform plate (*red solid and dotted lines*) forms the olfactory fossa (*asterisk*) and the roof of the horizontal central part of the nasal cavity. It consists of a medial lamella (*red solid line*) and a lateral lamella (*red dotted line*) that are separated by the vertical lamella of the middle turbinate (*arrowheads*). Laterally, the cribriform plate becomes contiguous with the roof of the ethmoid labyrinth, the fovea ethmoidalis (FE), formed by the orbital plate of frontal bone.

It should be noted that in addition to the lateral lamella of the cribriform plate, the anterior part of the ethmoid roof, in the area just behind the frontal recess, also represents a site of potential inadvertent breach during endoscopic surgery.[25]

The nasal cavity is divided into two compartments by the nasal septum. The nasal septum consists of a longer, posterior bony component and a shorter anterior cartilaginous component (▶ Fig. 1.7). The bony nasal septum is formed by the perpendicular plate of the ethmoid bone superiorly (descending from the cribriform plate) and the vomer inferiorly. The shape of the nasal septum is highly variable and, frequently, there is some degree of deviation from the midline. The septum can assume an **S**-shaped configuration and bony spurs may project from the septum (▶ Fig. 1.7).

Laterally, the nasal cavity consists of the lateral nasal wall and the attached turbinates, whereas the floor of the nasal cavity is formed by the hard and soft palate.[3,4] The lateral nasal cavity is formed by multiple bones, including the maxilla, the ethmoid bone, the perpendicular plate of the palatine bone, the lacrimal bone, the medial pterygoid plate, and the inferior nasal concha. The inferior nasal concha is a separate bone, whereas the superior and middle turbinates are extensions of the ethmoid bone, as is the uncinate process. The bony labyrinth of the ethmoid is at the superolateral boundary of the nasal cavity.

There are three nasal conchae arising from the lateral or superior nasal cavity margins.[3,4,9,23] Together, the bony nasal conchae and the vascular mucosa and submucosa lining them are referred to as turbinates. The three main turbinates are the superior, middle, and inferior turbinates, with the inferior turbinate being the largest among them (▶ Fig. 1.8). Some, but not all, individuals also have small supreme turbinates (arising from the ethmoid bone), but these have little clinical or radiologic significance. The nasal concha/turbinates curve inferomedially and form a roof for a groove, or meatus. As such, the meati are the nasal cavity airspaces inferior and lateral to their respective turbinates (▶ Fig. 1.8). These airspaces represent the ultimate site of drainage of the paranasal sinuses as well as the nasolacrimal duct.

The superior concha or turbinate is a small, curved osseous lamina posterosuperior to the middle turbinate (▶ Fig. 1.8). The superior turbinate is an important landmark during endoscopic surgery for the identification of the sphenoid sinus and its natural ostium. In a majority of patients, the sphenoid sinus ostium is located medial relative to the posterior part of the superior turbinate, between the superior turbinate and nasal septum. In a very small percentage of patients (2% in one study), the natural ostium can be located laterally.[26]

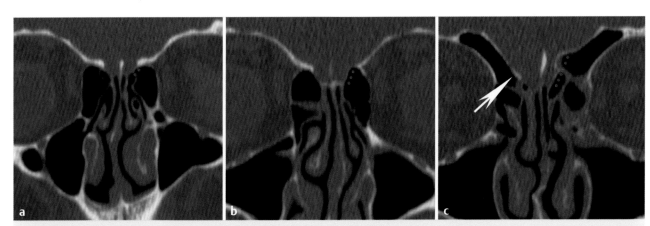

**Fig. 1.6** Keros classification and other important variants of the fovea ethmoidalis—examples on sinus CT. Coronal reformats from sinus CT scans of three different patients demonstrate variations in the depth of the olfactory fossa, as defined by the height of the lateral lamina of the cribriform plate (*red dotted line*). Based on the Keros classification, there are three types: (**a**) 2 mm (type 1: 1–3 mm); (**b**) 4 mm (type 2: 4–7 mm); and (**c**) 10 mm (type 3: 8–16 mm). Greater depth corresponds to a greater risk of iatrogenic injury. In addition to variations in the olfactory fossa depth, there is asymmetry of the ethmoid roof as well as a flat sloping shape of ethmoid roof on the right (**c**; *arrow*), with an increase in the angle between the fovea ethmoidalis and the lateral lamina of the cribriform plate approaching 180 degrees. Both of these variants can be associated with an increased risk of iatrogenic injury and complications during endoscopic surgery.

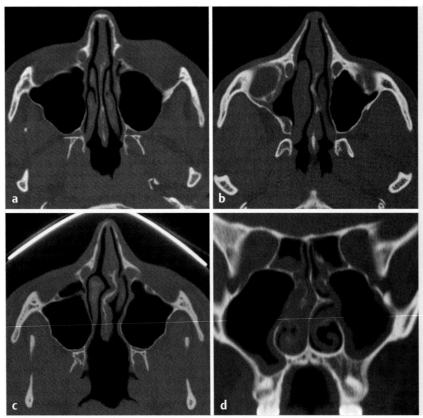

**Fig. 1.7** Anatomy and variations of the nasal septum. The nasal septum consists of a longer posterior bony component and an anterior cartilaginous component, as demonstrated on the axial high-resolution sinus CT images from different patients (**a–c**). The nasal septum can have various shapes and frequently deviates from the midline (**a–c**). It may also have bony projections or nasal septal spurs, as demonstrated on the coronal reformatted image (**d**).

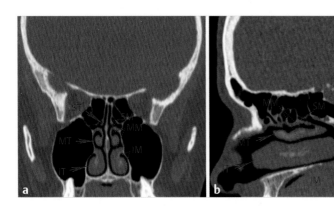

**Fig. 1.8** Nasal turbinates. (**a**) Coronal and (**b**) sagittal reformats from a sinus CT demonstrating the superior (ST), middle (MT), and inferior (IT) nasal turbinates and their respective meati (SM, superior meatus; MM, middle meatus; IM, inferior meatus). On the sagittal image (**b**), the superior turbinate is not seen because it is medial to the plane of the section.

The middle turbinates have a particularly complex anatomy and understanding this anatomy is key for understanding the functional units and drainage pathways in the paranasal sinuses.[27,28] The attachment of the middle turbinates to adjacent bones has components in all three planes (▶ Fig. 1.9). There is variation in the terminology used which can cause confusion, but according to some descriptions, the basal lamella of the middle turbinate can be divided into three portions.[27,28] An anterior vertical portion lies in a near sagittal plane and attaches to the cribriform plate, between the medial and lateral lamella of the cribriform plate (▶ Fig. 1.5, ▶ Fig. 1.9). More posteriorly, the middle portion lies in a nearly coronal plane and attaches to the lamina papyracea (▶ Fig. 1.9). The most posterior portion lies in a nearly horizontal plane and attaches to the lamina papyracea, medial maxillary sinus wall, or both (▶ Fig. 1.9). As would be expected, the anterior part of the basal lamella is best seen on the coronal plane, whereas the middle

and posterior parts are best seen in the sagittal plane (▶ Fig. 1.5, ▶ Fig. 1.9). The latter are also the landmark for separation of the anterior from the posterior ethmoid air cells (▶ Fig. 1.9). As discussed earlier, there is variation in the terminology used for different parts of the middle turbinate, and some consider the anterior vertical part attaching to the cribriform plate the vertical lamella and the more posterior parts the basal lamella.[3]

One of the most common anatomic variations of the middle turbinate is pneumatization of that turbinate (▶ Fig. 1.10), with significant variation in extent of pneumatization seen in different patients. In one study, 53% of patients examined had some degree of middle turbinate pneumatization.[29] Pneumatization may be limited to the upper vertical lamella or extend more caudally to the bulbous portion of the turbinate. There is again variation in the use of terminology, but when the pneumatization is limited to the vertical lamina, some refer to it as partial pneumatization, whereas some reserve the term concha bullosa

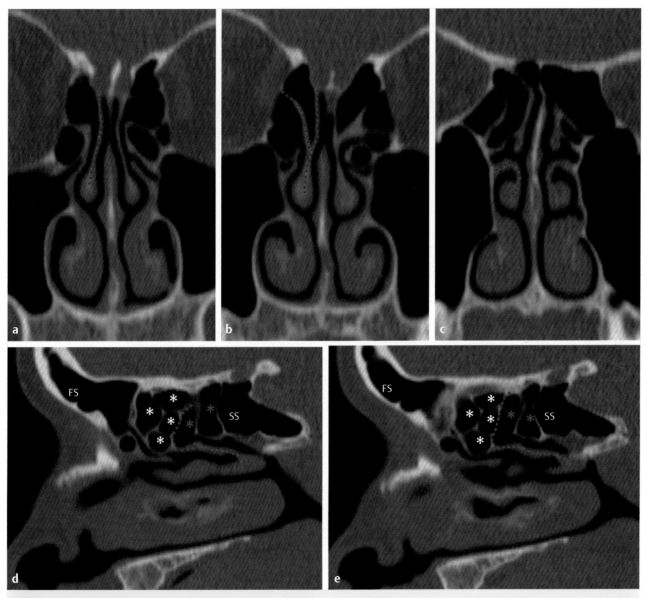

**Fig. 1.9** Attachments of the middle turbinate. (**a–c**) Coronal reformats (anterior to posterior) and (**d,e**) sagittal reformats from a sinus CT demonstrate the complex anatomy of the middle turbinate with attachments to adjacent bones that has components in all three planes (*red dotted lines*). There is variation in terminology used, some referring to all parts as the basal lamella of the middle turbinate and others referring to the anterior part as the vertical lamella and the middle and posterior parts as the basal lamella. Regardless, there is an anterior vertical portion in a near sagittal plane that attaches to the cribriform plate between the medial and lateral lamella of the cribriform plate (**a,b**). More posteriorly, the middle portion lies in a nearly coronal plane and attaches to the lamina papyracea and the most posterior portion lies in a nearly horizontal plane and attaches to the lamina papyracea, medial maxillary sinus wall, or both (**b–e**). It should also be noted that the basal lamella of the middle turbinate is the landmark used for separating anterior (*white asterisks*) from posterior (*blue asterisks*) ethmoid air cells (**d,e**). FS, frontal sinus; SS, sphenoid sinus.

only when the pneumatization extends to the caudal bulbous portion of the turbinate.[6] Middle turbinate pneumatization is commonly an incidental finding of no clinical significance. However, some believe that concha bullosa may become clinically significant when they are large and result in obstruction of drainage pathways and air cells. Another common variation of middle turbinates is paradoxical curvature. This refers to cases where the middle turbinate has a convex curvature on its lateral side rather than the more common medial side. This is typically considered to be of no clinical significance unless it obviously obstructs an air channel.[6,30] Unlike the middle

turbinates, pneumatization of the inferior turbinates is a rare finding.[31]

The superior meatus is a narrow passage between the superior and middle turbinates (▶ Fig. 1.8). Posterior ethmoidal air cells drain via a variable number of ostia into the anterior portion of the superior meatus and then into the sphenoethmoidal recess (the recess between the superior concha and the body of the sphenoid; ▶ Fig. 1.11). The sphenoethmoidal recess represents the site of drainage of the sphenoid sinus via the sphenoid ostium and leads to the superior meatus anteriorly. Drainage is ultimately into the posterior nasal cavity and nasopharynx.

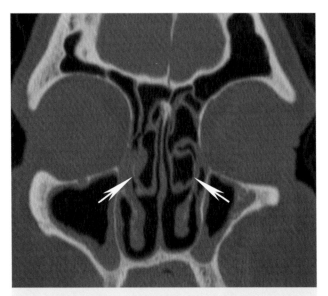

**Fig. 1.10** Pneumatization of the middle turbinate (or concha bullosa). Coronal reformat from a sinus CT demonstrates bilateral middle turbinate pneumatization affecting both the vertical lamella and the caudal bulbous portion of the turbinate (*arrows*). Some reserve the term concha bullosa only for cases where the pneumatization involves to the caudal bulbous portion of the turbinate, as in this case.

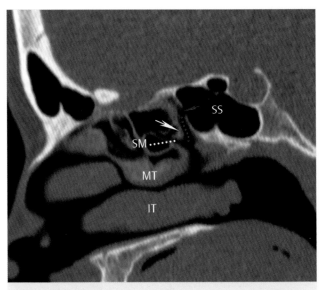

**Fig. 1.11** Sphenoethmoidal recess and related drainage pathways. The sphenoethmoidal recess (*red dotted line*), the recess between the superior concha (*white arrow*) and the body of the sphenoid, receives drainage from the sphenoid sinus as well as from the posterior ethmoidal air cells (via the superior meatus). The *red arrow* marks the sphenoid ostium. IT, inferior turbinate; MT, middle turbinate; SM, superior meatus; SS, sphenoid sinus.

The middle meatus is wider than the superior meatus (▶ Fig. 1.8). It receives drainage from the frontal sinus, anterior ethmoid air cells, and the maxillary sinus (▶ Fig. 1.12; discussed in greater detail in the following sections). The middle meatus contains a rounded elevation called the bulla ethmoidalis (▶ Fig. 1.12), representing the curved surface covering the anterior medial ethmoid air cells.[6] Inferior to this, there is a curved cleft known as the hiatus semilunaris (▶ Fig. 1.12). The inferior margin of the hiatus is formed by the uncinate process (▶ Fig. 1.12). The ostium of the maxillary sinus is normally located lateral to the uncinate process. Pertaining to frontal sinus drainage, anatomic variations of the uncinate process determine the pathway for the drainage of the frontal sinus in this region and are discussed in greater detail later. The functional anatomy of the inferior meatal region is more straightforward. The inferior meatus is the largest of the meati (▶ Fig. 1.8) and the ostium of the nasolacrimal canal is located at the junction of its anterior and middle thirds.

Much of the nasal cavity and paranasal sinuses are lined by pseudostratified ciliated (respiratory) epithelium containing goblet cells. The olfactory cleft and adjacent regions are lined by olfactory epithelium, and there is stratified squamous epithelium anteroinferiorly in continuity with the nares. The mucosa is adherent to the adjacent periosteum or perichondrium, sometimes referred to as the mucoperiosteum. Seromucous glands of the nasal mucosa secrete a mucous film which is moved posteriorly into the nasopharynx by ciliary action. The lamina propria also contains cavernous venous vascular tissue, thickest over the conchae. Paranasal sinus mucosa is thinner, less vascular, contains fewer goblet cells, and is more loosely attached to underlying bones.

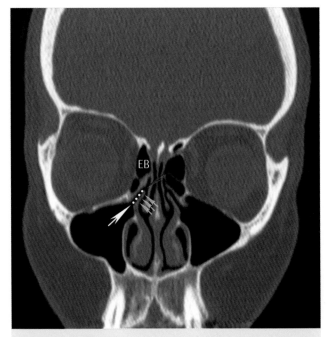

**Fig. 1.12** Ostiomeatal unit (OMU). Coronal reformat from a sinus CT demonstrating the main components of the OMU as seen in the coronal plane. The OMU refers to a functional unit of structures draining the frontal, anterior ethmoid, and maxillary sinuses. It includes the middle meatus, the ethmoid bulla (EB), the uncinate process (*blue arrows*), hiatus semilunaris (*red arrow*), the infundibulum (*dotted line*), and the superomedial maxillary sinus/maxillary sinus ostium (*white arrow*).

The arterial supply of the nasal cavity is derived from branches of the ophthalmic, maxillary, and facial arteries which ramify to form anastomotic plexuses within and deep to the nasal mucosa. Venous drainage of the cavernous tissue involves the sphenopalatine vein, veins accompanying the anterior ethmoidal arteries which lead to the cavernous sinuses, and, in cases of a patent foramen caecum, a nasal vein communicating with the superior sagittal sinus as discussed earlier. Lymphatic drainage from the anterior nasal cavity joins that of the skin, and the primary nodal groups draining this area are those in the submandibular region (level IB lymph nodes). The primary nodal drainage areas for the posterior two-thirds of the nasal cavity and paranasal sinuses are the retropharyngeal lymph nodes and the level II and III lymph nodes.[32] The posterior aspect of the nasal floor may also drain into parotid lymph nodes.[11]

Nasal cavity general sensory innervation is mediated by branches of the ophthalmic (V1) and maxillary (V2) divisions of the trigeminal nerves, including anterior ethmoidal, infraorbital, anterior superior alveolar, greater palatine, nasopalatine, and Vidian nerves. Autonomic innervation occurs by sympathetic vasomotor fibers following the distribution of blood vessels. Parasympathetic secretomotor functions are mediated by branches of the maxillary nerves. This includes contributions from the Vidian nerve, which provides parasympathetic innervation to the nose and lacrimal gland. This is clinically important and if this nerve requires sacrifice as part of the patient's surgery, it can result in an ipsilateral dry eye. As such, when at risk, this will have to be discussed with the patient during the consenting procedure. The olfactory nerves form a plexiform network in the subepithelial lamina propria of the superior septal and turbinate mucosa. This network coalesces into as many as 20 separate bundles which traverse the cribriform plate in lateral and medial groups to form the olfactory bulbs. At this level, the dura is continuous with the nasal periosteum.

## Paranasal Sinuses

### Frontal sinus

The paired frontal sinuses are located between the cortical tables of the frontal bone. Each frontal sinus usually underlies a triangular portion of the face, though rarely in a symmetrical configuration. The frontal sinuses on either side are separated from one another by the intersinus septum, although frequently the septum is not exactly midline and the larger sinus crosses the midsagittal plane to the contralateral side. The majority of time, the intersinus septum is complete, but occasionally there may be focal defects allowing intercommunication between the sinuses. The septum may also have an intersinus septal cell. These are believed to arise from the frontal sinuses themselves, rather than migration of anterior ethmoid air cells. The sinuses may, in addition, be divided into numerous interconnected recesses by incomplete bony septa or intrasinus septa. The primary ostium of the frontal sinus is located medially and drains through the frontal recess into the middle meatus, discussed in detail in the section on sinus drainage and frontoethmoidal recess later.

The pneumatization of frontal sinuses is variable. These sinuses typically extend a short distance above the medial aspect of the eyebrow and, posteromedially, they may reach into the orbital roof as far as the lesser wing of the sphenoid.

Occasionally, one or both frontal sinuses are hypoplastic or absent.[6] The arterial supply to the frontal sinuses is through the supraorbital and supratrochlear branches of the ophthalmic artery as well as the anterior ethmoidal artery (also supplying anterior ethmoid air cells), a branch of the ophthalmic artery.[6,11] Their venous drainage is primarily through the superior ophthalmic veins. The primary lymphatic drainage of the frontal sinuses is to the submandibular (level IB) lymph nodes. Innervation is mainly through the supraorbital branch of the frontal nerve (a distal branch of the ophthalmic [V1] division of the trigeminal nerve).

### Ethmoid sinus

The ethmoid sinuses or air cells are formed of numerous thin-walled spaces within the ethmoidal labyrinth, varying in number from 3 to 18 per side. These cells are located between the superolateral margin of the nasal cavity and the medial aspect of the orbit, separated from the latter by a thin osseous plate, the lamina papyracea. Given this relationship, the presence of defects such as from prior lamina papyracea fractures or developmental defects or dehiscence,[33] particularly those with herniation of orbital fat into the sinus (▶ Fig. 1.13), should be reported to avoid misinterpretation as inflammatory disease or unintended surgical manipulation. The smaller anterior part of the lateral ethmoid wall is formed by the lacrimal bone. In the adult, the ethmoid labyrinth is usually pyramidal shaped, with its base directed posteriorly. Therefore, it becomes wider posteriorly. Less commonly, it may have similar dimensions anteriorly and posteriorly. This is important to recognize because the operative field will not get wider as one proceeds posteriorly during surgery.

The ethmoid air cells are functionally divided into anterior and posterior groups by the basal lamella of the middle turbinate as discussed earlier (▶ Fig. 1.9). Within each group, the

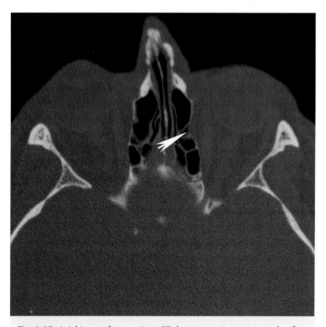

**Fig. 1.13** Axial image from a sinus CT demonstrating an example of an old left lamina papyracea fracture with mild herniation of extraconal fat into the ethmoidal labyrinth (*arrow*).

sinuses are divided by incomplete osseous septations. Broadly, the anterior group of ethmoid air cells drain via one or more orifices into the ethmoid bulla and the hiatus semilunaris (also discussed later) and then to the middle meatus (▶ Fig. 1.12). More specifically, the anterior ethmoid air cells can be subdivided into frontal recess cells (draining into the frontal recess), infundibular cells (draining into the infundibulum and hiatus semilunaris), and bullae cells (draining into a groove on the bulla ethmoidalis).[6] Ultimately, these drain into the middle meatus. The drainage of the posterior ethmoid air cell group typically is through the superior meatus and the sphenoethmoidal recess and then into the nasopharynx (▶ Fig. 1.11).

Virtually any part of the ethmoid bone can be pneumatized and depending on the location, the pneumatization may have significance for treatment planning or contribute to sinus pathology and obstruction. In addition, there can be expansion of ethmoid air cells outside the ethmoid, known as extramural expansion. These can encroach on adjacent structures such as frontal, maxillary, and sphenoid sinuses. While these represent anatomic variations and not anomalies per se, certain specific patterns of extramural expansion can contribute to disease or represent potential surgical risks and therefore must be recognized.

The anterior ethmoid air cells constitute approximately two-thirds to three quarters of the ethmoid air cells.[6,34] The ethmoid bulla is usually the largest and most constant anterior ethmoid air cell (▶ Fig. 1.12), although it can vary significantly in extent of pneumatization. If very large, this could theoretically impinge on the ostiomeatal unit (OMU), although typically it is incidental and it is not clear whether this can have a true effect or relation to sinusitis. As discussed earlier, there can also be pneumatization of the middle turbinate, and some have proposed that when large enough a concha bullosa (▶ Fig. 1.10) may result in sinus obstruction. However, the majority of time these are incidental and the association with sinusitis is not clear-cut.[35]

Ethmoid air cells may pneumatize the frontal process of the maxilla adjacent to the anterior attachment of the middle turbinate to the ethmoid crest of the ascending process of the maxilla. These are known as agger nasi cells (▶ Fig. 1.14). The reported incidence of these cells varies considerably between different studies (3–100%).[6,36] When present, these are the most anterior ethmoid air cells, located anterior, inferior, and lateral to the frontal recess. They are deep to the lacrimal bone and also serve as a landmark for the nasofrontal duct. The majority of time, these are of no clinical significance, although some have suggested a potential association with frontal sinusitis.[36,37] Anterior ethmoid air cells may pneumatize the roof of the orbits, known as supraorbital ethmoid cells (▶ Table 1.1). On axial and sagittal images, these are posterior to and separated from the frontal sinus by an intact wall. Preoperative identification of these cells is important to avoid mistaking them for the frontal ostium during endoscopic surgery.[34]

An ethmoid air cell may invade the medial orbital floor, known as a Haller's cell or infraorbital ethmoid cell (▶ Fig. 1.15). Some believe that Haller's cells may contribute to rhinosinusitis by narrowing the infundibulum, but there is controversy and inconsistent reports regarding this association.[36,38,39,40] Regardless,

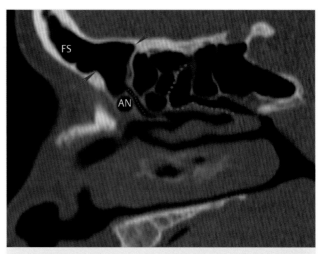

Fig. 1.14 Frontal sinus drainage pathway (FSDP) or recess. Sagittal reformat from a sinus CT demonstrates an example of the FSDP. The FSDP has a superior compartment communicating with the frontal sinus ostium (*between red arrows*) and a narrower inferior compartment communicating with the middle meatus. Depending on the anatomy and site of insertion of the uncinate process anteriorly, the inferior compartment may either be formed by the ethmoid infundibulum or by the middle meatus. In the current example, it is formed by the ethmoid infundibulum (*red dotted line*). This occurs when the anterior portion of the uncinate process extends superiorly and attaches to the skull base. In these cases, the ethmoid infundibulum drains into the middle meatus via the hiatus semilunaris. On the other hand, in cases where the anterior part of the uncinate process attaches to the lamina papyracea instead of the skull base, the inferior compartment is formed by the middle meatus itself (not shown). The basal lamella of the middle turbinate, separating anterior from posterior ethmoidal air cells, is marked by the *blue dotted line*. AN, agger nasi cell; FS, frontal sinus.

Table 1.1 Types of air cells around the frontal sinus drainage pathway or recess

| Type | Description |
| --- | --- |
| Supraorbital ethmoid cell | Anterior ethmoid air cell that extends superiorly and laterally over the orbit from the frontal recess and drain into the frontal recess; separated from the frontal sinus by a bony septum; it should not be mistaken for a septated frontal sinus |
| Frontal cells | Type 1: Single air cell above the agger nasi cell that does not extend into the frontal sinus<br>Type 2: Two or more air cells above the agger nasi cell<br>Type 3: Single large air cell above the agger nasi cell that extends into the frontal sinus<br>Type 4: Isolated air cell in the frontal sinus |
| Suprabullar cell | Air cell above the ethmoid bulla whose anterior wall does not extend into the frontal sinus |
| Frontal bullar cell | Air cell above the ethmoid bulla that extends into the frontal sinus |
| Inter–frontal sinus septal cell | Pneumatized frontal sinus septum |

Source: Modified from Huang et al[34]

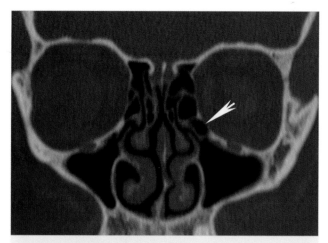

**Fig. 1.15** Example of a Haller cell (or infraorbital ethmoid cell; *arrow*) on a coronal reformat from a sinus CT.

optic nerves, at risk for inadvertent surgical injury.[39,41,42] Sphenoid septations are typically not in the horizontal plane and the presence of horizontal or near-horizontal septations in the sphenoid area on coronal images suggests the presence of Onodi cells. These can be present unilaterally or bilaterally and may coexist with other anatomic variations of importance (▶ Fig. 1.16). Some reports describe the sphenomaxillary plate, referring to a thin bony partition between the maxillary sinus and the sphenoid sinus.[42] If present, there is the potential for the sphenoid sinus to be mistaken for posterior ethmoid cells during the transantral ethmoidectomy.[42]

As discussed earlier, the roof of the ethmoid labyrinth is formed by the orbital plate of the frontal bone and is referred to as the fovea ethmoidalis. The Keros's classification for cribriform plate and ethmoid roof configuration was discussed earlier (▶ Fig. 1.6) and it is worth emphasizing that the fovea ethmoidalis is at a slight angle and descends as it extends posteriorly. Therefore, anteriorly, it can be higher than the cribriform plates (▶ Fig. 1.5, ▶ Fig. 1.6). In addition to its depth, it is also important to note any ethmoid roof asymmetry as this predisposes to intracranial penetration during endoscopic sinus surgery, usually on the side where the ethmoid roof is lower (▶ Fig. 1.6).[43] However, other than absolute differences in height, asymmetry in shape, including a flat sloping shape of ethmoid roof (▶ Fig. 1.6), may also predispose to skull base injury.[44]

Other anatomic structures worth evaluating during preoperative planning are the canals for the anterior and posterior ethmoidal arteries (▶ Fig. 1.17). The anterior ethmoidal artery crosses from the orbit through the ethmoidal labyrinth and through the lateral lamella of the cribriform plate at the anterior ethmoidal sulcus and can serve as a surgical landmark.[45]

awareness of this variant is important because its presence can increase the risk of intraorbital injury during surgery.[36,39,40] A posterior ethmoid air cell may also extend posterior to the maxillary sinus, resulting in a double maxillary antrum. If that cell is infected, this must be recognized because it will require opening of the posterior maxillary sinus wall for access to that cell.

Posterior ethmoid cells can also extend into the sphenoid sinus, typically located superiorly and laterally and partly surrounding the optic nerve canal. This is referred to as an Onodi cell (▶ Fig. 1.16). The importance of the Onodi cell is that there is potential for misidentification during endoscopic surgery. This puts closely related critical structures, in particular the

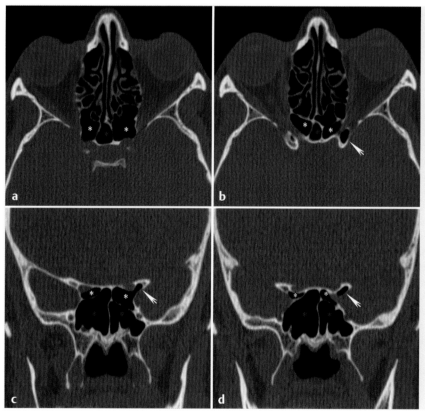

**Fig. 1.16** Onodi cell configuration and other important anatomic variations of posterior ethmoidal air cells and the sphenoid sinus. **(a,b)** Axial and **(c,d)** coronal reformats from a sinus CT demonstrate multiple important variants in the same patient. In this case, there is bilateral Onodi cell configuration (*white asterisks*), representing extension of posterior ethmoid cells into the sphenoid sinus (*red asterisks*). Note the resultant exposure of optic nerves, putting them at risk for inadvertent surgical injury. In this case, this is further exacerbated by anterior clinoid pneumatization, asymmetric on the left (*white arrows*). There is in addition thinning and dehiscence of parts of the bony covering of the optic **(c)** and carotid **(a,d)** canals. In this particular case, the combination of anatomic variants also results in asymmetric exposure of the left carotid canal (*red arrow*; **d**).

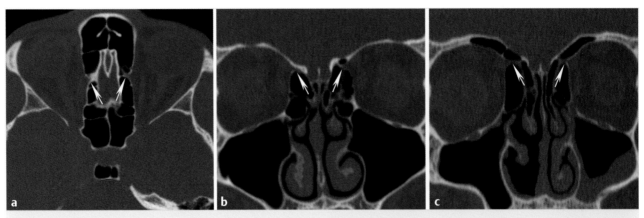

**Fig. 1.17** Variations in the course of the canals for the anterior ethmoidal arteries (AEA). (**a**) Axial and (**b**) coronal reformats from a sinus CT demonstrating the canals for AEAs coursing through the ethmoidal labyrinth (*arrows*). The relation to the ethmoid roof is best appreciated on coronal images. In this case, the canal for the AEA abuts the ethmoid roof on the right side, but on the left, the canal for the AEA travels below the ethmoid roof. Some refer to this configuration as the canal being on a mesentery. (**c**) Coronal reformatted sinus CT image from another patient demonstrating canals for AEA on a mesentery bilaterally.

In addition, this is the area where the bone is thinnest in the anterior skull base. There are also close adhesions of dura mater to the sinus walls in the anterior ethmoidal region. As such, this is considered a high-risk area.[45] In some patients, the canals for the anterior ethmoidal arteries may travel below the ethmoid roof (▶ Fig. 1.17). Some refer to this configuration as the canal being on a mesentery. This results in increased exposure of the artery and increases the risk of an iatrogenic injury during endoscopic sinus surgery that could lead to hematoma, including intraorbital hematoma, CSF leak, or infection.[23]

The posterior ethmoidal artery travels along the roof of the posterior ethmoid sinus. This artery usually courses within the bony roof that is thicker than that of the anterior ethmoid sinus. However, occasionally although much less commonly than with the anterior ethmoidal artery, this artery may also course below the roof and if so, this should be noted. Because it tends to be larger, damage to this artery may cause more bleeding than damage to the anterior ethmoidal artery.[23]

The arterial supply to the ethmoid derives from the nasal branches of the sphenopalatine artery as well as the anterior and posterior ethmoidal arterial branches from the ophthalmic artery. As such, the arterial supply is both from branches of the internal and external carotid arteries. The venous drainage of the ethmoid air cells is through the nasal veins into the nose or through the ethmoidal veins into the ophthalmic veins. Thrombophlebitis of these valveless veins may result in cavernous sinus thrombosis as a complication of ethmoid sinusitis. Lymphatics follow the functional anterior and posterior mucociliary drainage divisions, leading to the submandibular (level IB) and retropharyngeal lymph node groups,[11] respectively. Sensory innervation of the anterior ethmoid air cells is via the anterior ethmoidal nerve (arising from the nasociliary branch of the ophthalmic [V1] division of the trigeminal nerve). The posterior ethmoid air cells are innervated by branches of the posterior ethmoidal nerve (arising from ophthalmic division [V1] of the trigeminal nerve) and the posterolateral nasal branches of the sphenopalatine nerve (arising from the maxillary division [V2] of the trigeminal nerve).[6]

## Maxillary sinus

The maxillary sinuses or antra are the largest of the paranasal sinuses, filling the bodies of the maxilla. They have roughly pyramidal shapes with bases directed medially, paralleling the lateral walls of the nasal cavities. The floors are formed by the maxillary alveolar and palatine processes. The roofs of the maxillary sinuses are composed of the orbital floors and are traversed by the infraorbital groove posteriorly. The groove becomes a canal more anteriorly. Occasionally, parts of these canals may project within the sinus or in a partial septation in the sinus. Laterally, the apex of the pyramidal configuration is capped by the zygomatic process of the maxilla. The anterior superior alveolar nerve and associated vessels pass inferiorly from the infraorbital foramen resulting in a groove in the anterior wall of the sinus. Posterolaterally, the wall of the sinus abuts retromaxillary fat and contains a canal for the posterosuperior alveolar nerve to the molar dentition. The posterior wall of the maxillary sinus forms the anterior margin of the pterygopalatine fossa (PPF), discussed in greater detail later.

Most commonly, the maxillary sinuses develop symmetrically with minor common variations of unilateral or bilateral hypoplasia present in less than 10% of cases.[6] Maxillary sinus hypoplasia should not be confused with an atelectatic sinus, discussed later in the section on the OMU. Other variants that may be seen include internal septa. If the septum results in complete compartmentalization, this should be noted and the site of drainage (e.g., through an accessory maxillary ostium) should be identified. Compartmentalization by extension of an ethmoid air cell posterior to the maxillary sinus was discussed earlier. Dental roots may form conical elevations in the floor of the maxillary sinus. Less commonly, dental roots may project into the antrum. Occasionally, the overlying bone may be dehiscent only with sinus mucosa separating the roots from the sinus cavity.

Medially, the maxillary bone has a large hole or defect called the maxillary hiatus. However, this defect is partially covered by parts of the ethmoid bone, the perpendicular plate of the palatine bone, the lacrimal bone, and the inferior turbinate.

The main drainage of the maxillary sinus is through the maxillary ostium medially opening into the infundibulum (▶ Fig. 1.12; also discussed in greater detail later in the section on paranasal sinus drainage). The location of the main, natural maxillary sinus ostium can vary but is typically high, just below the floor of the orbit. Depending on the specific location, the surgeon may elect to enter the sinus at a lower level.

Between the inferior part of the uncinate process and the insertion of the inferior turbinate, the medial maxillary hiatus is covered by opposing nasal and sinus mucosa. This membranous area is referred to as the fontanelle and is divided into a posterior and an anterior fontanelle by the ethmoidal process of the inferior turbinate, which extends superiorly to contact the uncinate process.[6] This membranous area can break down and result in the formation of accessory maxillary ostia. In cases where the natural maxillary ostium cannot be cannulated because of a large uncinate process or because it would put the orbit at risk, this represents an alternate site of penetration into the middle meatus.[6,46]

The arterial supply to the maxillary sinus is through the maxillary artery including the infraorbital, greater palatine, posterosuperior alveolar, and anterior superior arteries. Venous drainage is via the anterior facial vein anteriorly or the maxillary vein posteriorly. The maxillary vein connects to the pterygoid venous plexus which in turn connects to the dural venous sinuses and this represents a potential pathway for spread of infection from maxillary sinusitis to result in meningitis. The maxillary vein also joins the superficial temporal vein to form the retromandibular vein, ultimately draining into the internal and external jugular veins. The main lymphatic drainage of the maxillary sinus is into the submandibular (level IB) lymph nodes, although there can also be drainage to other nodal stations, including the lateral retropharyngeal lymph nodes.[6,47] Innervation to the maxillary sinus is through multiple branches of the superior alveolar nerve (anterior, middle, posterior), the anterior palatine nerve, and the infraorbital nerve. The posterosuperior alveolar nerve pierces the posterior maxillary sinus wall and travels anteriorly and inferiorly to supply the molar teeth.[6]

## Sphenoid sinus

The sphenoid sinuses are located within the body of the sphenoid bone, posterior to the upper nasal cavity. There is considerable variation in the degree of pneumatization on the left and right sides of the sphenoid sinus. The sphenoid sinus septum is usually midline anteriorly, aligned with the nasal septum. However, posteriorly, it frequently can deviate far to one side, creating two unequal sinus cavities. The sphenoid septations are vertical in orientation. Therefore, if horizontal septations are seen on coronal or sagittal images, then ethmoid air cell septations or Onodi cells should be suspected (▶ Fig. 1.16).

Because of extensive variation in the degree of pneumatization of the sphenoid sinus and its potential impact on preoperative planning, different classification systems have been introduced to describe the degree of pneumatization. There is no universally accepted classification system, but generally the sphenoid sinus may be classified as conchal or non-pneumatized (rare; describing cases where the posterior wall of the sinus lies anterior to the sella turcica), presellar (the posterior limit of the sinus cavity extends only to the anterior wall of the sella turcica), or sellar (the sinus cavity extends posterior to the anterior sella turcica wall and lies under the sella floor, such that the sella bulges into the sinus).[6,48] Some may also include a fourth type, the postsellar type, referring to cases where the posterior boundary of the sinus extends to or more posterior to the posterior part of the sella, with pneumatization completely surrounding the sella.[48] The conchal type is relatively rare, constituting as little as 2% of cases in some studies.[48] In this group of patients, the thick bony posterior sinus wall makes the transsphenoid approach to the pituitary particularly challenging and this anatomy may be considered a relative contraindication to transsphenoidal hypophysectomy.

In addition to variable posterior pneumatization, there is also variable lateral pneumatization and extent of the sphenoid sinus. There can be extension of the lateral recesses from the main sphenoid sinus cavity into the greater sphenoid wing, where it forms the floor of the middle cranial fossa and the posterior orbital wall, the lesser sphenoid wing, or the pterygoid process. When present, the lateral extension almost always goes between the foramen rotundum and the Vidian canal (▶ Fig. 1.18). Therefore, depending on sphenoid pneumatization, the foramen rotundum may either be completely outside the sinus or bulge into the lower lateral sinus wall (▶ Fig. 1.18). The Vidian canal may be within the sphenoid bone proper, bulge into the sphenoid sinus, or occasionally be elevated on a septum within the sinus cavity (▶ Fig. 1.18). The combination of prominent arachnoid granulations and widely pneumatized, thin adjacent bone could predispose to an osteodural defect resulting in a CSF leak (▶ Fig. 1.19). Therefore, when evaluating CT scans for CSF leaks, these areas should be carefully scrutinized.

Awareness of the anatomic variations and configurations that could predispose to optic nerve or carotid injury during endoscopic sinus surgery is essential for preoperative planning and well demonstrated on high-resolution CT scans of the sinuses. One such variation is the Onodi cell, discussed earlier in the section on the ethmoid sinus (▶ Fig. 1.16). However, there are other anatomic configurations that may result in increased exposure of the optic nerves to injury. This includes the extent

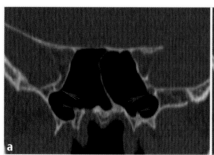
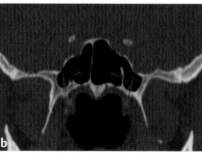

**Fig. 1.18 (a,b)** Examples of lateral pneumatization of the sphenoid sinus extending lateral to the foramen rotundum (*arrows*) and Vidian canals (*small arrowheads*). Coronal reformats from sinus CT scans of two different patients demonstrate prominent inferolateral sphenoid sinus pneumatization and variable extension of the Vidian canal within the sinus. **(b)** The left Vidian canal travels within a septation extending deep within the sinus.

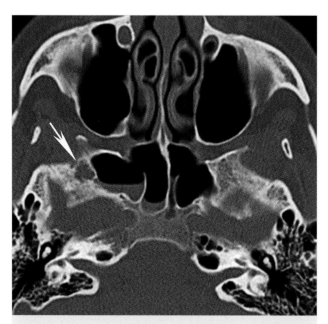

**Fig. 1.19** The combination of prominent arachnoid granulations (*arrow*) and pneumatized, thin adjacent bone could predispose to an osteodural defect resulting in a CSF leak, as shown in this case. Note the air fluid level in sphenoid sinus secondary to a CSF leak (rather than sinusitis).

of protrusion of the optic nerves into the sphenoid sinus, classified by DeLano et al into four types (▶ Table 1.2).[49] Regardless of whether the actual classification is used in routine clinical practice, awareness of these variations and potential exposure of the optic nerve by the otolaryngologist on preoperative scans is essential to help avoid complications. In addition to Onodi cell configuration, other anatomic variants resulting in increased exposure of the optic nerve as well as dehiscence of the bony covering of the optic nerve canal are potential predisposing factors for catastrophic injury and should be noted on preoperative scans. One of these is anterior clinoid pneumatization (▶ Fig. 1.16), which has been found to have an increased association with optic nerve dehiscence and considered an indicator of optic nerve vulnerability during endoscopic sinus surgery.[6,49]

**Table 1.2** DeLano's classification of the relationship of the optic nerve to the posterior paranasal sinuses[49]

| Type | Description | Contact with posterior ethmoid air cells |
|------|-------------|-------------------------------------------|
| 1 | Course adjacent to the sphenoid sinus without indentation of the sphenoid sinus wall | No |
| 2 | Course adjacent to the sphenoid sinus, causing indentation of the sphenoid sinus wall | No |
| 3 | Course through the sphenoid sinus[a] | No |
| 4 | Course immediately adjacent to the sphenoidal sinus and the posterior ethmoidal air cells | Yes |

[a]This may be defined as at least 50% of the nerve being surrounded by air/pneumatized sinus.[6]

The sphenoid sinus roof, the planum sphenoidale, is thin and vulnerable to perforation during surgery. The other sinus walls are of variable thickness, depending on the degree of pneumatization. As discussed earlier, when the sphenoid sinuses are well developed, many important neighboring structures can be identified by their indentation into the sinus cavity, including Vidian canal and the foramen rotundum (maxillary nerve [V2]), optic nerve, and the internal carotid artery, among others. In some cases, bony ridges or septations may be present on some of these structures (▶ Fig. 1.16). Areas with dehiscent walls are potentially susceptible to perforation during surgery. This is especially so with regard to the planum sphenoidale, the lateral sinus wall, and the medial roof of a lateral sinus recess into the greater sphenoid wing or pterygoid process. The latter area is also frequently the site of spontaneous CSF leak secondary to slow erosion resulting in an osteodural defect, as discussed earlier (▶ Fig. 1.19).

The posterior ethmoid surface and the anterior face of the sphenoid sinus share a common wall that is divided by the perpendicular attachment of the superior turbinate.[6] The ostium of the sinus lies in the upper portion of the intranasal surface and drains into the sphenoethmoidal recess, as discussed earlier. Because of its position and location, the normal drainage of the sphenoid sinus in the erect posture relies entirely on ciliary action. The sphenopalatine artery crosses the face of the sphenoid below the ostium. As such, during procedures aimed at enlarging the natural sphenoid sinus ostium, this artery may have to be cauterized. Air cells may be present within the posterosuperior part of the nasal septum and, when present, usually communicate with the sphenoid sinus. These can become inflamed like other sinus air cells and should be recognizable on CT and if necessary using MRI to distinguish from other pathology.

Arterial supply to the sphenoid sinus is derived from the posterior ethmoidal branches of the ophthalmic arteries (supplied by the internal carotid arteries) and the sphenopalatine branches of the maxillary artery (supplied by the external carotid arteries). Venous drainage is through the maxillary vein (and therefore there is a communication with the pterygoid plexus of veins) and the posterior ethmoidal veins into the superior ophthalmic veins. The lymphatics drain into the retropharyngeal lymph nodes. Innervation of the sphenoid sinus is through the posterior ethmoidal nerve, a branch of the nasociliary nerve (supplied by the ophthalmic [V1] division of trigeminal nerve) as well as the sphenopalatine branches (from the maxillary [V2] division of the trigeminal nerve) to the floor of the sinus.[6]

## Paranasal sinus drainage pathways

### Overview of paranasal sinus drainage pathways

Normal paranasal sinus drainage is through the coordinated ciliary action of its mucosal lining, propelling secretions toward the natural ostia. Given the location of the sinus ostia, in the erect position, drainage is largely accomplished by intact ciliary action. Successful drainage also requires intact/patent drainage pathways. As such, understanding the main drainage pathways and associated landmarks is key for the evaluation of sinus anatomy and these may best be considered as functional units. Obstruction at key sites within these functional units results in a predictable pattern of sinus obstruction.

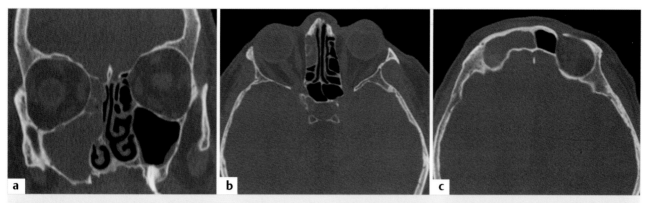

**Fig. 1.20** Coronal reformatted **(a)** and axial **(b,c)** images from a sinus CT demonstrate an example of obstruction of the ostiomeatal unit or complex (OMU) at the convergence of the drainage of the frontal, anterior ethmoid, and maxillary sinuses resulting in a predictable pattern with opacification of those sinuses.

The main drainage for the maxillary sinus is via the maxillary ostium into the infundibulum, hiatus semilunaris, and then the middle meatus (▶ Fig. 1.12). The frontal sinus drains through the frontoethmoidal recess (▶ Fig. 1.14) into the middle meatus, where it joins flow from ipsilateral maxillary sinus. The anterior ethmoid complex drains via the ethmoid bulla and hiatus semilunaris into the middle meatus. The posterior ethmoid complex and sphenoid sinus drain into sphenoethmoidal recess, then into superior meatus and subsequently nasopharynx (▶ Fig. 1.11). The inferior meatus receives drainage from nasolacrimal duct.

## Ostiomeatal unit

The ostiomeatal unit or complex (OMU) refers to a functional unit of structures draining the frontal, anterior ethmoid, and maxillary sinuses (▶ Fig. 1.12). It includes the middle meatus, the ethmoid bulla, the uncinate process, hiatus semilunaris, the infundibulum, and the superomedial maxillary sinus/maxillary sinus ostium.[3] The hiatus semilunaris is the area between uncinate process and ethmoid bulla that receives drainage from anterior ethmoid air cells and maxillary sinus (via the infundibulum; ▶ Fig. 1.12). Familiarity with this functional unit and pattern of drainage is important and obstruction of the unit can result in a predictable pattern of sinus opacification (▶ Fig. 1.20).

Based on the structures constituting and surrounding the OMU, different anatomic variants can be important for preoperative assessment and planning of procedures involving this drainage pathway. Haller cells, ethmoid bulla, and concha bullosa were discussed previously. Pneumatization of uncinate process or uncinate bulla represents an additional potential predisposing factor for impaired sinus ventilation. It is believed to be caused by extension of the agger nasi cell within the anterosuperior portion of the uncinate process.

When encountering an OMU pattern of obstruction, one important entity that should be recognized and distinguished is the atelectatic sinus or silent sinus syndrome.[50] This occurs when the free edge of the uncinate process is rotated laterally or adherent to the orbital floor or inferior part of the lamina papyracea. This configuration, possibly combined with superimposed inflammation, results in occlusion of the infundibulum (▶ Fig. 1.21). This in turn is believed to result in negative pressure

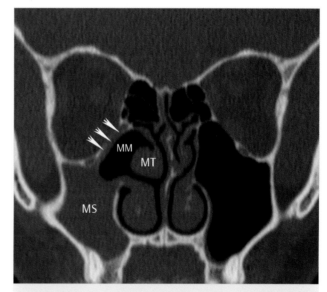

**Fig. 1.21** Atelectatic maxillary sinus. Characteristic imaging findings are shown including a retracted adherent uncinate process with absence of patent infundibulum (*arrows*), retracted maxillary sinus walls, and an enlarged ipsilateral middle meatus (MM) secondary to a retracted medial maxillary sinus wall. MS, maxillary sinus; MT, middle turbinate.

formation in the sinus that could in turn result in further rotation and retraction of the infundibulum, exacerbating and propagating the obstruction. The characteristic imaging findings are a retracted, adherent uncinate process with the absence of patent infundibulum, retracted maxillary sinus walls, and an enlarged ipsilateral middle meatus secondary to the retracted medial maxillary sinus wall (▶ Fig. 1.21).[50] Clinically, this can lead to painless spontaneous enophthalmos, hypoglobus, and facial deformities and asymmetries. When encountered, it is important to recognize this entity and not confuse with a developmentally hypoplastic maxillary sinus. For surgical planning, it is also important to note that in these cases the ipsilateral orbital floor can be low-lying, increasing the risk of inadvertent penetration of the orbit during surgery.[6]

## Frontal recess

Each frontal sinus drains through an inferiorly located ostium into the frontal recess or frontal sinus drainage pathway (▶ Fig. 1.14). The frontal recess is a somewhat hourglass-shaped narrowing between the frontal sinus and the anterior middle meatus providing the pathway for drainage of the frontal sinus. Its relations are the lamina papyracea laterally, the middle turbinate medially, the posterosuperior wall of the agger nasi cell (if present) anteriorly, and the anterior wall of the ethmoid bulla posteriorly.[6]

The frontal sinus drainage pathway can be thought of as having a superior and an inferior compartment (▶ Fig. 1.14).[26] The superior compartment is formed by the union of adjacent air spaces at the anteroinferior portion of the frontal bone and the anterosuperior portion of the ethmoid bone. The frontal ostium is at the upper border of the superior compartment. The superior compartment directly communicates with the inferior compartment.

The anatomy of the inferior compartment of the frontal sinus drainage pathway can vary depending on the site of insertion of the uncinate process anteriorly.[28] When the anterior portion of the uncinate process extends superiorly to attach to the skull base, this results in formation of the ethmoid infundibulum (constituting the inferior part of the frontal sinus drainage pathway) (▶ Fig. 1.14). The ethmoid infundibulum communicates with the middle meatus through the hiatus semilunaris. On the other hand, when the anterior portion of the uncinate process attaches to the lamina papyracea rather than the skull base, the inferior compartment of the frontal sinus drainage pathway becomes the middle meatus itself.

A number of anatomic variants and air cells may be present along the frontal sinus drainage pathway. Some are incidental and of no clinical significance, whereas others could be important

for surgical planning and/or potentially result in narrowing of the pathway depending on their exact location and size. Agger nasi cells were discussed earlier. There are also other air cells in this area that could be important and should be recognized on preoperative scans, including four types of frontal cells.[34] These are summarized in ▶ Table 1.1.

## Pterygopalatine Fossa

We will finish the section on the clinical anatomy of the anterior skull base and paranasal sinuses with a discussion of the PPF because of its important relationship to the skull base and paranasal sinuses. The PPF is an important site of anatomic convergence of multiple neural pathways. Familiarity with this area is critical, particularly for the evaluation of tumors where there is potential for perineural spread of tumor affecting treatment planning and management. The PPF is an elongated, vertically oriented, predominantly fat-filled region located lateral to the posterior aspect of the nasal cavity (▶ Fig. 1.22, ▶ Fig. 1.23).[51,52] The posterior wall of the maxillary sinus forms the anterior margin of the PPF. The posterior boundary of this space is composed of the fused pterygoid plates and the base of the sphenoid bone. The perpendicular plate of the palatine bone forms the majority of the medial margin of the PPF with the exception of the sphenopalatine foramen superiorly (▶ Fig. 1.22). The lateral boundary is the pterygomaxillary fissure, an elongated vertical communication with the infratemporal fossa (▶ Fig. 1.22). The superior aspect is in continuity with the inferior orbital fissure (▶ Fig. 1.22). Inferiorly, the PPF tapers into the greater palatine canal ultimately leading to the greater and lesser palatine foramina (▶ Fig. 1.22).

The neurovascular contents of PPF include the maxillary division of the trigeminal nerve, the pterygopalatine ganglion, and terminal branches of the internal maxillary artery. As alluded

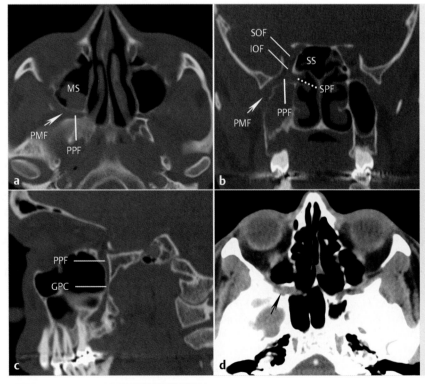

**Fig. 1.22** Major imaging landmarks for the pterygopalatine fossa (PPF). **(a,d)** Axial images with **(b)** coronal and **(c)** sagittal (from the normal left side) reformats from a contrast-enhanced neck CT are shown from a patient with perineural spread of adenoid cystic carcinoma to the right PPF. On the reconstructions using soft-tissue windows **(d)**, at a level slightly higher than in **(a)**, note normal fat-filled left PPF containing normal vascular and neural structures. The right PPF, on the other hand, is infiltrated and mildly expanded (*black arrow*; **d**). Perineural spread of tumor can be subtle or not detectable on CT and is most accurately evaluated using MRI. GPC, greater palatine canal; IOF, inferior orbital fissure; MS, maxillary sinus; PPF, pterygopalatine fossa; PMF, pterygomaxillary fissure; SOF, superior orbital fissure; SPF, sphenopalatine foramen; SS, sphenoid sinus.

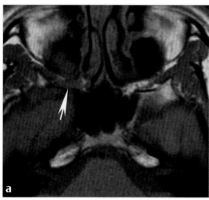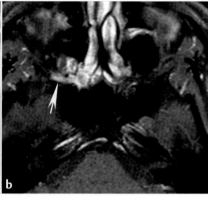

**Fig. 1.23** Pterygopalatine fossa (PPF) and perineural spread of tumor (adenoid cystic carcinoma) on MRI. Axial (**a**) T1-weighted and (**b**) fat-suppressed postcontrast T1-weighted images from the same patient as in ▶ Fig. 1.22 demonstrate perineural spread of tumor in the right PPF (*arrow*). Also note the appearance of the normal contralateral PPF.

earlier, the PPF communicates with multiple adjacent spaces.[3] Laterally, the pterygomaxillary fissure opens into the infratemporal fossa. Medially, the sphenopalatine foramen opens just posterior to the superior or middle meatus where the foramen is covered by mucosa. The sphenopalatine foramen transmits the sphenopalatine artery as well as the nasopalatine and superior nasal nerves from the PPF. Posteriorly, the foramen rotundum communicates with the middle cranial fossa, transmitting the maxillary (V2) branch of the trigeminal nerve. Inferior and medial to the level of the foramen rotundum, the Vidian (pterygoid) canal is located posteriorly and extends to the foramen lacerum. This canal transmits the Vidian nerve. Superolaterally, the inferior orbital fissure transmits the infraorbital nerve and artery. Inferiorly, the pterygopalatine canal leads to the greater and lesser palatine foramina and then the oral cavity.[3] The greater palatine foramen transmits the greater palatine nerve and descending palatine vessels. The lesser palatine foramen transmits the lesser palatine nerves. Although commonly single, there can be two or rarely more than two lesser palatine foraminas.[53]

# 1.4 Pathology of the Anterior Skull Base and Paranasal Sinuses

## 1.4.1 Tumors

### Squamous Cell Carcinoma

Sinonasal cancers constitute a small percentage, approximately 5%, of all head and neck cancers with an estimated worldwide incidence of 1 per 100,000 annually.[54] Among these, 50 to 80% are squamous cell carcinomas (SCCs). In the nasal cavity, males are affected more frequently than females and patients most commonly present between the ages of 55 and 65 years.[55] Multiple occupational risk factors have been identified for SCC and sinonasal adenocarcinoma, including those resulting in exposure to nickel, wood furniture and leather production, chromium, mustard gas, isopropyl alcohol, formaldehyde, arsenic, and radium.[55,56,57] Additional risk factors include a history of previous radiation therapy as well as immunosuppression and smoking.[58,59] Thorotrast exposure is an established etiologic agent for maxillary sinus carcinoma, although practically no longer seen as the contrast agent has long been discontinued.[55] SCC may develop concurrently within an inverted papilloma or subsequent to resection. Synchronous or metachronous SCCs of

the same histologic type occur in 15%, most often outside of the head and neck. The most common tumor location is the maxillary antrum, followed by the nasal cavity and ethmoid sinuses. Much less commonly, the sphenoid and frontal sinuses are the sites of tumor origin.

## Imaging characteristics

On CT, SCC of the sinonasal cavities has the appearance of a soft-tissue mass with variable contrast enhancement (▶ Fig. 1.24, ▶ Fig. 1.25, ▶ Fig. 1.26). Aggressive and relatively extensive osseous destruction is often present, while bone remodeling and/or sclerosis are less common (▶ Fig. 1.24, ▶ Fig. 1.25, ▶ Fig. 1.26).[55] Corresponding with osseous destruction, there may be alteration of fat attenuation or frank soft-tissue extension in adjacent regions such as the retromaxillary fat and the extraconal orbit. CT also directly delineates the cribriform plate, lateral lamella, fovea ethmoidalis, and orbital walls (▶ Fig. 1.27). It should be noted that the appearance of the normal cribriform plate can include small focal lucencies and these do not imply erosion secondary to tumor or invasion.[60] In cases of early focal invasion, the difference can be subtle and requires careful evaluation. Intracranial transgression can be determined by identification of tumor density or intensity tissue extending through the defect to the intracranial aspect of the bone (▶ Fig. 1.28). In this regard, MRI is superior for tumor delineation and evaluation of intracranial extension and should be performed if there is ambiguity regarding skull base invasion and intracranial extension.

Perineural extension may be apparent as evidenced by effacement and infiltration of normal fat in key neurovascular conduits such as the PPF (▶ Fig. 1.23). In advanced cases, tubular soft-tissue structures may be visible extending along adjacent neural pathways (▶ Fig. 1.29), sometimes with associated osseous destruction or remodeling at the sites of skull base foramina including the Vidian (pterygoid) canals, foramen rotundum, and foramen ovale. In advanced and longstanding cases, unilateral denervation changes such as muscular atrophy and fatty replacement in the territory of an involved motor nerve such as the mandibular division of the trigeminal nerve can be present (▶ Fig. 1.29). Denervation changes should not be confused with direct tumor spread and invasion. Apart from differences in signal intensity depending on the stage of denervation, one clue for identifying denervation change is that while the signal in the muscles may be abnormal, their overall architecture and shape is preserved, unlike muscle invaded by tumor.

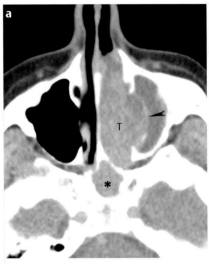
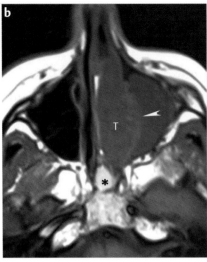

**Fig. 1.24** Squamous cell carcinoma of the nasal cavity and ethmoid air cells: secretions versus tumor on CT and MRI. (a) Axial contrast-enhanced CT and (b) T1-weighted MRI without contrast demonstrate tumor (T) filling the left nasal cavity and invading the medial maxillary sinus wall with a bulging contour (*arrowhead*). (a) On CT, the attenuation of the enhancing tumor can be similar to that of obstructive or inflammatory secretions, depending on their protein concentration. In this case, the secretions in the left maxillary sinus have mildly lower attenuation compared to the tumor, but there is opacification of the sphenoid sinus with similar attenuation to tumor (*asterisk*) making distinction impossible. (b) MRI is superior to CT for distinguishing tumor from obstructive secretions. In this case, the sphenoid sinus contents have high signal on T1-weighted images (*asterisk*), consistent with proteinaceous secretions and clearly distinguishable from the intermediate signal tumor.

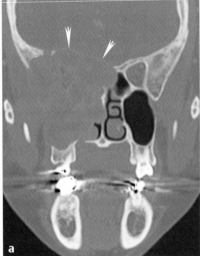
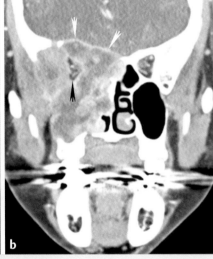
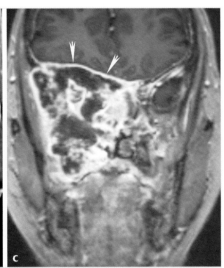

**Fig. 1.25** Large invasive sinonasal squamous cell carcinoma (spindle cell variant) with bone destruction and invasion of adjacent structures and spaces. Coronal reformats from a contrast-enhanced CT displayed in bone (a) or soft-tissue (b) windows as well as a coronal contrast-enhanced T1-weighted MRI (c) demonstrate a large heterogeneously enhancing mass with areas of internal cystic change and necrosis. There is extensive bone erosion and destruction with tumor extending lateral to the maxillary sinus and medially into the nasal cavity, ethmoidal labyrinth, and part of the nasal septum. Superiorly, there is extension into and encasement of the posterior right orbital structures (*short black arrow*; b), and anterior cranial fossa (*short white arrows*). Large aggressive tumors can exhibit significant heterogeneity and necrosis.

On MRI, SCC typically has intermediate signal on T1-weighted images and is mildly hyperintense on T2-weighted images (▶ Fig. 1.24, ▶ Fig. 1.28).[55] Tumor texture can be homogeneous, especially for smaller tumors but tends to be heterogeneous for larger tumors, in which case there may be evidence of necrosis, hemorrhage, and/or surface ulceration (▶ Fig. 1.25, ▶ Fig. 1.28). In the absence of necrosis, tumor tissue can often be best differentiated from reactive inflammation and obstructive secretions on T2-weighted images, with excellent contrast between the intermediate to high signal tumor and the very high signal of obstructed secretions and mucosal inflammatory changes (▶ Fig. 1.30). However, the signal of secretions varies depending on their protein content, and on occasion, their signal may

approach that of the tumor on T2-weighted images. In those cases, the signal on the other sequences, including the unenhanced T1-weighted image, typically enables a reliable distinction (▶ Fig. 1.24, ▶ Fig. 1.30). On postcontrast T1-weighted images, solid nodular tumor enhancement is typically distinguishable, but there are pitfalls. The inherent T1-weighted hyperintensity often manifested by chronically obstructed secretions can make detection of superimposed enhancement and therefore delineation of the sinonasal margin of enhancing tumor more challenging (▶ Fig. 1.30). In these cases, subtraction images or comparing pre- and post-contrast images can be helpful. It should also be noted that inflamed sinus mucosa can demonstrate robust enhancement. However, the relatively thin

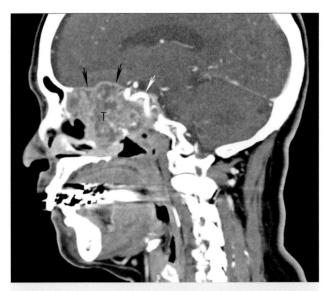

**Fig. 1.26** Squamous cell carcinoma (SCC) with extensive bone erosion, ICA encasement, and intracranial extension. Sagittal reformat from a contrast-enhanced CT demonstrates extensive skull base involvement from a sinonasal spindle cell variant SCC (T) with encasement of the cavernous internal carotid artery (*small white arrow*) as well as invasion and breach through the orbital plate of the frontal bone (*small black arrows*).

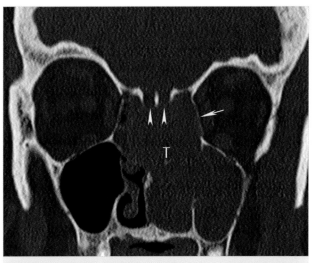

**Fig. 1.27** Squamous cell carcinoma (SCC) of nasal cavity and ethmoid air cells: assessment of the cribriform plate and periorbita. Coronal reformat from a sinonasal CT displayed in bone windows demonstrates diffuse opacification of the left nasal cavity crossing to the right as well as left maxillary sinus secondary to tumor (T). Note erosion of cribriform plates bilaterally (*arrowheads*), superior part of the nasal septum, and medial maxillary sinus wall. There is also smooth remodeling of the left medial orbital wall (*arrow*) without break-through, suggesting that the periorbita remains intact. As discussed in the earlier figures, some of the sinonasal opacification could represent retained secretions and inflammatory changes, and when in doubt these are best delineated by MRI.

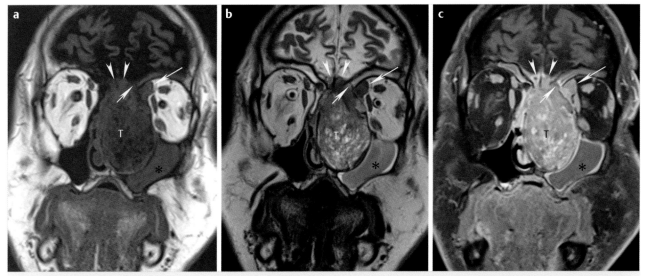

**Fig. 1.28** Squamous cell carcinoma (SCC) intracranial extension and orbital invasion on MRI. Coronal T1 (**a**), T2 (**b**), and contrast-enhanced fat-suppressed T1-weighted (**c**) images of a SCC of the nasal cavity and ethmoid air cells are shown. There is a heterogeneous mass (T) that remodels the nasal cavity margins but also has focal areas of erosion, including the cribriform plates and inferior margin of the left frontal sinus. There is enhancing tissue extending into the olfactory fossae bilaterally with contiguous dural enhancement extending laterally (*arrowheads*). Enhancing tissue enters the inferomedial aspect of the left frontal sinus (*short arrow*). There is invasion of the medial left orbital wall superiorly with loss of fat plane medial to the superior oblique muscle and enlargement of the superior oblique muscle (*long arrow*), consistent with orbital and extraocular muscle invasion. Note the difference between the mass (T) and obstructive inflammatory changes of the left maxillary sinus (*asterisk*). Incidentally, there are gliotic changes in the inferomedial frontal lobes, suggestive of unrelated prior traumatic injury.

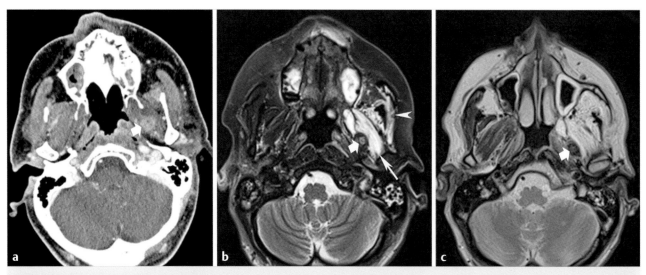

**Fig. 1.29** Mandibular nerve (V3) perineural spread from squamous cell carcinoma of the lower lip shown on contrast-enhanced CT (**a**), fat-suppressed T2-weighted MRI (**b**), and standard T2-weighted MRI (**c**) in the axial plane. Perineural spread is seen manifesting as cordlike thickening of V3 (*thick arrows*), located along the medial aspect of the lateral pterygoid muscle belly (*thin arrow*; **b**). There is increased signal in the lateral pterygoid (*thin arrow*; **b**) and temporalis muscles (*arrowhead*; **b**) that is best seen on the fat-suppressed T2-weighted image, in keeping with denervation edema. These denervation changes are much less conspicuous on CT. Without fat suppression, the involved muscles are indistinguishable from fat and could be confused with fatty infiltration from more chronic denervation.

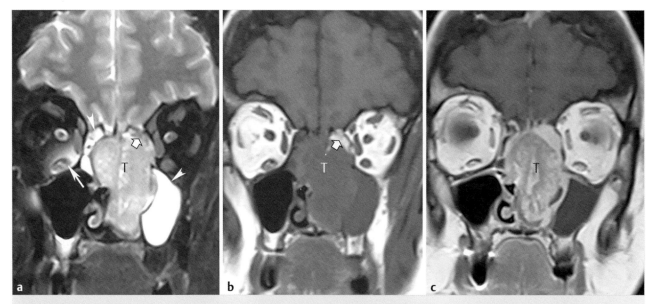

**Fig. 1.30** Squamous cell carcinoma of the nasal cavity and ethmoid air cells versus obstructive inflammatory paranasal sinus changes. T2-weighted MRI with fat-suppression (**a**), unenhanced T1-weighted MRI (**b**), and contrast-enhanced T1-weighted MRI (**c**) in the coronal plane are shown. There is very good differentiation of the intermediate to high signal tumor centrally (T) from the very high signal secretions in the left maxillary sinus and right ethmoid air cells (*arrowheads*; **a**). Small areas with lower signal on T2-weighted images in some uninvaded left ethmoid air cells have corresponding high signal on precontrast T1-weighted images, consistent with inspissated secretions rather than tumor (*thick arrow*; **a,b**). The distinction is less clear on the postcontrast images due to tumoral and mucosal enhancement as well as the intrinsically high signal of those secretions on T1. The low-signal lamina papyracea and periorbita appear intact on the T1-weighted images, and there is preservation of normal extraconal fat and extraocular muscle signal in the adjacent retrobulbar orbit. Note artefactual signal abnormality in the inferomedial right orbit on the fat-suppressed T2-weighted image (*thin arrow*; **b**), related to inhomogeneous fat suppression resulting from magnetic susceptibility artifact at the air–bone interface of the normal right maxillary sinus. This is not present on the left, possibly in part due to the presence of secretions and absence of air–bone interface on that side.

linear mucosal enhancement associated with obstructive changes is typically distinguishable from solid and nodular tumoral enhancement.

Tumor spread outside of the sinus is well depicted on MRI. In cases of spread to predominantly fat-containing areas, such as the retromaxillary fat, tumor spread is well depicted on precontrast T1-weighted images by virtue of the intrinsic contrast between intermediate signal intensity of tumor versus inherently high signal intensity of normal fat on this sequence (▶ Fig. 1.31, ▶ Fig. 1.32). However, tumor spread and invasion of soft tissues is often best depicted overall on fat-suppressed postcontrast T1-weighted images and all sinus and neck protocols should include a postcontrast acquisition with fat suppression.

CT and MRI are complementary for the evaluation of bone invasion. CT is excellent for demonstrating fine bone detail and for the evaluation of cortical bone destruction or destruction of thin bony septae that may not be individually distinguishable on MRI (▶ Fig. 1.27). MRI, on the other hand, is superior to CT for identifying early bone marrow invasion. Once again, one can leverage the intrinsic signal differences between tumor and fat to help identification of marrow invasion. On MRI, loss of high signal of marrow fat on T1-weighted images without contrast is an important early clue for marrow invasion (▶ Fig. 1.31,

▶ Fig. 1.32, ▶ Fig. 1.33). Bone marrow invasion will appear relatively hyperintense on T2-weighted images and will enhance, resulting in a high signal, after administration of contrast. However, it is important to be aware that although MRI is more sensitive for the detection of early marrow invasion, signal changes on MRI may also overestimate marrow invasion or even give a false-positive result. This is because reactive marrow edema will appear hyperintense on T2-weighted images and enhance. Therefore, when evaluating marrow invasion on MRI, it is important to evaluate the signal on all sequences and make sure that it is similar to that of the native tumor. Reactive edema will not necessarily follow that pattern on all sequences and on T2-weighted images; it may have higher signal than the native tumor. Cortices and thin osseous lamina such as the walls of the paranasal sinuses, lamina papyracea, cribriform plate, and fovea ethmoidalis are represented on MRI as well-defined, hypointense structures on T1- and T2-weighted imaging but may sometimes be better evaluated on CT as discussed earlier.

Although the most common route of spread of SCC is direct invasion of nearby structures, there is also a less common but important route of spread for head and neck cancer along nerve bundles, referred to as perineural spread of tumor. Distant perineural spread of tumor refers to cases where the tumor appears to use the nerve as a conduit to spread away from the primary

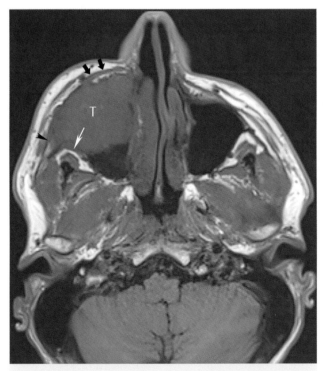

Fig. 1.31 Sinonasal undifferentiated carcinoma located anteriorly in the right maxillary sinus on axial T1-weighted MRI without contrast. Tumor (T) fills much of the sinus, and has intermediate signal nearly isointense to skeletal muscle. There is lobular, irregular extension of the mass into the premaxillary soft tissues, including the expected location of the infraorbital nerve, deep to the levator labii superioris alaeque nasi muscle (*thick black arrows*). There is obliteration of the normal high marrow signal in the right zygoma (*black arrowhead*) secondary to tumor invasion, as well as encroachment of intermediate-signal tumor into the high-signal retromaxillary fat (*white arrow*).

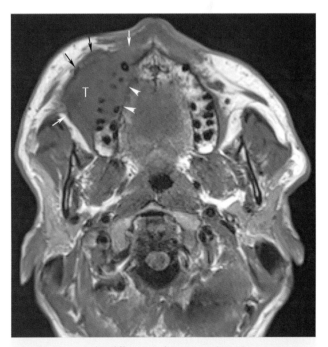

Fig. 1.32 Sinonasal undifferentiated carcinoma (SNUC), extrasinus extension. Axial T1-weighted MRI without contrast of a right maxillary sinus SNUC is shown at the level of the maxillary alveolus. Tumor (T) extends outside the sinus with extensive involvement of the subcutaneous tissues and muscles of facial expression (*white and black thin arrows*) as well as the maxillary alveolus marrow (*white arrowheads*).

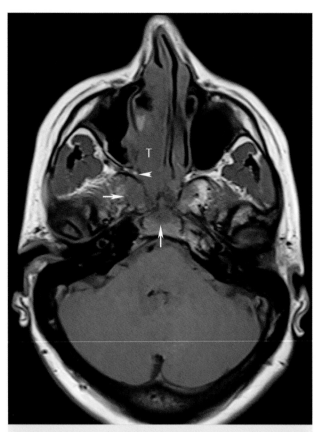

**Fig. 1.33** Sinonasal neuroendocrine carcinoma (T) invading adjacent spaces and bone on T1-weighted axial MRI without contrast. Note loss of normal high-signal fat in the marrow of the sphenoid body (*white arrows*) as well as early extension into the right pterygopalatine fossa (*arrowhead*).

site. This should be distinguished from local perineural invasion by the tumor mass. Most commonly, perineural spread of tumor along nerve bundles is in a central direction toward the skull base, although there can also be retrograde spread of tumor.

Although perineural spread, especially when advanced, can be detectable on CT, MRI is the optimal modality for evaluation when perineural spread of tumor is suspected (▶ Fig. 1.22, ▶ Fig. 1.23, ▶ Fig. 1.29). MRI is the optimal test both for early detection of perineural spread of tumor and for delineation of its extent. Early signs of perineural spread of tumor are differential enhancement of major nerve bundles relative to the contralateral side and early asymmetry secondary to infiltration of tumor density or signal tissue. Because of the venous plexus around the nerves, some degree of nerve enhancement is normal and should not be misinterpreted as perineural spread of tumor. In this regard, comparison with the contralateral side is essential and can be very helpful. When more advanced, the nerve bundle can be grossly enlarged and if large enough there can be remodeling and expansion of the bony foramen. Postcontrast images are key in the identification of perineural tumor spread, demonstrating hyperenhancement and/or enlargement of neural structures beyond what can be attributed to adjacent or contralateral normal nerve or abnormal infiltration of spaces such as the PPF (▶ Fig. 1.22, ▶ Fig. 1.23,

▶ Fig. 1.29). Fat-suppressed T1-weighted images are an important sequence for the evaluation of all head and neck cancer on MRI. However, postcontrast T1-weighted images without fat suppression also play an important complementary role, particularly for the evaluation of perineural spread of tumor. Even though there is controversy regarding their necessity in the literature, it should be noted that there is propensity for image distortion at air–bone interfaces in the paranasal sinuses and skull base that can obscure small neural foramina. Fat-suppressed images have a higher propensity for this type of susceptibility artifact (▶ Fig. 1.30). As such, some groups routinely perform at least one set of postcontrast but non–fat-suppressed T1-weighted images, typically in the coronal plane, in all studies evaluating the skull base and paranasal sinuses.

In addition to the evaluation of perineural spread of tumor, MRI is also the optimal modality for the evaluation of intracranial extension of sinonasal tumors. It should be noted that thin linear dural enhancement alone is insufficient to diagnose dural invasion and can be reactive. Dural thickening exceeding 5 mm, focal dural nodularity, and/or leptomeningeal enhancement have been suggested as imaging criteria for dural invasion[61,62] (▶ Fig. 1.28). When there is evidence of dural invasion, diagnosis of parenchymal brain invasion can be challenging. Findings of vasogenic edema in the white matter of displaced portions of the adjacent frontal lobes are not well correlated with histopathologic evidence of brain invasion.[60] Frontal lobe invasion can generally be confirmed only on imaging by disruption of the cortical ribbon secondary to encroachment by tumor.

The orbital periosteum, also known as the periorbita, is continuous with the dura and the optic nerve sheath at the orbital apex. This robust layer is loosely adherent to the osseous orbit and provides a displaceable barrier to tumor spread.[63] The integrity of the periorbita can be assessed indirectly on CT and directly on MRI.[60] CT findings of intact periorbita in the context of adjacent osseous destruction include broad, smooth displacement of a well-defined margin with orbital fat (▶ Fig. 1.27).[64] On MRI, the periorbita can be evaluated directly. It normally has the appearance of a thin, smooth, T1- and T2-hypointense line (▶ Fig. 1.30, ▶ Fig. 1.34).[60] Loss of this structure, especially when accompanied by signal changes or abnormal nodular tissue extending in the adjacent orbital fat and/or extraocular muscles, is concerning for transgression (▶ Fig. 1.25, ▶ Fig. 1.28, ▶ Fig. 1.35).[65,66,67]

Fat-suppressed T2-weighted images can increase conspicuity of small abnormal lymph nodes. While level IB and retropharyngeal lymph nodes are the primary drainage site for the paranasal sinuses and the nasal cavity, the retropharyngeal route may be disrupted by infection in childhood.[55] As a result, frequent sites of initial nodal metastatic spread are levels I, II, and III. Lymphatic spread is associated with the extension of the primary tumor to the skin surface, alveolar buccal sulcus, or pterygoid musculature.

Currently, MRI is considered the gold standard imaging test for the evaluation of sinonasal cancer. Unless contraindicated, MRI should be performed for the evaluation of sinonasal cancer after the administration of gadolinium-based contrast agents. In addition, MRI should be performed when perineural spread of tumor or intracranial extension of tumor is suspected. CT also plays an important role in the evaluation of sinonasal cancer. As discussed earlier, CT is complementary for the

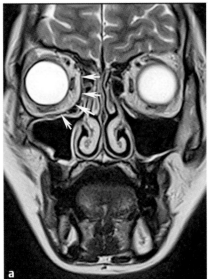
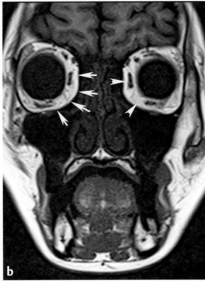

Fig. 1.34 Normal periorbital tissues. Normal orbits, paranasal sinuses, and nasal cavity on T2-weighted (**a**) and T1-weighted (**b**) MRI images in the coronal plane. Note the smooth, low-signal orbital margins on both sequences, representing orbital cortex and adjacent orbital periostium (also referred to as periorbita, *white arrows*). T1-weighted images in particular demonstrate normal high-intensity extraconal fat (*arrowheads*; **b**) in contrast to sinonasal mucosa, cortex, periorbita, and extraocular muscle tissue.

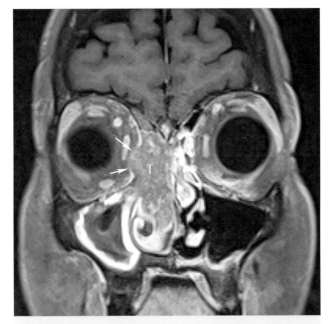

Fig. 1.35 Orbital invasion (neuroendocrine tumor). Sinonasal neuroendocrine tumor (T) of the superior nasal cavity and ethmoid air cells on a fat-suppressed contrast-enhanced T1-weighted image in the coronal plane is shown. A focal area of nodular tumor tissue protrudes into the medial right orbit (*white arrows*), suggesting orbital invasion.

evaluation of certain structures, such as bone invasion. Furthermore, CT better demonstrates variations in sinonasal and skull base anatomy that are important for preoperative planning and intraoperative guidance. In patients who have had a contrast-enhanced MRI, a CT scan could be performed without contrast for preoperative planning and intraoperative guidance. However, the role of CT is not limited solely for complementing the MRI. In most cases, CT will adequately define the extent of tumors, although as discussed earlier some features, such as distinction from secretions, can be more challenging on CT.

If CT is performed to stage the tumor because of contraindications to MRI or accessibility, optimally the CT should be performed without and with contrast. This could be helpful for the identification of enhancing tumor and the distinction from intermediate to high attenuation secretions, although there is variation in practice and protocols used. Fluorodeoxyglucose-positron emission tomography (FDG-PET) metabolic imaging is not routinely performed for the initial staging of sinonasal tumors. However, for the detection of disease recurrence, FDG-PET CT is superior to conventional CT and MRI, although with moderate specificity as it pertains to the inflammatory effects of therapy.[68] Utilization of this modality is increasing, based on availability.

## Staging

In the primary tumor component of the TNM classification[69] for maxillary sinus tumors, T1 lesions are limited to the sinus mucosa. Limited bone erosion, with the exception of involvement of the posterior wall of the maxillary sinus and the adjacent pterygoid plates, denotes T2. T2 tumors tend to be confined to infrastructure components as defined by Ohngren's line—the oblique plane extending from the medial canthus of the eye to the angle of the mandible.[69] These tumors are more often surgically resectable compared with more advanced tumors and those that invade structures superolateral of this plane (i.e., in the suprastructure). T3 tumors involve the posterior wall of the maxillary sinus, the subcutaneous tissues, the orbital floor or medial wall, the PPF, or ethmoid sinuses. T4a, moderately advanced local disease, is distinguished by invasion of anterior orbital contents, skin of the cheek, pterygoid plates, infratemporal fossa, cribriform plate, sphenoid, or frontal sinuses. In stage T4b, very advanced local disease, there is involvement of the orbital apex, dura, brain, middle cranial fossa, cranial nerves other than the maxillary division of the trigeminal nerve, nasopharynx, or clivus.

T staging for nasal cavity and ethmoid sinus lesions is determined with a separate categorization system. T1 lesions are restricted to a single subsite, irrespective of bone invasion.

Ethmoid subsites are right and left ethmoid labyrinths. Subsites of the nasal cavity include the septum, floor, lateral wall, and vestibule. T2 tumors can invade two subsites in a single region or a single subsite with the involvement of an adjacent region in the nasoethmoidal complex. Involvement of the medial wall or floor of the orbit, maxillary sinus, palate, or cribriform plate denotes T3. T4a tumors invade anterior orbital contents, skin, pterygoid plates, sphenoid, or frontal sinuses. These lesions may also minimally extend into the anterior cranial fossa. T4b lesions, similar to maxillary sinus tumors, may invade the orbital apices, dura, brain, middle cranial fossa, cranial nerves other than V2, the nasopharynx, or the clivus. There is no standard staging for frontal or sphenoid sinus tumors.

In regional lymph node staging, N1 denotes a single ipsilateral lymph node metastasis measuring 3 cm or less in greatest dimension. N2a is a solitary lymph node measuring between 3 and 6 cm in greatest dimension. Multiple ipsilateral lymph nodes measuring no more than 6 cm are considered to reflect stage N2b, while bilateral or contralateral lymph nodes measuring up to 6 cm are characterized as stage N2c. N3 is assigned when a lymph node measures more than 6 cm in greatest dimension. Metastasis to distant sites, including lymph nodes beyond the cervical chain or to other organs, defines stage M1.

## Prognosis and treatment

Five-year survival rates for sinonasal SCC are reported to range from 40 to 70%.[70,71] Human papillomavirus (HPV) association is emerging as an important etiologic factor in sinonasal SCC, although the impact on prognosis and optimal treatment is not yet defined.[72] Surgery combined with adjuvant radiotherapy is the treatment of choice.[73] One of the most important positive prognostic factors for SCC, along with other sinonasal malignancies, is the achievement of clear surgical margins.[59] Adjuvant chemotherapy may also sometimes be provided; however, there is as of yet no established role for adjuvant chemotherapy in the routine management of sinonasal malignancies. Endoscopic endonasal surgical approaches have recently been employed in a piecemeal fashion for curative resection, symptom palliation, and debulking before definitive chemoradiotherapy.[74]

In general, anterior skull base curative surgical resection is contraindicated when clear margins cannot be obtained. Additional contraindications include tumor surrounding the optic chiasm, perineural spread to Meckel's cave or the cavernous sinus, involvement of the carotid arteries, extensive brain parenchymal involvement, metastatic disease, or limiting comorbid illnesses. Successful resection may be difficult when there is evidence of central skull base involvement, tumor extension into the nasopharynx, or PPF.[73,75] There are data supporting the use of adjuvant radiation therapy when there are positive margins on final pathologic testing.[76] Neurologic function including vision and olfaction is preserved when possible. Operative complications are reduced by minimizing brain retraction, control of CSF, and segregation of intracranial contents from extracranial tissues. In cases extending to the lateral nasal wall, the lamina papyracea may be resected and the periorbita may also be resected if invaded to achieve clear margins.[74] Infiltration of orbital fat usually necessitates orbital exenteration. Skull base erosion is treated with skull base and

dural resection with subsequent duraplasty and flap reconstruction. Limited brain involvement can be managed with endoscopic or transcranial frontal lobe resection to achieve negative margins.

Various forms of maxillectomy are performed depending on the extent of tumors involving the maxillary sinus, floor of the nose, or hard palate, typically via a combined transoral, lateral rhinotomy procedure referred to as the Weber-Ferguson approach. Lateral extension of tumor into or through the PPF may be approached endoscopically via a transpterygoid route. For tumors involving the frontal sinuses, the midpoint of the orbital roof is considered the point of maximum lateral access for an endoscopic endonasal approach.[60] Resections extending lateral to this point necessitate an external transfrontal approach, as do those involving the anterior wall of the frontal sinus. Contraindications to a purely endoscopic approach include dural involvement beyond the mid-orbit, invasion of skin, orbital invasion, maxilla involvement beyond the medial wall, or significant brain involvement.

Following resection, adjuvant radiotherapy is often delivered to the operative bed and/or draining lymph nodes, depending on specific risk factors. Treatment of the operative bed is indicated for close or positive margins, T3/T4 stage, and can be considered for tumors with perineural invasion, lymphovascular invasion, or high histologic grade. A typical postoperative clinical target volume encompasses both halves of the nasal cavity and the ipsilateral maxillary sinus. The ethmoid sinuses and the ipsilateral medial orbital wall are also included if tumor involves the ethmoid air cells. Any tumor with documented perineural extension necessitates generous coverage of the skull base with extension of the clinical target volume to the appropriate neural foramina. Sixty to 63 gray (Gy) is typically prescribed to the clinical target volume at 1.8 to 2 Gy daily fractions, with a boost delivered to involved margins or gross residual tumor.[75] Regions at risk of microscopic tumor spread that have not been surgically manipulated may receive a lower dose equivalent to approximately 50 Gy in 2 Gy daily fractions. Treatment to the regional lymph nodes is indicated for node-positive disease and can be considered in the setting of a T3/T4 primary tumor. An additional margin is added to all clinical target volumes in order to account for daily setup variation, and the final volumes are referred to as the planning target volumes.

In cases in which radiotherapy is expected to be a component of a multimodality treatment approach, preoperative radiotherapy is sometimes employed as an alternative to postoperative radiotherapy.[77] Potential advantages of preoperative over postoperative radiotherapy include (1) smaller target volumes and (2) lower dose (typically 50 Gy in 2 Gy daily fractions to the entire clinical target volume) due to better oxygenation of the tissues. Regions that are expected to have close or microscopically positive surgical margins may receive a boost. Frankly unresectable disease would be inappropriate for this approach.

Unresectable lesions can be treated with definitive radiotherapy alone or in combination with systemic chemotherapy. The clinical target volume, which includes the gross tumor volume derived from CT and MR imaging as well as areas of potential microscopic extension, is typically treated to the equivalent of 70 Gy in 2 Gy daily fractions.[78] If chemotherapy cannot be delivered concurrently, the radiotherapy may be delivered with an alternative fractionation scheme (e.g., moderate acceleration) in order to improve the likelihood of control.

For the purposes of radiotherapy planning, critical, dose-limiting organs include the optic nerves, chiasm, eyes, lacrimal glands, auditory apparatus, parotid glands, pituitary, brainstem, and spinal cord. If critical structures cannot be excluded, a hyperfractionated regimen (1–1.2 Gy twice-daily fractionation) may be considered. If there is extensive orbital involvement by tumor and radiotherapy is delivered primarily, the involved eye is included in the treatment volume. If possible, the contralateral eye and the lacrimal glands are protected. Reduced doses to critical structures can often be achieved while maintaining target tumor dose with intensity-modulated radiotherapy (IMRT). The use of image-guided radiotherapy with volumetric CT data acquired at the time of each daily treatment can also be used to minimize dose to critical structures, particularly when employed in combination with IMRT. Proton beam therapy may be capable of treating deep-seated tumors such as those of the sinonasal cavities with improved sparing of adjacent normal tissues by virtue of the proton beam Bragg peak.[79] To date, however, there appears to be little clinical outcome data supporting the use of proton beam therapy at this site, likely related to limited availability.

## Adenocarcinoma

### Overview

Adenocarcinoma accounts for approximately 13% of all sinonasal malignancies and is the second most common histologic subtype in this location.[54,80] Sinonasal adenocarcinomas can be subclassified into salivary and nonsalivary types, with the nonsalivary group further divided into intestinal-type and non–intestinal-type lesions.[81] In some published series, occupation exposure to woodworking has been described in up to 90% of patients with sinonasal adenocarcinomas,[82] whereas others have shown the highest association with cigarette smoking and alcohol use.[83] Other occupational exposures include tanning and nickel. Cigarette smoking and alcohol use are the most commonly reported exposures in North American populations. Most patients are male and there is a wide age range at presentation. The most common primary location is the ethmoid sinuses, followed closely by nasal cavity. Cases related to industrial wood exposure have a particularly strong predilection for the ethmoid sinuses, while sporadic cases are more often seen in the maxillary sinuses.[80] Presenting symptoms are nonspecific, including nasal obstruction, rhinorrhea, and epistaxis.[81]

### Imaging characteristics

Sinonasal adenocarcinomas, in general, have characteristics on CT and MRI that are similar to and cannot be readily distinguished from the more common SCCs (▶ Fig. 1.36).[80] Both of these tumors have the appearance of an enhancing soft-tissue mass with variable degrees of necrosis, invasion, and bone destruction. Please refer to the section on SCC for a more detailed description.

## Prognosis and treatment

There is conflicting evidence regarding the effect of histologic subtype and degree of differentiation on survival.[80,81,83] In small primary tumors with low-grade histology, favorable outcomes have been achieved with wide surgical resection alone[83] (▶ Fig. 1.37). Multimodal therapy with surgery and radiotherapy results in improved survival for advanced lesions, sometimes with the addition of chemotherapy. Endoscopic surgery can be considered, most often for T1 and T2 lesions.[83] The local recurrence rate in a recent series was 29% with 5-year overall survival of 66%.[83]

## Sinonasal Undifferentiated Carcinoma

### Overview

Sinonasal undifferentiated carcinoma (SNUC) is a rare, aggressive malignancy typified by extensive disease at presentation and poor overall survival.[84] Patients most often present with advanced disease (Kadish group C, with extension beyond the sinonasal cavities), making identification of the site of origin difficult.[55] Histologically, the tumor has characteristics of an undifferentiated epithelial malignancy; however, it may be part of a spectrum of diminishing differentiation, including olfactory neuroblastoma (ONB), sinonasal neuroendocrine carcinoma, and SNUC.[84] Patients often present with a short history of epistaxis, obstruction, and/or neurological symptoms.[85] In one recent systematic review that included 167 patients, the mean patient age was 53 years with a wide range[84] and fewer than three-fourths were male.

### Imaging features

Imaging findings of SNUC resemble those of SCC.[55] The tumor typically has the appearance of an aggressive soft-tissue mass (▶ Fig. 1.31, ▶ Fig. 1.32) with erosion rather than remodeling of the adjacent bone (unlike ONB). Small lesions are often polypoid and unilateral in the nasal cavity with involvement of adjacent ethmoid or maxillary sinuses. Larger lesions commonly extend into the orbit and/or anterior cranial fossa. Lymphovascular and neural invasions are common.[86]

### Prognosis and treatment

Overall survival is poor and available evidence guiding therapy is limited. In one large systematic review, overall disease-free survival at last follow-up was 26%.[84] Cervical lymph node metastases are a particularly poor prognostic sign. Multimodal therapy appears better than single-modality therapy. However, surgical-based approaches have not been clearly demonstrated to be superior.[85] In one analysis, chemotherapy and/or radiation in addition to surgery conferred benefit, although there was no statistical difference with the addition of one, the other, or both in patients with advanced stages of disease.[84] Surgical intervention typically involves extensive craniofacial resection, maxillectomy, orbital exenteration, and sometimes dural or brain resection.[85] Reported chemotherapeutic agents used include carboplatin, cisplatin, and etoposide. Fractionated radiotherapy doses should be at least 60 Gy.[87,88]

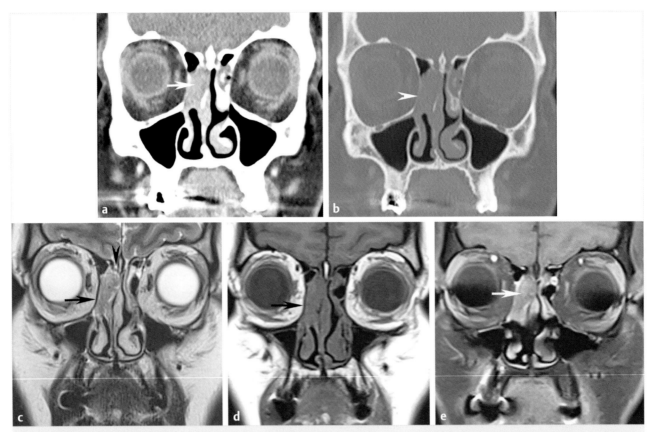

**Fig. 1.36** Small recurrent adenocarcinoma of the right ethmoid labyrinth and superior nasal cavity. Coronal reformatted contrast-enhanced CT displayed using soft-tissue window and algorithm (**a**) or bone window and algorithm (**b**), T2-weighted MRI (**c**), T1-weighted MRI (**d**), and fat-suppressed contrast-enhanced T1-weighted MRI (**e**) are shown. The recurrent lesion demonstrates mild, relatively homogeneous enhancement on CT and MRI (*white arrows*; **a,e**). The adjacent right lamina papyracea appears at most mildly attenuated (*white arrowhead*; **b**). Tissue signal is intermediate on T1 and T2, mildly hypointense to mucosa and secretions on T2-weighted images. The periorbita and extraconal orbital fat appear intact on T1- and T2-weighted images (*black arrows*; **c,d**). The tumor is in close proximity to the right cribriform plate; however, there is preservation of a low-signal line on T2WI (*black arrowhead*; **c**).

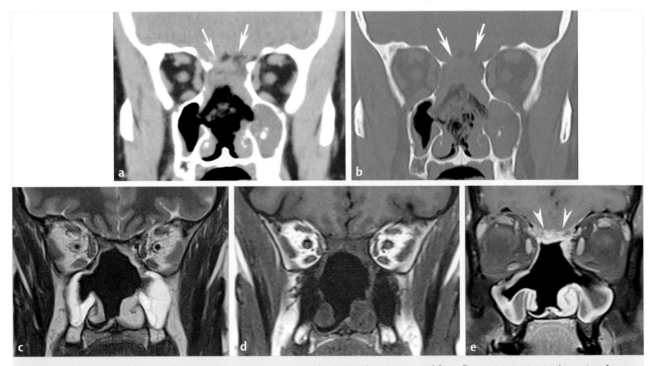

**Fig. 1.37** Postsurgical appearance following endoscopic re-resection and nasoseptal anterior cranial fossa flap reconstruction in the patient from ▶ Fig. 1.36. Unenhanced coronal reformatted CT displayed using soft-tissue window and algorithm (**a**) or bone window and algorithm (**b**) as well as T2-weighted (**c**), T1-weighted, (**d**) and contrast-enhanced fat-suppressed T1-weighted (**e**) MRI images are shown. There is intermixed fat and soft-tissue attenuation filling the anterior cranial fossa osseous defect on CT (*arrows*; **a,b**). The region contains mixed signal intensity enhancing material without focal nodularity. There is thin adjacent dural enhancement which is likely reactive (*arrowheads*; **e**).

## Adenoid Cystic Carcinoma

### Overview

Adenoid cystic carcinoma (ACC) is the most common salivary gland tumor histology in the sinonasal region, accounting for approximately 7% of sinonasal cancers. It is among the top three to six histologic types affecting the sinsonasal region.[54] The lesions can arise anywhere in the sinonasal cavity but most commonly, they originate in the palate and extend secondarily into the nasal fossa or paranasal sinuses.[55] Among primary sinonasal lesions, just less than half arise in the maxillary sinus followed closely by the nasal fossa, with ethmoid, sphenoid, and frontal sinus locations being much less common.[89] Patients are usually Caucasian, nonsmokers, and nondrinkers. Females are affected more often than males. Clinical features at presentation are similar to those of chronic benign sinonasal pathologies and commonly include nasal obstruction, facial pain, and epistaxis. Facial numbness in the distribution of the second division of the trigeminal nerve has also been reported as a common presenting symptom.

### Imaging features

Low-grade ACC can mimic a simple polyp on CT and MRI.[90] However, a spherical polypoid lesion should, in particular, raise concern for a salivary or nerve sheath tumor.[55] Bone remodeling may be present. In larger lesions, tumor signal intensity is highly variable on MRI (▶ Fig. 1.38). ACC, while not unique in this regard, has a particular propensity for perineural spread (▶ Fig. 1.23, ▶ Fig. 1.39, ▶ Fig. 1.40, ▶ Fig. 1.41) and, to a lesser degree, perivascular spread,[89] sometimes with macroscopic skip lesions.[91] On CT, early perineural spread can manifest as subtle infiltration and obliteration of fat-containing spaces such as the PPF. In more advanced cases, there is neurovascular thickening with adjacent osseous changes including bone remodeling, erosion, or sclerosis resulting in widening of foramina, fissures, and canals. On MRI, findings include replacement of normal high-signal fat on T1-weighted images with intermediate-signal tumor that has a grayish hue on postcontrast images, nerve enlargement, and increased enhancement that is most conspicuous on fat-suppressed images in regions not obscured by susceptibility artifact (▶ Fig. 1.23, ▶ Fig. 1.41). In one study, perineural spread was seen in 66% of 26 consecutive patients with head and neck ACC.[91] The sensitivity and specificity were 88 and 89% for CT versus 100 and 85% for MRI, respectively. ACC is classically not FDG avid.[92]

### Prognosis and treatment

Surgery with postoperative radiation provided the best overall and disease-specific survival in one large series.[89] Surgical interventions include total maxillectomy, medial maxillectomy, craniofacial resection, and orbital exenteration. Neck dissection is uncommonly performed. Adjuvant radiotherapy is almost always indicated for ACC due to the propensity for perineurovascular invasion and spread.[93] Radiotherapy clinical target volumes include paths of perineural spread toward skull base neural foramina, with the risk of subsequent osteonecrosis in these regions (▶ Fig. 1.42, ▶ Fig. 1.43). Typical radiotherapy doses are 60 Gy to the at-risk operative bed and 66 to 70 Gy to the gross or unresectable disease. Chemotherapy is most commonly reserved for palliation or clinical trials.

Lymph node and distant metastases are uncommon at presentation. Overall survival at 5 years has been reported to range from 50 to 86%.[83] Skull base invasion has been identified as a significant factor for overall survival. More than half of patients experience local recurrence (▶ Fig. 1.44). A significant number of locoregional recurrences occur as many as 10 to 15 years after primary therapy,[94] resulting in progressively diminishing long-term survival and a need for long-term surveillance. In some patients, slowly progressive lung metastases may also develop which are not immediately life threatening.

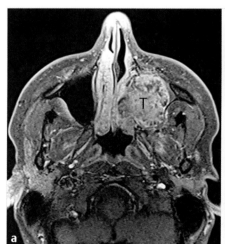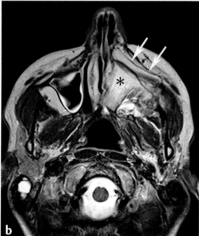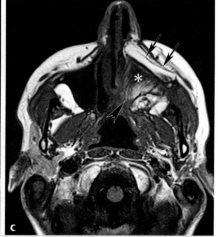

**Fig. 1.38** Adenoid cystic carcinoma involving the left maxilla before and after resection and osteomuscular flap reconstruction. Preoperative fat-suppressed contrast-enhanced T1-weighted MRI (**a**), as well as postoperative T2-weighted (**b**) and T1-weighted (**c**) MRIs are shown. (**a**) Heterogeneously enhancing tumor (T) occupies virtually the entire left maxillary sinus with expansile changes to the walls and extension into the nasal cavity. Following tumor resection, the maxilla has been reconstructed with an osteomuscular flap. There is high signal on T1- and T2-weighted images in the marrow of the osseous component (*white and black arrows*; **b,c**). Striations are present in the muscular component (*asterisk*; **b,c**) and help distinguish the flap from residual or recurrent tumor. There are areas of T1-hyperintense fatty infiltration within the striated muscular component, reflecting denervation change (*black arrowhead*; **c**).

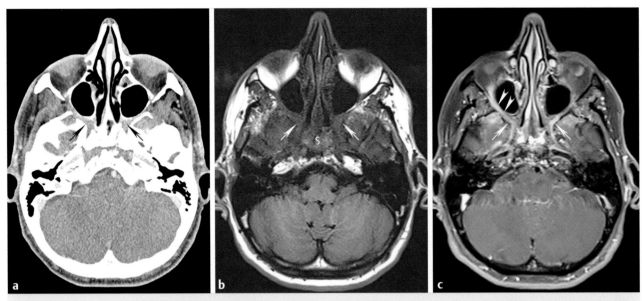

**Fig. 1.39** Bilateral perineural tumor spread from adenoid cystic carcinoma of the palate to the pterygopalatine fossae (PPF) and Vidian canals. Axial contrast-enhanced CT (**a**), T1-weighted precontrast MRI (**b**), and fat-suppressed contrast-enhanced T1-weighted MRI (**c**) are shown. Enhancing tissue replaces normal fat in the involved spaces bilaterally (*black and white arrows*). There is also loss of expected T1-hyperintense marrow fat in the surrounding sphenoid body (S) on the unenhanced T1-weighted image (**b**). An asymmetrical band of enhancement extends from the right PPF through the inferior orbital fissure into the orbit (*arrowheads*; **c**), along the expected course of V2.

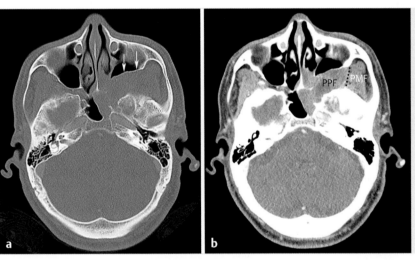

**Fig. 1.40** Adenoid cystic carcinoma of the left sinonasal cavity with extensive perineural extension into the left pterygopalatine fossa (PPF) and pterygomaxillary fissure (PMF). Axial contrast-enhanced CT images displayed in bone (**a**) and soft-tissue windows (**b**) are shown. There is marked widening of the PPF and PMF (*dotted line*) with remodeling of the posterior margin of the left maxillary sinus (*arrows*).

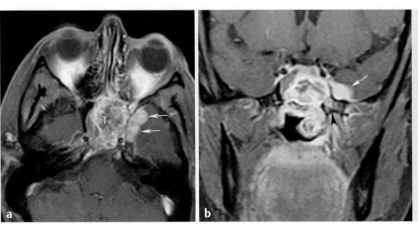

**Fig. 1.41** Adenoid cystic carcinoma (T) of the sphenoid sinuses with extension to the left cavernous sinus (*arrows*) on fat-suppressed contrast-enhanced T1-weighted MRI in the axial (**a**) and coronal (**b**) planes. There is also increased marrow enhancement in the base of the pterygoid processes on the left (*arrowhead*; **b**) with loss of the adjacent sphenoid sinus cortex, consistent with invasion.

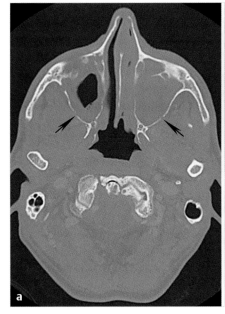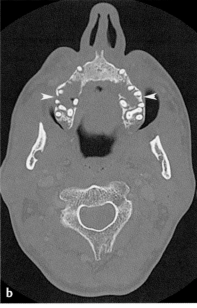

**Fig. 1.42 (a,b)** Osteonecrosis of the maxilla following radiotherapy for adenoid cystic carcinoma of the palate with perineural spread. Axial CT images displayed with bone window settings show heterogeneous areas of demineralization and lysis in the posterolateral (*black arrows*; **a**) and medial maxillary walls as well as the maxillary alveolus (*arrowheads*; **b**) bilaterally.

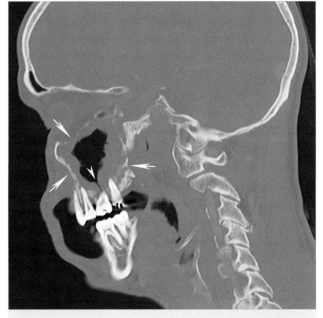

**Fig. 1.43** Osteonecrosis of the maxilla following radiotherapy for adenoid cystic carcinoma of the palate with perineural tumor spread. Sagittal reformatted CT image displayed using bone window settings shows heterogeneous lytic changes in the walls of the maxillary sinus and the maxillary alveolus (*arrows*). An air-filled tract extends to the roots of one of the molar teeth, suggesting oral-antral fistulization (*arrowhead*).

## Mucoepidermoid Carcinoma

### Overview

Mucoepidermoid carcinoma (MEC) is a rare disease entity, accounting for less than 0.1% of primary malignancies in the sinonasal tract.[95] The mean patient age at presentation is approximately 57 years. There is no clear gender predilection. Clinical presentation is most often nonspecific, including obstructive symptoms, epistaxis, soft-tissue mass, or ophthal-

mological symptoms which were present for about 10 months. The most common sites of origin are the nasal cavity followed by the maxillary sinuses and ethmoid sinuses.

### Imaging characteristics

MEC, like other salivary gland tumors, has a nonspecific appearance on imaging. Low-grade tumors typically remodel bone, but high-grade lesions result in more aggressive changes.[55] Salivary gland tumors in general can form spherical masses rather than polypoid or diffuse lesions and this may suggest the etiology on imaging. CT appearances may be homogeneous if the tumor is cellular or inhomogeneous due to necrosis, cystic degeneration, calcification, or accumulation of glandular secretions (▶ Fig. 1.45). The tumors typically have intermediate signal on T1-weighted images and variable signal on T2-weighted images.

### Prognosis and treatment

Most patients present with low-grade tumors and early-stage disease.[95] Wide surgical resection is the treatment of choice.[55] Surgical approaches can include endoscopic or open approaches (including orbital exenteration, if necessary), depending on the extent of the tumor and in order to achieve clear margins.[95] Adjuvant radiotherapy may be given postoperatively, typically in the context of incomplete resection of low-grade lesions and for most high-grade tumors.[55] Chemotherapy is not a common treatment.[95] Less than half of patients experience local recurrence, usually within 2 years of primary treatment. Five-year disease-free survival is estimated at approximately 40%.

## Olfactory Neuroblastoma/ Esthesioneuroblastoma

### Overview

Olfactory neuroblastoma (ONB, historically referred to as esthesioneuroblastoma) is believed to arise from the olfactory

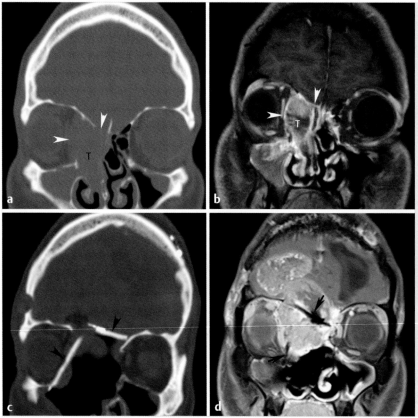

**Fig. 1.44** Adenoid cystic carcinoma of the sinonasal cavity before and after resection and recurrence. Coronal reformatted CT displayed with bone window settings (**a**) and coronal fat-suppressed contrast-enhanced T1-weighted MRI (**b**) prior to surgery shows a heterogeneous tumor (T) with medial orbital wall and cribriform plate erosion and invasion (*white arrowheads*). Coronal reformatted image early after surgery (**c**) shows early postoperative appearance of anterior cranial fossa and orbital wall reconstruction with osseous flaps (*black arrowheads*). Fat-suppressed contrast-enhanced T1-weighted MRI (**d**) obtained later shows extensive recurrence with enhancing tumor extending through the reconstruction flaps (*black arrows* point to residual low signal bone flap) with large intracranial as well as intraorbital components.

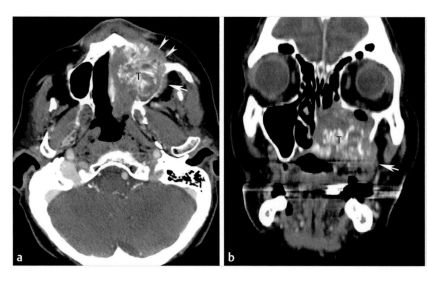

**Fig. 1.45** Mucoepidermoid carcinoma. Axial (**a**) and coronal reformatted images (**b**) from a contrast-enhanced CT show a tumor (T) in the left maxillary sinus extending to the nasal cavity, palate, premaxillary (*arrowheads*), and retromaxillary (*white arrows*) soft tissues. The tumor exhibits extensive internal heterogeneity with areas of marked increased attenuation which are suggestive of calcification.

epithelium lining the superior nasal fossa.[96] The precise cell of origin is controversial. ONB accounts for approximately 5 to 7% of sinonasal cancers, likely affecting males and females in equal proportion. Age distribution is broad and is often described as bimodal, with peaks in the third and sixth decades.[97] The most common presenting symptoms are unilateral nasal obstruction and epistaxis.

No clear etiological agents or risk factors have been documented in humans. In animals, exposure to nitrosamine compounds has been shown to induce ONB,[98] and there is also an association with the presence of retroviral particles in animal models.[99] In humans, there are a wide variety of documented biological activities, ranging from indolent growth and multidecade survival with known tumor to highly aggressive courses with widespread metastases and survival limited to months.[100]

## Imaging features

On CT, ONB has the appearance of a homogeneous, moderately enhancing mass, typically located unilaterally in the superior nasal cavity (▶ Fig. 1.46). Extension into adjacent ethmoid and maxillary sinuses is common, and advanced lesions may cross

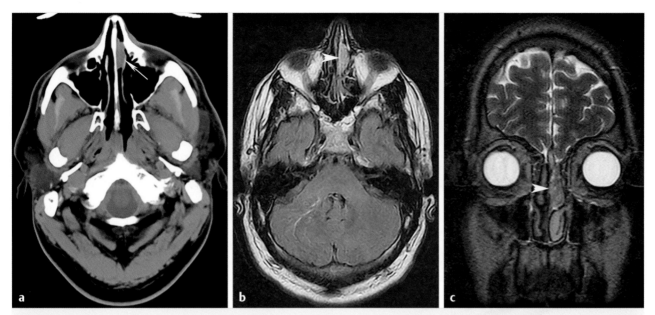

**Fig. 1.46** Early-stage olfactory neuroblastoma. Axial unenhanced CT (**a**), axial T2-weighted FLAIR MRI (**b**), and coronal T2-weighted MRI (**c**) are shown. On CT, the lesion has the appearance of an ovoid opacity in the superior left nasal cavity (*white arrow*). The lesion has intermediate- to high-signal intensity on the FLAIR and T2-weighted images (*arrowheads*). The cribriform plate does not appear breached and there is no clear involvement of the ethmoid air cells, in keeping with a Kadish A or T1 tumor.

into the contralateral nasal cavity.[55] Frequently, there is opacification of adjacent sinuses due to inflammation and retention of secretions. These processes may be difficult to differentiate from tumor extension on CT but usually are clearly distinguishable on MRI, similar to what was discussed for SCC in the earlier section. The lesions are further characterized by osseous remodeling and areas of amorphous tumor calcification (▶ Fig. 1.47).[101] Owing to the location of origin in the superior nasal cavity, in large tumors, extension through the cribriform plate into the anterior cranial fossa is common (▶ Fig. 1.47). Other structures to be evaluated for signs of osseous invasion and transgression with relevance to disease staging include the fovea ethmoidalis and lamina papyracea. In one imaging study, involved lymph nodes, when present, were typically solid, hyperenhancing, and FDG avid.[102] Level II lymph nodes were involved in almost all of these node-positive patients. Levels I and III were abnormal in greater than 50% with nodal disease, while retropharyngeal lymph nodes were involved in more than 40%.

On MRI, ONB typically presents as intermediate-signal intensity enhancing tissue, often with slightly high signal on T2-weighted images.[55] On T1-weighted images obtained prior to contrast administration, the tumor is often hypointense to gray matter. Adjacent obstructed secretions often have distinct but variable signal characteristics (▶ Fig. 1.48), and are associated with inflammatory peripheral mucosal hyperenhancement. This differentiation is highly significant for surgical planning. MRI-based delineation of dural involvement influences the extent of surgical resection and also can affect the decision to undertake endoscopic versus open craniofacial resection. If possible, intracranial tumor extension with isolated dural involvement should be differentiated from true brain parenchymal invasion, as this characteristic also alters surgical management.[55] Larger tumors may demonstrate cystic areas at the

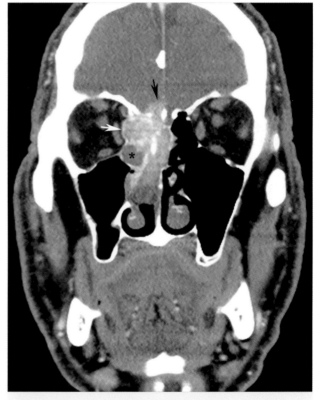

**Fig. 1.47** Olfactory neuroblastoma of the right nasal cavity with intracranial and right ethmoid involvement on coronal reformatted image from a contrast-enhanced CT. Enhancing tissue extends intracranially beyond the right olfactory fossa (*black arrow*). Internally, there are areas of higher attenuation secondary to amorphous tumor calcification. The right medial orbital wall is remodeled by tumor (*white arrow*). Of note, at the inferomedial margin of the right orbit, there are low-attenuation entrapped secretions in an ethmoid air cell (*asterisk*).

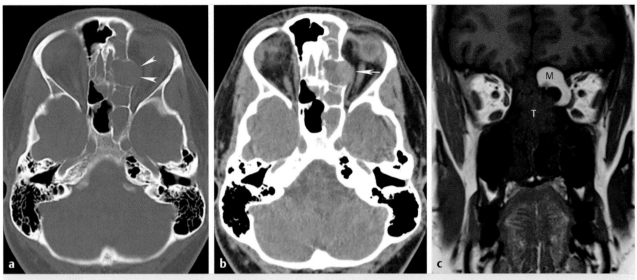

**Fig. 1.48** Olfactory neuroblastoma of the superior nasal cavity resulting in an ethmoid mucocele protruding into the left orbit. Axial unenhanced CT images displayed with bone (**a**) or soft-tissue window settings (**b**) and coronal T1-weighted MRI without contrast (**c**) are shown. There is focal remodeling and attenuation of the left lamina papyracea (*arrowheads*; **a**). The corresponding high-attenuation material underlying these changes (*white arrow*; **b**) protruding focally into the left orbit could be mistaken for orbital tumor invasion on CT. However, on MRI (**c**), the intrinsically high signal on T1-weighted MRI confirms that this represents inspissated proteinaceous secretions within a secondary mucocele (M) rather than orbital invasion, clearly distinguishing it from the intermediate signal tumor (T).

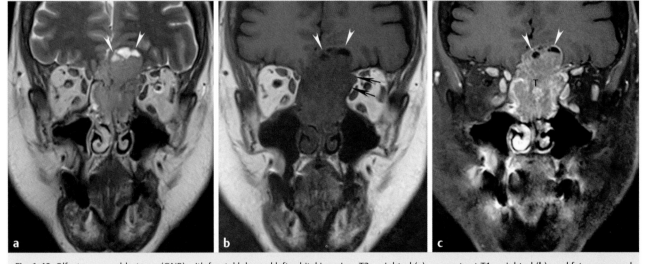

**Fig. 1.49** Olfactory neuroblastoma (ONB) with frontal lobe and left orbital invasion. T2-weighted (**a**), precontrast T1-weighted (**b**), and fat-suppressed contrast-enhanced T1-weighted MRI (**c**) images are shown. Note avid tumor enhancement on the postcontrast image (T; **c**). There are cysts at the margin of the tumor and the invaded frontal lobe forming a broad base with the intracranial extent of the tumor (*arrowheads*), a finding that is classic for ONB when present. Tumor invades the medial left orbit, infiltrating the superior oblique muscle (*black arrows*; **b**).

intracranial margins (▶ Fig. 1.49).[103] This is not a frequent finding but, when present, such cysts have broad bases of contact with the tumor. In these cases, the diagnosis of ONB is strongly suggested.

Staging of ONB was historically performed with Kadish staging but, more recently, a more detailed TNM system has been made available. Kadish staging is divided into groups A, B, and C.[104,105] Kadish group A describes tumors contained by the nasal cavity. Group B tumors involve the paranasal sinuses and group C is distinguished by extension beyond the paranasal sinuses. In the TNM system,[100] stage T1 ONB involves the nasal cavity and/or paranasal sinuses, with sparing of the most superior ethmoidal air cells and the sphenoid sinuses. T2 tumors extend to or erode the cribriform plate and may involve the sphenoid sinuses. When there is evidence of extension into the orbit or protrusion into the anterior cranial fossa without clear dural invasion, stage T3 is assigned. In advanced cases, involvement of the brain indicates that the tumor has reached stage T4. Cervical lymph node or distant metastases are denoted as N1 or M1, respectively.

## Prognosis and treatment

In a meta-analysis of patients with ONB, overall mean survival at 5 years was 45%.[96] The majority of tumors were Kadish group C. Cervical lymph node metastases were seen in an average of 5% at presentation, and less than one-third of these patients were successfully treated. Distant metastases were seen in 17%. Local recurrence was found in 29% of patients and 16% had regional recurrence. While most lymph node recurrences occur in the first 5 years following presentation, lifelong clinical and radiologic follow-up is often suggested.[97] Treatment most commonly consists of surgical resection, often with adjuvant radiotherapy.[97] In some centers, preoperative radiotherapy is delivered in place of postoperative radiotherapy.[77] The role of chemotherapy is uncertain. For centrally located tumors that do not invade the orbit, optic nerve/chiasm, carotid artery, or skin, an endoscopic approach is commonly performed in centers with available expertise. A limiting factor for expanded endonasal resection is dural involvement beyond the midline of the orbit, where access is difficult for endoscopic resection and reconstruction. In these cases, or when there is extensive intracranial involvement, an open craniofacial approach is used with a bicoronal or subfrontal craniotomy providing access from above the tumor and via an endonasal or transfacial approach from below. When tumor does not penetrate the orbit, the resection margin may include the lamina papyracea and, in some cases, small segments of periorbita. A variety of local, regional, and free grafts may be used to reconstruct the resultant defect which is important to recognize on postoperative surveillance imaging.

## Rhabdomyosarcoma

### Overview

Rhabdomyosarcoma (RMS) is the most common soft-tissue malignancy in childhood, accounting for 6% of all childhood cancers.[106] Thirty-five percent of cases occur in the head and neck region. The average age at diagnosis is 7 to 8 years, though it may occur at any time after birth including, rarely, in adulthood. The embryonal subtype is the most frequent form, most commonly occurring in patients younger than 10 years.[107] Adolescents and adults tend to develop alveolar or pleomorphic histologies. Incidence in males is approximately 1.5 times greater than in females.[108] The most common category of tumor locations in the head and neck is referred to as "parameningeal," accounting for 25% of all RMS tumors (▶ Fig. 1.50).[109] This category includes regions such as the nasopharynx, paranasal sinuses, nasal cavity, middle ear, temporal fossa, and PPF. Orbital and other head and neck locations are less common than those involving parameningeal sites (▶ Fig. 1.51).

### Imaging characteristics

On CT, small tumors are homogeneously isoattenuating to muscle and exhibit moderate to marked enhancement.[106,110] They are usually well defined and lack bone destruction. Larger RMSs tend to be less well defined, exhibiting bone erosion and infiltration of surrounding tissues. They may also be heterogeneous in density, due in part to areas of focal hemorrhage. On MRI, the lesions are of intermediate to low signal on T1-weighted images and intermediate to high signal on T2-weighted images. Hemorrhagic foci, when present, can result in foci with reversal of this pattern, such as high signal on T1-weighted images without contrast. In the orbit, globe deformity and extraocular muscle displacement are common (▶ Fig. 1.51).

### Staging

The Intergroup Rhabdomyosarcoma Study Group staging system combines site of primary tumor with tumor size, lymph node status, and the presence or absence of distant metastases.[111] Orbital and non-parameningeal head and neck tumors have better prognoses than parameningeal lesions. As a result,

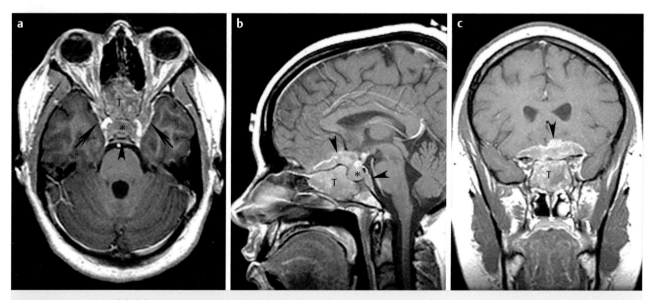

**Fig. 1.50** Parameningeal rhabdomyosarcoma (T) centered in the sphenoid sinuses with invasion of the dura (*arrowheads*) over the planum sphenoidale, tuberculum sella, and clivus, as well as the cavernous sinuses (*black arrows*; **a**) and pituitary gland (*asterisk*; **a,b**) on contrast-enhanced T1-weighted MRI in the axial (**a**), sagittal (**b**), and coronal (**c**) planes.

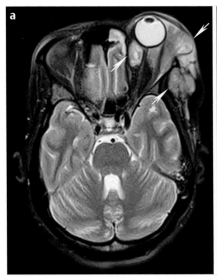
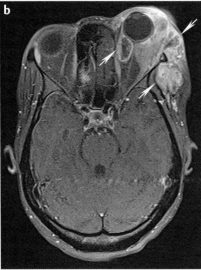

Fig. 1.51 Rhabdomyosarcoma of the left orbit. Axial fat-suppressed T2- (a) and contrast-enhanced T1-weighted (b) images demonstrate a heterogeneous enhancing mass in the intraconal and extraconal left orbit (*arrows*) that extends along the superficial aspect of the lateral orbital rim posteriorly, with resultant severe left-sided proptosis.

in the absence of distant metastases, these lesions are considered stage 1 at any size. Parameningeal tumors less than or equal to 5 cm in size are assigned stage 2. Stage 3 parameningeal tumors include those with nodal metastases regardless of size or, in the absence of nodal metastases, those tumors greater than or equal to 5 cm in diameter. Any lesion with a distant metastasis at diagnosis is stage 4.

## Prognosis and treatment

Maximal surgical resection is performed when technically feasible, followed by chemoradiotherapy. The orbit lacks lymphatics[106] and, as a result, regional lymph node metastases are rare unless the primary tumor is locally advanced. When there is little or no residual tumor after surgery, 5-year survival is at least 90%.[106] With significant residual tumor, this figure decreases to 35%. Outcomes in adult patients are generally poor, with an overall 5-year survival of 30%.[107]

## Melanoma

### Overview

Malignant melanoma of the sinonasal mucosa is rare, representing less than 4 to 7% of sinonasal neoplasms.[54,55] The location is also uncommon among melanomas as a whole, encompassing less than 2% of these lesions.[112] The nasal cavity is a much more common primary site than the paranasal sinuses, most often involving the lateral nasal wall and nasal septum. Eighty percent of sinus cases affect the maxillary antra, usually in conjunction with the nasal cavity, followed by the ethmoid sinuses.[55] Gender distribution is equal.[112] The mean age at presentation is greater than 60 years. Presenting complaints are most often related to obstruction, epistaxis, and, occasionally, pain.[55,112]

### Imaging characteristics

Melanoma is often a hypervascular tumor. As a result, they characteristically demonstrate avid enhancement (▶ Fig. 1.52).[55] Signal characteristics on unenhanced sequences are usually

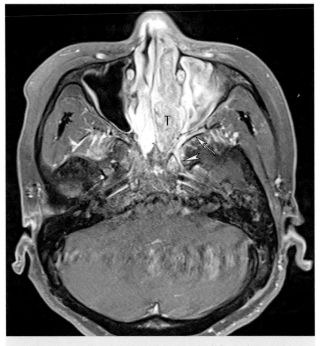

Fig. 1.52 Sinonasal melanoma centered in the left nasal cavity (T) on an axial postcontrast T1-weighted MRI. There is also asymmetrical enhancement in the left pterygopalatine fossa (*arrow*) and Vidian canal (*arrowhead*), suggesting perineural extension.

homogeneously intermediate signal on all sequences. Some cases may have intrinsically high signal on T1-weighted images performed without contrast (▶ Fig. 1.53, ▶ Fig. 1.54). This is believed to be secondary to the presence of hemorrhagic products and/ or the paramagnetic effects of melanin. When present, this is helpful in suggesting the diagnosis. In such cases, the tumor may have components with low signal on T2-weighted images. The tumors can be well defined, with nonaggressive appearing margins on imaging, belying their aggressive biological behaviors (▶ Fig. 1.55). Associated osseous changes typically are bone remodeling rather than frank erosion and destruction. Satellite

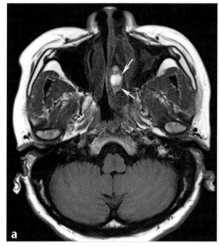
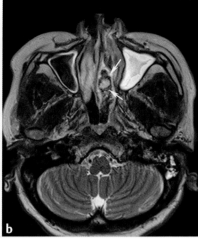

Fig. 1.53 Sinonasal melanoma of the nasal cavity. Axial T1-weighted MRI without contrast (**a**) and T2-weighted MRI (**b**) are shown. There is an area of intrinsically high signal on the T1-weighted image within the tumor with corresponding heterogeneous high and partly low signal intensity on the T2-weighted image, likely reflecting blood products (*arrows*). Tumor production of melanin could also present as high signal on T1-weighted images.

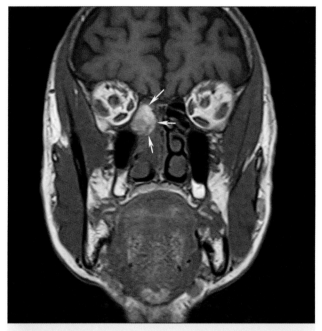

Fig. 1.54 Sinonasal melanoma of the right ethmoid region exhibiting high intrinsic signal (*arrows*) on T1-weighted MRI image without contrast. High signal on T1-weighted images could be due to hemorrhage from hypervascular tumor and/or melanin accumulation.

tumor nodules are common. These can be identified with FDG-PET, as can residual or recurrent disease.[113] Although rare, melanoma can be associated with perineural spread of tumor (▶ Fig. 1.52), especially with the uncommon desmoplastic variant.[114]

## Staging

Multiple staging systems have been proposed for the staging of melanoma. Beginning in 2010, the American Joint Committee on Cancer (AJCC) staging manual included a separate TNM system for mucosal melanoma of the head and neck.[69] T-staging begins at T3, denoting lesions limited to the mucosa. T4a tumors involve deep soft tissue, cartilage, bone, or skin. T4b

lesions involve the skull base, dura, brain, lower cranial nerves, masticator space, carotid artery, prevertebral space, or mediastinal structures. N1 and M1 stages encompass regional lymph node and distant metastases, respectively. Reflecting the aggressive behavior and poor prognosis, the earliest-stage tumors, mucosal lesions without lymph node or distant metastases, are considered stage III.

## Prognosis and treatment

The treatment of choice is wide local excision, sometimes combined with adjuvant radiotherapy.[112] Chemotherapy can be provided, typically for palliation. New treatments including biologic and targeted therapies have shown promise in clinical trials.[115] Up to one-third of patients present with cervical lymphadenopathy and/or distant metastases.[116] Many patients experience local recurrence within the first year following surgery. Median survival is 18 to 34 months,[55] with lesions of the nasal cavity carrying a better prognosis than those of the paranasal sinuses. Overall 5-year survival is less than 25%.[90]

## Lymphoma

### Overview

Sinonasal lymphoma (SNL) is rare, representing only 1.5% of all lymphomas.[117,118] SNLs can be classified histopathologically as Hodgkin's, non-Hodgkin's B-cell or T-cell/natural killer phenotypes, as well as other rarer entities, such as T/null cell.[119] Overall, they are more common in Asian than in Western populations, where they are the second most common extranodal group after gastrointestinal lymphoma.[55] Previous terminology for these lesions included lethal midline granuloma, malignant midline reticulosis, and polymorphic reticulosis. B-cell SNL typically involves the paranasal sinuses and is slightly more common in Western populations.[55] Of the paranasal sinuses, maxillary and ethmoid involvement predominates over the sphenoid and frontal sinuses.[119] T-cell SNL occurs most frequently in Asian and South American countries and is more frequently localized in the nasal cavity.[55] Patients with T-cell phenotypes are typically younger and more often female in comparison with B-cell disease. Epstein-Barr virus is strongly associated with NK/T-cell SNL. Presenting symptoms are

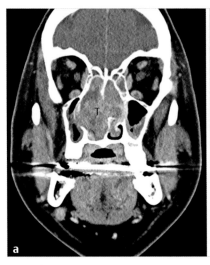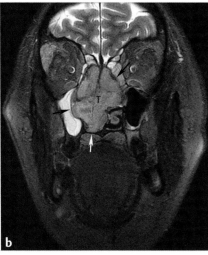

**Fig. 1.55** Sinonasal melanoma (T) centered in the right nasal cavity on coronal contrast-enhanced CT (**a**) and fat-suppressed T2-weighted MRI (**b**). Despite the aggressive nature of melanoma, some lesions which rapidly enlarge can have less aggressive appearances on imaging with well-defined margins and findings of bone remodeling (*arrows*) rather than frank destruction.

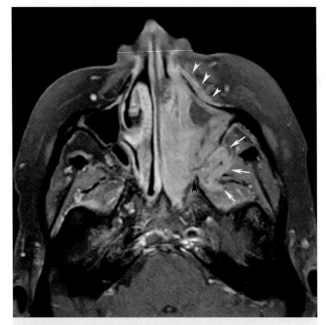

**Fig. 1.56** Sinonasal lymphoma. Axial fat-suppressed contrast-enhanced T1-weighted MRI demonstrates extensive infiltration of the left pterygopalatine fossa (*black arrowhead*), pterygomaxillary fissure, retromaxillary fat, and infratemporal fossa masticator space structures (*white arrows*) secondary to sinonasal lymphoma. There is also a rind of abnormal enhancing tissue extending across the anterior wall of the maxillary sinus to involve the premaxillary soft tissues (*white arrowheads*).

similar to other tumors of the region and can mimic chronic obstructive disease.

## Imaging characteristics

On CT and MRI, SNL most often manifests as a bulky soft-tissue mass with variable, often moderate enhancement (▶ Fig. 1.56).[55,90] In some cases, there is diffuse tumor infiltration along the walls of the nasal cavity.[90] Bilateral presentations can occur.[120] Signal intensity is usually intermediate on all sequences, and CT attenuation is similar to muscle.[55] In some cases, MRI reveals features of high cellularity, including relatively low signal on T2-weighted images and findings of diffusion restriction (▶ Fig. 1.57). These tumors tend to remodel bone or can sometimes permeate osseous structures, extending across them without obvious macroscopic destruction (▶ Fig. 1.58). NK/T cell lesions are typified by a more aggressive growth pattern, frequently presenting as locally destructive disease with the involvement of adjacent bones, large soft-tissue masses, and bone erosion.[55,121] Angioinvasive forms can manifest with necrosis. Spread to the meninges, cavernous sinuses, and CNS disease have been reported in approximately 5% of patients with non-Hodgkin's lymphoma.[122] These lesions can also have associated perineural spread of tumor.

## Prognosis and treatment

Lymphomas of the sinonasal cavities have worse outcomes than those of other regions.[90] Their biological behaviors range broadly from chronicity and indolence to very rapid growth over a period of days. Rarely, indolent lesions can clinically mimic fungal rhinosinusitis.[90,119] Therapy is nonsurgical, most often with chemotherapy.[119] Radiotherapy in combination with chemotherapy is sometimes utilized for more aggressive lesions, particularly T-cell/natural killer forms. T/NK-cell SNL is typically less responsive to therapy in comparison with B-cell tumors, but prognoses are sometimes reported to be similar.[119] Survival is generally determined by tumor stage and grade rather than cellular phenotype.[55] In one recent series, 5-year overall survival for a Western population was approximately 50%.[119]

## Osteosarcoma

### Overview

Osteosarcoma accounts for less than 1% of all head and neck cancers.[123] Less than 10% of all osteosarcomas arise in the head and neck, typically in the mandible or maxilla. Less common sites of origin include the calvarium and paranasal sinuses.[124] The median age of head and neck lesions is in the fourth decade, with a broad age range and an equal gender distribution. Retinoblastoma is a risk factor.[125] Prior radiotherapy

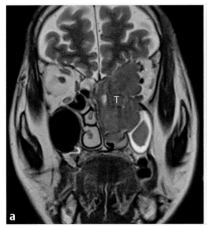
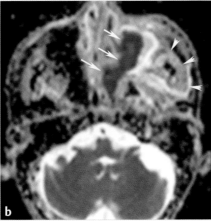

**Fig. 1.57** Sinonasal lymphoma (T) involving the left nasal cavity, maxillary sinus, ethmoid air cells, and left orbit. Coronal T2-weighted MRI (**a**) and axial apparent diffusion coefficient (ADC) map (**b**) are shown. Classic features of tumor hypercellularity are demonstrated, including relatively low T2 signal intensity as compared with other sinonasal tumors and also relatively low ADC values (*arrows*) that are similar to brain parenchyma or lower than the temporalis muscle (*arrowheads*), suggestive of diffusion restriction related to high tumor cellularity and high nucleus-to-cytoplasm ratios.

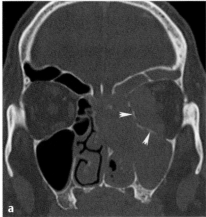
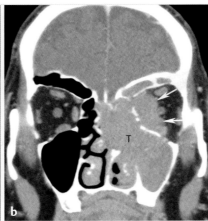

**Fig. 1.58** Sinonasal lymphoma (T). Coronal reformats from a contrast-enhanced CT displayed in bone window (**a**) and soft-tissue windows (**b**) are shown. Despite extensive infiltration of the extraconal and intraconal orbit (*white arrows*; **b**) by the homogeneously enhancing sinonasal mass (T), there is relative preservation of the inferior and medial orbital walls (*arrowheads*; **a**).

predisposes to the development of osteosarcoma in the radiation field, with treatment typically preceding presentation by nearly a decade.[126] More than 50% of osteosarcomas presenting in the head and neck have high-grade features at histopathology.[123]

## Imaging characteristics

A typical, though not invariant, feature of osteosarcoma is the "sunburst" aggressive periosteal reaction arising at the site of a bone-centric soft-tissue mass.[55] Localized cortical and trabecular erosion is often present, although an alternative manifestation is dense, sclerotic bone accompanying a contiguous soft-tissue mass. This appearance is sometimes seen in the maxillary alveolus. Tumor matrix, when present, is suggestive of irregular, disorganized calcification or ossification (▶ Fig. 1.59, ▶ Fig. 1.60).

On MRI, the soft-tissue lesions enhance and are variable in signal intensity, most often heterogeneously low signal on T1-weighted images and intermediate signal on T2-weighted images.[55] Marrow infiltration manifests as loss of normal high signal fat on T1-weighted images.

## Staging

In the AJCC TNM staging system, tumors less than or equal to 8 cm in their maximum dimension are considered T1.[69] T2 lesions are larger and T3 refers to locally discontinuous lesions

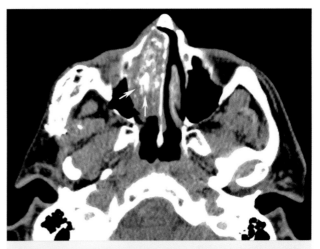

**Fig. 1.59** Osteosarcoma of the right nasal cavity following radiotherapy for retinoblastoma shown on unenhanced axial CT displayed using soft-tissue window and algorithm. Note internal areas of amorphous heterogeneous calcification/ossification (*arrows*).

within the primary osseous site. Lymph node and distant metastases are denoted as N1 and M1, respectively. The latter is divided into M1a and M1b subclassifications, where the former is limited to the lungs.

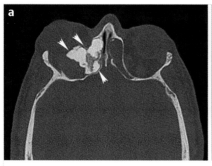

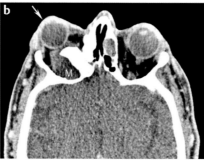

**Fig. 1.60** Osteosarcoma of the right frontal and ethmoid sinus with a secondary mucocele formation. Axial CT image displayed with bone window settings (**a**) and a contrast-enhanced axial CT displayed using soft-tissue window settings (**b**) are shown. Expansile areas of dense amorphous calcification and ossification (*arrowheads*; **a**) are seen representing osteoid matrix typical of osteosarcoma. The low attenuation area protruding into the orbit is in keeping with secretions within a secondary mucocele (M; **b**). The combined result is right-sided proptosis (*arrow*; **b**).

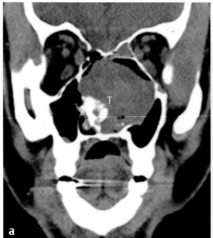

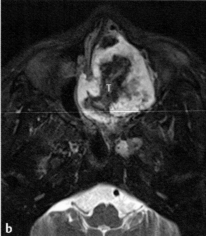

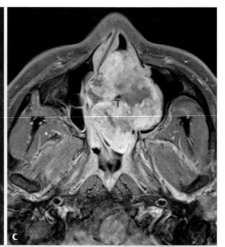

**Fig. 1.61** Chondrosarcoma of the nasal cavity (T). Coronal reformatted CT image (**a**), axial fat-suppressed T2-weighted (**b**), and postcontrast fat-suppressed T1-weighted (**c**) MRI images demonstrate a large mass arising from the nasal septum and occupying the nasal cavity with remodeling of adjacent bony margins such as the left maxillary sinus wall. On CT, the mass has a large soft-tissue density component and also a bone density mineralized component. On MRI, the lesion is heterogenous with areas of very low as well as very high signal on T2-weighted images and enhances heterogeneously after administration of contrast.

## Prognosis and treatment

Surgical resection is most often the primary treatment, followed by adjuvant radiotherapy for close or positive operative margins.[123] Adjuvant chemotherapy is of uncertain utility but may be of value in the context of poor prognostic factors.

Overall survival at 5 years is 60 to 70%, decreasing to 55% at 10 years.[123,124] Positive surgical margins predict a worse outcome at multivariate analysis.[123] When osteosarcoma develops in a region as a late complication of prior radiotherapy, the prognosis is often poor.[55]

## Chondrosarcoma

### Overview

Chondrosarcomas of the sinonasal cavity are rare tumors that mainly affect the nasal septum or other sites along the sinonasal tract, including the maxillary sinus and sphenoid sinus.[127,128]

### Imaging characteristics

There is limited literature describing the imaging appearance of these tumors in the sinonasal tract. When present, the presence of chondroid-type calcifications can be used to suggest the diagnosis. However, the appearance can be nonspecific and a typical chondroid matrix may not necessarily be present (▶ Fig. 1.61). This diagnosis should also be considered for masses that appear to arise from the nasal septum.[129]

### Prognosis and treatment

Surgical resection is most often the primary treatment, but may be supplemented with adjuvant radiation therapy.[128] Because chondrosarcoma may be difficult to identify on frozen sections, reoperation may be required to obtain satisfactory margins before definitive reconstruction. In general, these tumors are slow growing and locally invasive but rarely metastatic and have overall good long-term prognosis when successful and complete surgical resection has been achieved.[128] Based on one systematic review, local recurrence was relatively common, seen in 31% of patients.[128]

## Inverted Papilloma

### Overview

Inverted papilloma (IP) is the second most common benign polypoid tumor of the Schneiderian mucosa, following exophytic (everted) papilloma.[55] As a group, Schneiderian polyps are relatively uncommon, accounting for 0.4 to 4.7% of all sinonasal tumors, with IP comprising just less than half. Males between the ages of 40 and 70 years are most commonly affected. The characteristic location of origin is the lateral nasal wall near the middle turbinate, often with extension into maxillary and ethmoid sinuses. Presenting symptoms are similar to other tumors of this region and are nonspecific. There is evidence of human papilloma virus (HPV) involvement in approximately 25% of IP, and this rate is higher in dysplastic IP as well as SCC, the most common malignant disease arising in an inverted papilloma, with increasing ratios of high-risk to low-risk viral types.[130] The detection of high-risk viral-type HPV in IP is thought to affect recurrence rates and propensity for coexistent malignant disease.

## Imaging characteristics

A unilateral nasal mass located along the lateral nasal wall in the region of the middle meatus is suggestive of an IP.[55] Sinonasal papillomas in general can vary from small, nonspecific polypoid masses to expansile lesions with bone remodeling, intrasinus extension, and secondary obstruction. The surface of larger lesions is often lobulated. Areas of more aggressive-appearing bone destruction, as well as sites of necrosis and findings of adjacent tissue invasion, raise the possibility of coexistent malignant disease (most commonly SCC; ▶ Fig. 1.62). Calcific densities can be seen within IPs and could be helpful for suggesting this diagnosis when present. These are often thought to represent residual bone fragments. In addition, a

focal area of peripheral hyperostosis or ossification where the lesion abuts an osseous structure sometimes correlates with the site of origin and attachment (▶ Fig. 1.63). On MRI, IPs are classically characterized by a convoluted or cerebriform internal texture in cross-section on T2-weighted or contrast-enhanced T1-weighted images (▶ Fig. 1.64, ▶ Fig. 1.65). However, this pattern is not entirely specific, and has also been described for other tumors such as adenocarcinoma.

## Prognosis and treatment

Lateral rhinotomy with transfacial medial maxillectomy including en bloc resection of lateral nasal wall and mucosa was the conventional "gold standard" in the past.[131] However, this approach has largely been replaced by endoscopic resection, sometimes combined with an open approach. Recurrence rates of up to 20% are seen, usually in the first 2 years.[55,131] Synchronous or metachronous SCC may occur in around 10% of cases, although a wide range of rates have been described. Rarely, other carcinomas may be seen in association with IPs, such as adenocarcinoma.

## Juvenile Angiofibroma

### Overview

Juvenile nasopharyngeal angiofibroma (JNA) is a rare entity, accounting for 0.05% of all head and neck neoplasms.[55] It occurs

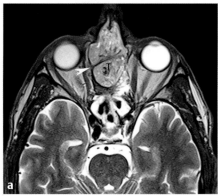
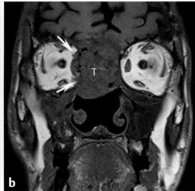

**Fig. 1.62** Inverted papilloma of the ethmoid air cells and superior nasal cavity as shown on an axial T2-weighted (**a**) and coronal T1-weighted MRI without contrast (**b**). On the T2-weighted image, the tumor (T) is heterogeneous and convoluted in appearance. There is a low-signal stalk (*arrowhead*; **a**) tethering the lesion to the right lamina papyracea, suggesting the location of origin of this large tumor. Abnormal low signal in the fat of the medial right extraconal orbit (*arrows*; **b**), best demonstrated on the T1-weighted image, is concerning for orbital invasion resulting from coexistent malignant disease (squamous cell carcinoma).

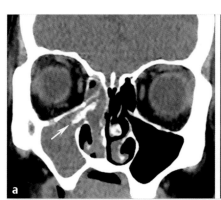
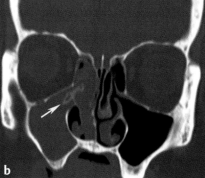
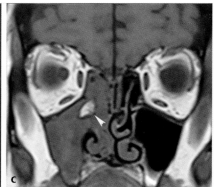

**Fig. 1.63** Inverted papilloma of the right nasal cavity and maxillary sinus demonstrating a focus of ossification and hyperostosis at the presumed site of origin of the tumor (the uncinate process of the infundibulum). Unenhanced CT displayed with soft-tissue (**a**) or bone window settings (**b**) and coronal T1-weighted MRI without contrast (**c**) are shown. The hyperdense region on CT (*arrows*; **a,b**) is well defined, containing central lucency with corresponding high signal on the T1-weighted image (*arrowhead*; **c**), consistent with marrow fat within the ossific focus.

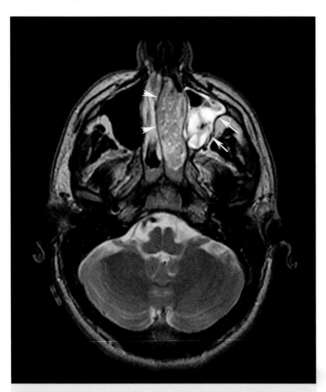

**Fig. 1.64** Inverted papilloma of the left nasal cavity on axial T2-weighted MRI. There is a lesion with heterogeneous, partly intermediate signal intensity tissue filling, expanding and remodeling the left nasal cavity with a convoluted (sometimes referred to as cerebriform) appearance that is classic for inverted papilloma (*arrowheads*). Higher signal material in the adjacent left maxillary sinus (*arrows*) likely reflects reactive mucosal thickening and fluid related to obstruction of mucociliary drainage resulting from the tumor.

## Imaging characteristics

Given the site of origin, these tumors can extend as an asymmetrical polypoid mass into the adjacent nasopharynx as well as the underlying PPFs (▶ Fig. 1.66, ▶ Fig. 1.67).[133] This results in characteristic widening of the PPF via anterior bowing and displacement of the posterior wall of the maxillary sinus. These osseous changes are accompanied by loss of normal fat attenuation on CT and fat signal in the PPF on MRI. When advanced, PPF extension may continue through the pterygomaxillary fissure into the infratemporal fossa. Other sites of extension, in decreasing order of frequency, include the adjacent sphenoid sinus, followed by the maxillary and ethmoid sinuses.[134] Intracranial extension primarily involves the middle cranial fossa via the PPF, followed by the inferior orbital fissure and the superior orbital fissure.[132] These fissures may appear widened on CT. Parasellar extension is usually extradural and more often reflects displacement rather than invasion. Advanced cases may demonstrate encasement of the internal carotid artery and cavernous sinus invasion.

On CT, JNA enhances avidly (▶ Fig. 1.66) but can diminish and "wash out" if imaging is delayed.[55] These enhancement characteristics are affected by the relative composition and distribution of vascular and fibrous tissue within the lesion. Lesions with a greater fibrous component can be indistinguishable from other benign sinonasal tumors. Adjacent osseous structures can be involved and this is believed to occur via two different mechanisms. One mechanism is believed to be demineralization by pressure, hypervascularity, and osteoclastic activation and the other by direct spread along perforating arteries into cancellous bone.[135] As a result, bone involvement by JNA can appear aggressive on imaging.

On MRI, the mass typically appears vascular, with numerous flow voids on a background of intermediate signal on T1- and T2-weighted images (▶ Fig. 1.66, ▶ Fig. 1.67). Alteration of normal marrow signal intensity may be seen, such as in the sphenoid body. When present, meticulous resection of involved cancellous bone is associated with a significantly reduced rate of tumor recurrence.[132] These tumors also have a propensity for filling the Vidian canal; therefore, at the time of surgery, it is important to recognize and remove tumor in this area if present.

almost exclusively in young males, most often in the second decade of life. Though histologically benign, the lesions are locally aggressive and infiltrative. Virtually all of these tumors originate near one of the sphenopalatine foramina. The most common presenting features are nasal obstruction and recurrent epistaxis.[132]

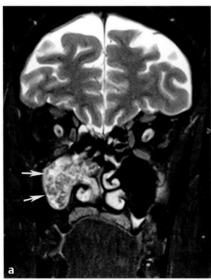
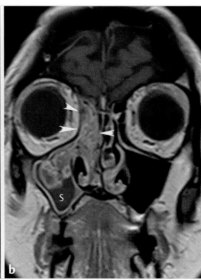

**Fig. 1.65** Inverted papilloma on coronal fat-suppressed T2-weighted (**a**) and contrast-enhanced T1-weighted MRI (**b**). There is a heterogeneous enhancing lesion with convoluted/cerebriform appearance within the right maxillary sinus (*arrows*; **a**), maxillary infundibulum, right nasal cavity, and right ethmoid air cells (*arrowheads*; **b**). Retained secretions (S) and reactive mucosal thickening are noted inferiorly in the right maxillary sinus, related to obstruction of the maxillary infundibulum.

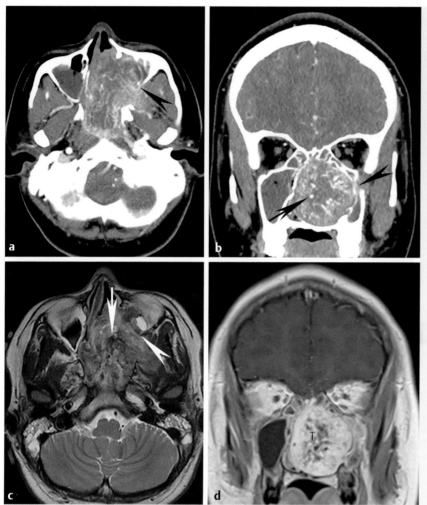

**Fig. 1.66** Juvenile nasopharyngeal angiofibroma filling and expanding the left pterygopalatine fossa, nasal cavity, and nasopharynx. Axial images (**a**) and coronal reformats (**b**) from a contrast-enhanced CT as well as axial T2-weighted (**c**) and coronal contrast-enhanced T1-weighted MRI without fat suppression (**d**) are shown. There is a large heterogeneous enhancing nasal cavity mass with marked widening of the left pterygopalatine fossa with remodeling of the posterior and medial walls of the left maxillary sinus (*arrowheads*; **a-c**). The lesion contains numerous enlarged enhancing vascular structures with corresponding low T2-signal flow voids (*arrows*; **b,c**) consistent with a highly vascular lesion. On MRI, the tumor (T; **d**) exhibits marked enhancement after administration of contrast, similar to or greater than sinonasal mucosa.

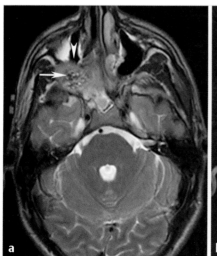

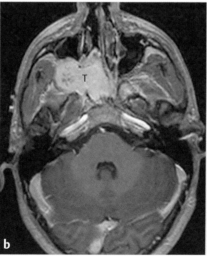

**Fig. 1.67** Juvenile nasopharyngeal angiofibroma. Axial T2-weighted (**a**) and contrast-enhanced T1-weighted MRIs without fat suppression (**b**) demonstrate marked widening of the right pterygopalatine fossa as well as tumor extending into the posterior nasal cavity, nasopharynx, and pterygomaxillary fissure. The posterior wall of the right maxillary sinus is bowed anteriorly (*arrowhead*; **a**). Flow voids are present within the tumor on T2-weighted images (*arrow*; **a**) and the tumor (T; **b**) has marked internal enhancement after administration of contrast, consistent with a highly vascular mass.

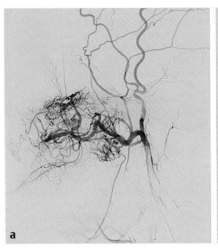
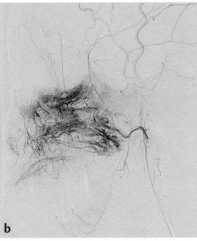

**Fig. 1.68** Conventional angiogram in arterial (**a**) and capillary (**b**) phases following internal maxillary artery injection showing extensive abnormal tumor vascularity in a juvenile nasopharyngeal angiofibroma.

Conventional angiography is sometimes employed for operative planning and preoperative embolization with the aim of reduction in surgical blood loss.[132] The ipsilateral internal maxillary and ascending pharyngeal arteries may be enlarged due to increased flow to these highly vascular lesions (▶ Fig. 1.68). The contralateral external carotid circulation can also be recruited.[55] Internal carotid branch supply can be associated with intracranial extension.

## Staging

Multiple JNA staging systems have been described. The most recent system, published by Radkowski et al, is divided into three categories, each with two to three subcategories.[136] Stage IA lesions are limited to the nose and/or nasopharynx. IB tumors involve one or more sinuses. Stage II lesions involve the PPF. IIA denotes minimal extension into the PPF, IIB describes full occupancy with or without orbital bone erosion, and IIC traverses the PPF to involve the infratemporal fossa. Stage III lesions erode the skull base, with minimal intracranial extension in stage IIIA and more extensive involvement with or without cavernous sinus invasion in stage IIIB.

## Prognosis and treatment

Preoperative embolization followed by complete surgical resection is the treatment of choice. Conventional surgical approaches include transpalatal, transmaxillary, and infratemporal fossa routes.[137] Endoscopic resection is useful in tumors limited to the nasopharynx and nasal cavity, as well as the ethmoid and sphenoid sinuses.[132] Radiotherapy is often reserved for cases that are considered unresectable. Gamma knife radiosurgery has been employed for treatment of residual or recurrent JNA, particularly when located near critical structures such as the cavernous sinus. Recurrence rates range from 20 to 40%, increasing with tumor stage and bone involvement.

## Meningioma

### Overview

Meningiomas are typically benign tumors that arise from arachnoid rests. They are overall two to four times more common in females and have a peak incidence near the age of 45 years.[55] Twenty to forty percent of intracranial lesions are located in the anterior cranial fossa,[138] most commonly in relation to the olfactory groove, planum sphenoidale, and tuberculum sellae.[139] These lesions most often present with visual impairment or an alteration in memory, personality, or executive functioning.[138] Less than 1% of meningiomas are primarily extracranial.[140] When the sinonasal cavities are involved by meningioma, the lesions may result from (1) direct extension of an intracranial tumor (representing approximately two-thirds of these cases), (2) extracranial metastasis from an intracranial lesion, (3) arachnoid rests located along suture lines or transosseous structures such as cranial nerves and blood vessels, or (4) none of the above, including primary intraosseous and other ectopic meningiomas.[55] Presenting features include pain, proptosis, and facial deformity.[141]

## Imaging characteristics

Sinonasal meningiomas most often have the appearance of an avidly enhancing mass with expansile bone remodeling and hyperostosis.[55] Most sinonasal lesions are located in the nasal vault. A pathway of direct extension from the anterior cranial fossa may be demonstrated, typically with the mass center located above the skull base (▶ Fig. 1.69). Lesions located entirely within the nasal cavity often lack the adjacent dural thickening and enhancement ("dural tail") seen in more common intracranial lesions. Reactive bone formation with sclerosis and hyperostosis adjacent to the tumor can often be seen, sometimes mimicking the ground-glass matrix appearance of fibrous dysplasia or other fibroosseous lesions. The calvarial diploe may be widened,[141] either due to bone invasion or "reactive" bone expansion.[142] As a result, radiotherapy treatment volumes often include regions of hyperostosis and bone expansion.[143] Longstanding lesions may be heavily calcified. Signal intensity on T1- and T2-weighted images in the absence of heavy calcification are similar to gray matter and vascular flow voids can occasionally be observed (▶ Fig. 1.70).

## Prognosis and treatment

Surgery is the mainstay of treatment, most often with a craniotomy approach to address lesions involving anterior cranial fossa

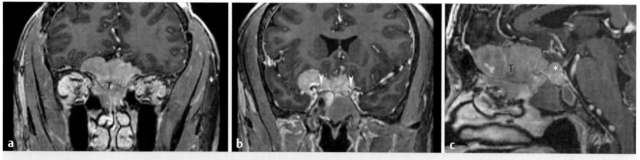

**Fig. 1.69 (a-c)** Anterior cranial fossa meningioma (T; **a,c**) extending into the superior nasal cavity and ethmoid sinuses as well as the sellar/suprasellar region (*asterisk*; **c**). Contrast-enhanced T1-weighted MRI in the coronal plane at the level of the orbits (**a**) and optic canals (**b**) as well as in the sagittal plane (**c**) show a large mass that also encases the canalicular segments of the optic nerves, greater on the right (*arrowheads*; **c**).

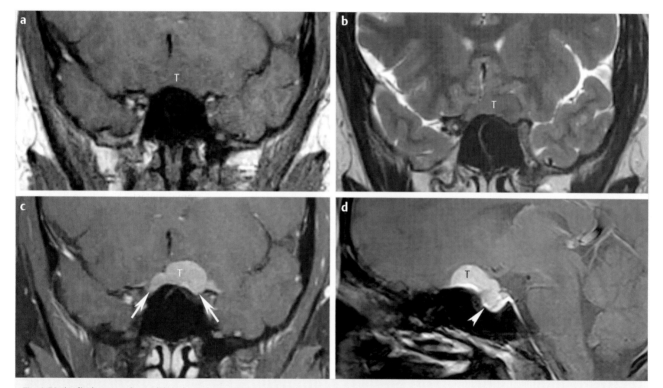

**Fig. 1.70 (a-d)** Planum sphenoidale/tuberculum sella meningioma extending into the optic canals (*arrows*; **c**), greater on the left, and the sella (*arrowhead*; **d**). Coronal T1-weighted (**a**), coronal T2-weighted (**b**), and fat-suppressed contrast-enhanced coronal (**c**) and sagittal (**d**) T1-weighted MRI are shown. The tumor (T) is isointense to brain on T1- and T2-weighted images and demonstrates homogeneous and avid enhancement after administration of contrast.

and an endoscopic (or transfacial) approach for the sinonasal component.[138] Pure endoscopic endonasal techniques are increasingly used, but there is often a lesser gross-total resection and a high incidence of postoperative CSF leakage.[144] Stereotactic radiosurgery (SRS) or fractionated radiotherapy is utilized primarily for high-risk surgical patients, as adjuvant therapy following surgery, or in the treatment of recurrence.[143] For primary radiotherapy of intracranial lesions, SRS is preferred for lesions less than 3 to 4 cm in diameter and when there is reasonable separation from critical structures such as the optic apparatus.[145] Five- and 10-year progression-free survival with

SRS are 95 and 89%, respectively,[146] while for fractionated radiotherapy, these figures range from 93 to 95% and 96 to 88%, respectively.[143]

## 1.4.2 Tumor Mimics

### Nasal Polyposis

### Overview

Nasal polyps represent the most common mass lesion of the nasal cavity.[147] They result from recurrent acute or subacute inflammatory processes involving the sinonasal mucosa, leading to the development hypertrophic, polypoid, atrophic, and fibrotic changes.[148]

## Imaging characteristics

On CT, polyps are often characterized by soft-tissue attenuation, although this can be altered by the contents of adjacent trapped secretions.[148] After administration of contrast, the surface mucosa of polyps enhances robustly. The center of the polyp may not enhance, although if there is sufficient fibrosis and neovascularization at their core there may also be enhancement centrally mimicking other lesions. When advanced, polyposis often results in smooth expansion of the nasal cavity with pressure atrophy of adjacent bone. MR signal is variable, reflective of the various stages of polyp evolution, including edematous, glandular, cystic, and fibrous, as well as changes in content and hydration of associated entrapped secretions (▶ Fig. 1.71).

## Prognosis and treatment

When patients are asymptomatic or minimally symptomatic, nasal polyps may be managed with observation or saline lavage.[149] Systemic or topical corticosteroid therapies can improve symptoms, and other anti-inflammatory treatments, including antihistamines and leukotriene inhibitors, may be used as adjuncts. In select patients, allergy testing and allergen avoidance can be of benefit. Endoscopic sinus surgery is commonly employed for the removal of gross polyp tissue and clearance of inspissated secretions, though recurrence is common and ongoing medical treatment is usually required.

## Mucocele

### Overview

Mucoceles are thought to arise as a consequence of obstruction of a main sinus ostium.[150] This may be the end result of numerous inflammatory and noninflammatory obliterative processes. More than half involve the frontal sinuses, followed in frequency by the ethmoid air cells.

## Imaging characteristics

The classic imaging features of mucoceles include enlargement of affected sinuses with thinning and dehiscence of the sinus walls. They result in remodeling and expansion rather than aggressive or invasive features seen with malignant tumors. Following contrast administration, there is usually peripheral mucosal enhancement and occasional calcification.[148] There should be no enhancing nodular component within the mucocele and central fluid contents do not enhance. Similar to what has already been described for paranasal sinus inflammatory and postobstructive secretions, mucocele contents can have variable signal on T1- and T2-weighted images depending on their protein content and inspissated components (▶ Fig. 1.71). When evaluating mucoceles, there may also be evidence of a neoplastic (▶ Fig. 1.48, ▶ Fig. 1.60) or inflammatory cause for sinonasal ostial obstruction and that needs to be specifically scrutinized for whenever a mucocele is encountered.

## Prognosis and treatment

When symptomatic, surgical decompression is the treatment of choice, including endoscopic approaches, when appropriate.[151] The recurrence rates are typically reported to be less than 10%.

## Fungal Sinusitis/Allergic Fungal Sinusitis
### Overview

Fungal sinus disease can be broadly divided into invasive and noninvasive categories.[152] Invasive forms are characterized by the presence of fungal hyphae both within and deep to the mucosa. Subtypes of invasive fungal sinus infection include acute invasive, chronic invasive, and chronic granulomatous invasive fungal sinusitis. In noninvasive forms, hyphae do not enter the mucosa. These subtypes include allergic fungal sinusitis (AFS) and fungal mycetoma.[153] While asymptomatic fungal colonization is common in individuals with intact immune systems, invasive fungal sinusitis is typically associated with abnormal immunity.[152] The most commonly implicated organisms include *Aspergillus*, *Bipolaris*, and *Rhizopus*. Pathological differentiation of invasive and noninvasive forms may require

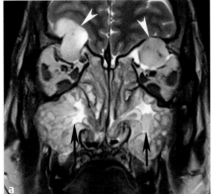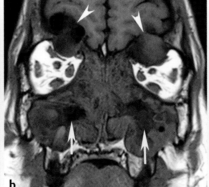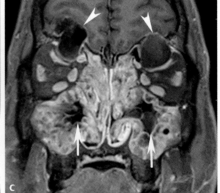

**Fig. 1.71** Sinonasal polyposis. Coronal T2-weighed (**a**), T1-weighted (**b**), and fat-suppressed contrast-enhanced T1-weighted MRI (**c**) images are shown. The nasal cavity and paranasal sinuses are almost completely filled with variable signal intensity polypoid tissue resulting in expansion and remodeling of the walls of these structures. The polyps themselves demonstrate variable appearances, and there are also additional interspersed areas of retained secretions (*arrows*). Bilateral frontal mucoceles are present (*arrowheads*).

large quantities of sinus contents and extensive biopsy specimens including diseased and adjacent healthy mucosa and bone.[153] AFS is the most common form of fungal sinusitis, estimated to be present in 5 to 10% of all patients undergoing surgery for chronic hypertrophic sinus disease.[154] AFS is particularly common in warm, humid climates, which promote fungal growth. Chronic sinonasal inflammation is thought to result from immediate and delayed hypersensitivity reactions to inhaled fungal organisms such as *Bipolaris*, *Curvularia*, *Alternaria*, *Aspergillus*, and *Fusarium*. Pathologically, AFS is characterized by the presence of eosinophil-containing "allergic mucin" within affected sinuses, with the consistency of peanut butter.[155] Sparse, noninvasive fungal hyphae are present.[156] Affected individuals are often immunocompetent and in the third decade of life. There are associations with atopy and previous sinus surgery. Clinical features include chronic headaches, nasal congestion, and chronic sinusitis.

Fungal mycetoma is relatively uncommon.[152] It is thought to result from reduced paranasal sinus mucociliary clearance of inhaled fungal organisms, which replicate and provoke an inflammatory response in the adjacent sinus mucosa. Pathologically, a mycetoma or fungal ball consists of tangled hyphae in the absence of allergic mucin or evidence of mucosal invasion. The most commonly implicated organism is *Aspergillus fumigatus*.[152] Older, immunocompetent patients are more often affected and there is a female predilection. Clinical symptoms are typically minimal or absent.[153] Acute invasive fungal sinusitis is rare in healthy individuals with normal immune systems.[152] It is seen predominantly in immunocompromised patients such as those with neutropenia and poorly controlled diabetes. Clinically, a painless, necrotic nasal septal ulcer is often seen in conjunction with sinusitis and rapid extramucosal spread over a timeframe of days to weeks. Angioinvasion and hematogeneous dissemination are frequent. Presenting symptoms include fever, facial pain or numbness, nasal congestion, serosanguinous nasal discharge, and epistaxis which can rapidly progress to include findings of orbital and intracranial spread, leading to death.

Chronic invasive fungal sinusitis can affect immunocompetent patients with a history of rhinosinusitis. Patients with diabetes or mildly immunocompromised individuals are more susceptible.[152] Symptoms include sinus pain, serosanguinous discharge, epistaxis, and fever. Symptoms attributable to invasion of the maxilla, orbits, or cranium develop over months to years. Chronic granulomatous invasive fungal sinusitis is a related disorder seen primarily in Africa and Southeast Asia[153] characterized by noncaseating granulomas within affected tissues. Clinical and imaging features resemble those of chronic invasive fungal sinusitis.

## Imaging characteristics

In AFS, many or all of the paranasal sinuses as well as the nasal cavity may be affected. Involved sinuses are typically almost completely opacified and expanded, resulting in smooth erosion of sinus walls, skull base distortion, and orbital erosion.[156] On CT performed without contrast, allergic mucin located centrally within the sinus lumen and nasal cavity is typically hyperattenuating (▶ Fig. 1.72).[157] This material demonstrates characteristic low or absent signal intensity on T2-weighted images,[158] usually attributed to fungal concentration of metal

ions including iron, magnesium, and manganese, as well as high protein and low free-water content. T1-weighted image signal is variable. Surrounding these areas there may be interspersed low attenuation nasal polyps with high signal on T2-weighted images.[156] Peripheral mucosal thickening characterized by enhancement and high signal on T2-weighted images is common.[152] Imaging findings of invasion of adjacent tissues and blood vessels are absent.

Fungal mycetomas typically manifest on imaging as a mass within the lumen of a single paranasal sinus, most often maxillary (▶ Fig. 1.73).[152] The mass is usually diffusely hyperattenuating on CT performed without contrast and may demonstrate punctate internal calcifications. The adjacent mucosa often appears inflamed, but the central sinus contents do not enhance. The sinus walls may demonstrate thickening and sclerosis or, if there is sinus expansion, the walls may demonstrate smooth thinning and erosion. On MRI, the mycetoma is typically hypointense on T1- and T2-weighted images for reasons similar to those listed earlier for AFS.

Acute invasive fungal sinusitis manifests with mucosal thickening or soft-tissue attenuation within paranasal sinuses and the nasal cavity, with a predilection for unilateral involvement of ethmoid and sphenoid sinuses.[152] Severe unilateral nasal cavity soft-tissue thickening is the most consistent early CT finding.[159] Abnormal MR signal or CT attenuation in normally homogeneous premaxillary or retroantral fat can be an important sign of invasion. It is therefore important to scrutinize these areas carefully in suspected cases for early diagnosis and treatment. Later, aggressive bone destruction is often seen with intracranial and intraorbital extension of inflammatory changes. Of note, bone erosion and mucosal thickening can sometimes be very subtle as angioinvasion results in extrasinus extension with intact bony walls (▶ Fig. 1.74).[152] Angioinvasion may also result in absence of mucosal enhancement. Acute fulminant invasive fungal sinusitis most commonly begins as mucosal inflammation in the region of the middle turbinate and can manifest on MRI as the "black turbinate sign," referring to a nonenhancing, hypointense turbinate. This has been described as an early sign of nasal mucormycosis on MRI.[160]

Chronic fungal sinusitis typically presents with a hyperattenuating soft-tissue attenuation structure within one or more paranasal sinuses which may be mass-like.[152] Destruction of sinus walls with mottled osseous lucency or irregular bone destruction and evidence of extrasinus extension can closely mimic malignancy. Alternatively, the walls of the affected sinuses may be thickened and sclerotic as a result of chronic sinus inflammation. Low signal on T1- and T2-weighted images may help differentiate this process from a neoplastic process.

## Prognosis and treatment

AFS is treated with endoscopic surgical drainage of allergic mucin from affected cavities in almost all cases, followed by removal of obstructing polyps and restoration of normal sinonasal drainage.[161] Osseous expansion, erosion, and mucocele formation can distort surgical landmarks and erode normal barrier structures, potentially increasing surgical risk and making imaging guidance even more valuable. A variety of medical therapies have been employed to obtain long-term symptom control and prevent the need for revision surgery.[156] Reported recurrence rates range from 10 to 100%.[161] Mycetoma treatment

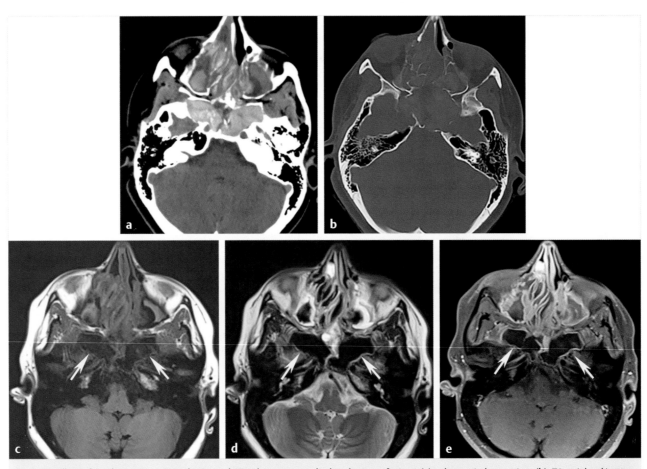

**Fig. 1.72** Allergic fungal sinusitis on CT and MRI. Axial CT without contrast displayed using soft-tissue (**a**) or bone window settings (**b**), T1-weighted images without contrast (**c**), T2-weighted (**d**), and contrast-enhanced fat-suppressed T1-weighted MRI (**e**) images are shown. On CT, the paranasal sinuses are diffusely opacified with variable attenuation material that includes a large component with spontaneous high attenuation. The sinuses are expanded and deformed. On MRI, some areas with corresponding high attenuation on CT (such as the expanded sphenoid sinuses, indicated by the *arrows*; **c,d**) have very low signal, most pronounced on T2-weighted images, simulating aerated sinus on this sequence. The low signal in this context is often attributed to a combination of chronically inspissated secretions with reduced hydration and accumulation of manganese within fungal elements.

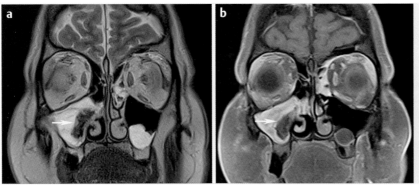

**Fig. 1.73** Mycetoma of the right maxillary sinus on coronal T2-weighted (**a**) and contrast-enhanced fat-suppressed T1-weighted MRI (**b**). The mycetoma (*arrows*) has low signal on both sequences, likely related to inspissated content and accumulation of manganese within fungal elements, resulting in magnetic susceptibility artifact. Surrounding is a component with predominantly high signal on T2 along with inflammatory changes and secretions.

when required involves more limited surgical sinus evacuation and drainage pathway restoration.[152] Adjunct treatments are not often required and recurrence is rare.

Invasive fungal sinusitis requires aggressive surgical debridement concurrent with systemic antifungal therapy and reversal of immunosuppression.[152] Extensive biopsy of suspicious areas is important for early diagnosis.[162] The reported mortality rate for acute invasive fungal sinusitis is 50 to 80%,[163] but with active surveillance of at-risk populations and early, aggressive

management, this has been reported to decrease to as little as 18%.[164]

## Fibrous Dysplasia

### Overview

Fibrous dysplasia is a benign osseous developmental anomaly in which the normal medullary space of an affected bone (or bones, in the case of polyostotic forms) is progressively replaced

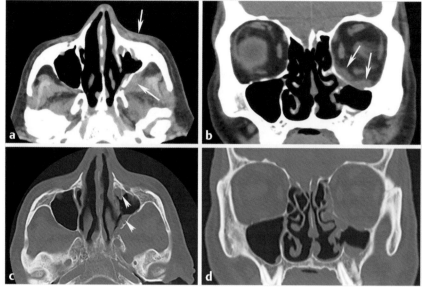

**Fig. 1.74** Invasive fungal sinusitis in an immuno-compromised patient. Axial and coronal reformats from a CT scan performed without contrast displayed using soft tissue (**a,b**) and bone window and algorithm settings (**c,d**) are shown. There is a small amount of peripheral opacification within the left maxillary sinus (*arrowheads*; **c**). There is abnormal attenuation within the fat surrounding the sinus, including within the retromaxillary and premaxillary fat and inferior aspect of the adjacent orbit (*arrows*; **a,b**), though the bony walls are intact. These findings are suggestive of angioinvasion.

by disorganized fibroosseous tissue.[165] Eighty percent of cases are monostotic, and 20% of these involve the head and neck region.[64] Polyostotic forms are associated with various syndromes and associated lesions, including McCune-Albright syndrome, primary hyperparathyroidism, tuberous sclerosis and soft-tissue myxomas (Mazabraud's syndrome) or, rarely, an aneurysmal bone cyst.[166] Craniofacial involvement in polyostotic forms ranges in frequency from 50 to 100%.[167] Most lesions are diagnosed prior to 30 years of age. There is no gender predilection. When the craniofacial bones are involved, the most common site is the skull base.[168] Patients are frequently asymptomatic and many lesions are detected incidentally on imaging. Presentation may occur as a result of cosmetic changes or neurological abnormalities such as visual or hearing loss. Symptoms of recurrent rhinosinusitis or trigeminal neuralgia are frequently reported.

## Imaging characteristics

Foci of fibrous dysplasia manifest on imaging as expansile, well-defined intramedullary lesions with variable thickness and mineralization of the surrounding cortical rim. CT frequently reveals a ground-glass matrix, but contents may range from cyst-like radiolucency to frank sclerosis (► Fig. 1.75, ► Fig. 1.76). Narrowing of traversing neurovascular foramina may be observed. Marrow signal intensity on MRI within affected bones is highly variable, often with areas of intense contrast enhancement. If encountered for the first time on MRI, fibrous dysplasia can mimic an aggressive neoplasm. If there is doubt, correlation with a CT scan will help make the correct diagnosis. Malignant transformation can be detected on serial imaging by a rapid increase in size, development of bone destruction, and/or soft-tissue invasion.

## Prognosis and treatment

Fibrous dysplasia has traditionally been described as self-limiting after puberty, though diagnosis can occur in adulthood and growth in pregnancy or after partial resection has been observed.[165] Owing to rarity of the diagnosis, no treatment

guidelines exist. Many cases do not require immediate intervention. Historically, surgical resection was the only potential therapeutic avenue. Recently, bisphosphonates have been found to be of potential value for reduction of pain and stabilization of morphology.[169] Malignant transformation is observed in 0.4 to 4% of cases,[170] more commonly in polyostotic forms or following radiation therapy. The most common resultant malignant histologies include osteosarcoma, fibrosarcoma, and chondrosarcoma.

## Granulomatosis with Polyangitis

### Overview

Granulomatosis with polyangiitis (GPA, formerly known eponymously as Wegener's granulomaosis) was first described in the late 1930s as a syndrome characterized by chronic rhinitis and renal failure with histologic features of granulomatous necrotizing inflammation.[171] Prevalence in the United States is estimated to be 3 cases per 100,000. Most new cases involve the head and neck, and many affect the central nervous system.[172,173] There is no gender predilection. Presentation may occur at any age, most commonly in the fourth or fifth decades with nasal involvement accompanied by pulmonary and renal disease. Elevated levels of antineutrophil cytoplasmic antibodies (ANCA) are important for diagnosis, although in 25% of cases this marker is not detectable[171] and the diagnosis may require nasal biopsy. Histopathology typically reveals necrotizing granulomas, tissue necrosis, and variable amounts of vasculitis involving small to medium vessels.

### Imaging characteristics

Sinonasal involvement by GPA is characterized on CT by osseous erosion and destruction, mucosal thickening, and neoosteogenesis (► Fig. 1.77, ► Fig. 1.78).[171] Bone erosion has a predilection for the anterior ethmoid region. Mucosal thickening most frequently affects the maxillary sinuses,[174] and can sometimes be distinguished from chronic sinusitis by a pattern of nodularity. Obliterative bone changes resulting from vasculitis-

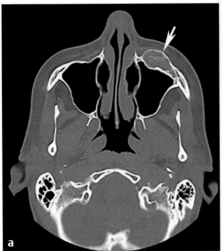
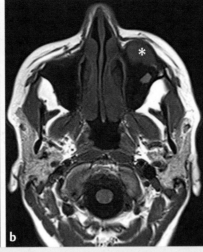
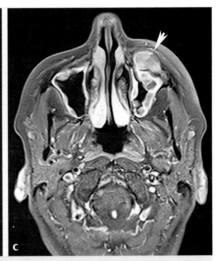

**Fig. 1.75** Fibrous dysplasia of the anterior wall of the left maxilla. CT scan displayed using bone window and algorithm settings (**a**), T1-weighted MRI without contrast (**b**), and fat-suppressed contrast-enhanced T1-weighted MRI (**c**) are shown. On CT, there is an expansile intraossoeus lesion with characteristic "ground-glass" matrix (*arrow*; **a**). The overlying cortices are preserved. On the T1-weighted image, there is a well-defined lesion with internal contents that are of intermediate signal and hypointense to fat (*asterisk*; **b**). The overlying subcutaneous fat has normal preserved high signal. Following contrast administration, the lesion exhibits mildly heterogeneous enhancement (*arrowhead*; **c**). If first encountered, the appearance of fibrous dysplasia can be misleading for more aggressive process or tumor and correlation with a CT scan can be very helpful for making the correct diagnosis.

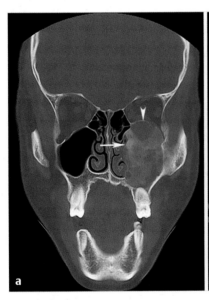
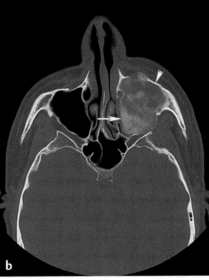

**Fig. 1.76** Fibrous dysplasia of the left maxillary sinus on coronal reformatted (**a**) and axial (**b**) CT images displayed using bone window and algorithm settings. A heterogeneous-density mass fills and expands the left maxillary sinus, with contents including areas of ground-glass attenuation (*arrows*) as well as more lucent regions (*arrowheads*).

induced avascular necrosis are common and localize initially to the midline septum and turbinates, spreading symmetrically to the antra and remaining sinuses with characteristic sparing of the hard palate.[175] Neoosteogenesis has the appearance of a well-corticated leading edge of bone paralleling the sinus wall overlaying less dense bone with corresponding T1-hyperintensity, suggestive of ossification and fatty marrow deposition.

Orbital involvement occurs in more than 50% of patients with GPA,[173] most commonly manifesting as orbital pseudotumor. Imaging commonly reveals a unilateral extraconal or diffuse inflammatory infiltrate conforming to the shape of the orbit.[171] Occasionally, there is extension to adjacent paranasal sinuses[176] or cavernous sinus (▶ Fig. 1.79).[177] In late stages, orbital socket contracture can occur as a result of fibrotic deposition.[171] This

fibrotic tissue has characteristic low signal on T1- and T2-weighted images.[178] Skull base involvement commonly results from direct extension of an adjacent sinonasal or orbital lesion. On MRI, inflammatory thickening and enhancement of adjacent cranial nerves can be seen, often unilaterally (▶ Fig. 1.79), and most commonly involving the olfactory and optic nerves.[179] Optic nerve atrophy can result from compression by an adjacent orbital granuloma. Rarely, GPA can produce acute optic neuritis,[180] with resultant T2-hyperintense enlargement of the involved optic nerve. Local pachymeningeal thickening and enhancement (▶ Fig. 1.79) can also extend contiguously from adjacent sinonasal or orbital disease, though diffuse, symmetrical dural thickening and enhancement can be observed independently.[181]

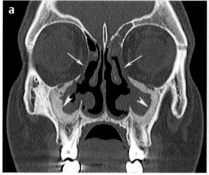 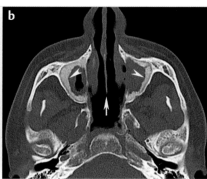

**Fig. 1.77** Granulomatosis with polyangiitis. Coronal reformat (**a**) and axial CT (**b**) image displayed using bone window and algorithm settings are shown. There is marked thickening and sclerosis/mucoperiosteal reaction of the superior, lateral, and inferior walls of the maxillary sinuses bilaterally (*arrowheads*) suggestive of chronic inflammatory process. In addition, there is irregular and nodular soft-tissue opacity lining the thickened walls associated with erosive changes. The medial walls of the maxillary sinuses and the inferior ethmoid air cells are eroded. The nasal septum is thinned and shortened posteriorly (*arrow*; **b**). The middle and inferior turbinates are also reduced in volume. The lamina papyracea are demineralized bilaterally (*thin arrows*; **a**).

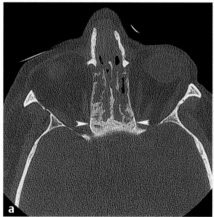 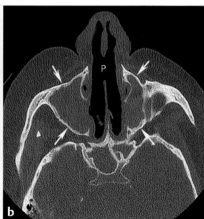

**Fig. 1.78** Granulomatosis with polyangiitis. Axial CT images displayed using bone window and algorithm settings at the levels of the ethmoid air cells (**a**) and maxillary sinuses (**b**) are shown. There is near-complete opacification of ethmoid air cells, extensive erosion of ethmoid septa, and new bone formation (*arrowheads*; **a**). The nasal septum is perforated (P; **b**). The maxillary sinuses are completely opacified, the medial walls are eroded, and the remaining walls exhibit hyperostosis (*arrows*; **b**). Similar changes of opacification and wall thickening and sclerosis are also seen in the sphenoid sinuses.

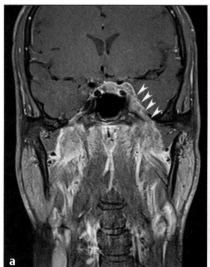 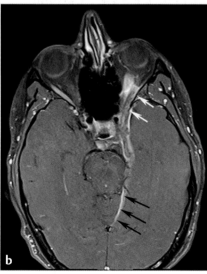

**Fig. 1.79** Granulomatosis with polyangiitis on MRI. Fat-suppressed contrast-enhanced T1-weighted MRI images in the coronal (**a**) and axial (**b**) planes are shown. The left cavernous sinus has an abnormally thick enhancing component extending to the foramen ovale (*arrowheads*; **a**). The thickening extends posteriorly along the left tentorial leaflet (*black arrows*; **b**) as well as anteriorly through the superior orbital fissure (*white arrows*; **b**).

## Prognosis and treatment

Early disease stages can reportedly be treated with corticosteroids and methotrexate.[182] Some authors suggest instituting systemic cyclophosphamide therapy for locally aggressive variants.[183] Systemic disease has been shown to respond to rituximab; however, the benefit in the head and neck is unclear.[184,185] In one recent series documenting patients with GPA treated in a head and neck clinical setting,[183] complete remission was seen in response to systemic therapy in 96% by an average of 15 months. The mean disease-free time prior to relapse was 21 months.

# 1.5 Summary and Conclusion

In this chapter, we have provided a broad overview of the wide array of pathology that can involve the anterior skull base, nasal cavity, and paranasal sinuses along with important anatomic landmarks and variants that may be important for surgical planning. Pathology affecting these regions was combined in one chapter, rather than discussed in isolation, because of their close anatomic relationship and the consequent overlap in disease or complications affecting adjacent anatomic regions.

Imaging has an essential and central role in the evaluation of pathology affecting these regions as well as preoperative staging and treatment planning in cases of neoplastic disease. In certain cases, imaging enables accurate diagnosis and identification of benign disease or "no touch" lesions that do not require any intervention. When evaluating malignant disease, certain imaging features can narrow the differential or occasionally suggest a specific histologic type. However, in general, the final diagnosis of malignant disease is based on biopsy and histopathology. For this group of diseases, one of the most important contributions of imaging is to accurately evaluate the extent of disease and upstage the initial clinical assessment by identifying disease spread to regions that cannot be reliably evaluated on clinical examination. Imaging identification of important anatomic variants is also important for preoperative planning and avoiding potential complications, particularly when minimally invasive endoscopic approaches are used. In this regard, the aim of this chapter was not only to review the imaging appearances of common and uncommon pathologies but also discuss relevant anatomic variants or spread patterns that are important and help optimize patient management.

# 1.6 High-Yield Summary

Imaging evaluation of anterior skull base, nose, and paranasal sinuses:

- CT is typically first-line test for the evaluation of inflammatory disease and is also used for preoperative identification of important anatomic landmarks and variants that may predispose to complications during endoscopic surgery.
- Extent of neoplastic disease is typically best evaluated with MRI; CT has a complementary role, especially for the evaluation of bone involvement; PET-CT has a more selective role, especially for the evaluation of recurrent disease.
- It is important to correctly recognize developmental variants and benign lesions in the skull base to avoid unnecessary invasive procedures or biopsy.

- Some benign bone lesions such as fibrous dysplasia can have a misleading aggressive appearance on MRI; if in doubt, perform a CT scan for better evaluation of bone architecture and typical findings such as a ground-glass matrix that can enable an accurate diagnosis.
- When evaluating and describing malignant disease, focus on features that will change staging and management; evaluate carefully for perineural spread of tumor, intracranial extension, and orbital involvement, best done with MRI.
- CT is excellent for identification of cortical bone invasion, whereas MRI has higher sensitivity for identification of early marrow invasion; MRI has the potential to overestimate marrow involvement because of signal changes from marrow edema and this pitfall can be avoided by ensuring that tumor within the marrow follows the signal of the native tumor on ALL sequences.
- When there is paranasal sinus involvement by tumor, obstruction of sinus drainage pathways can result in sinus opacification that may appear similar to tumor on CT; when in doubt, MRI has high accuracy for distinguishing secretions from tumor and should be used to accurately delineate and not overestimate tumor extent.
- The specific pathways involved with perineural spread depend on the anatomic site and extent of the primary lesion: carefully evaluate the major neural pathways supplying the area of involvement by the primary tumor.
- Perineural tumor spread may be seen on CT but is best evaluated with MRI; in addition to fat-suppressed contrast-enhanced sequences for improved visualization, include at least one series of non-fat suppressed postcontrast T1-weighted images in the coronal plane for better evaluation of foramina near air–bone interfaces that are prone to distortion from susceptibility artifact.
- Malignant tumors and aggressive infections may not always be distinguishable by imaging features alone; clinical information including patient risk factors and presentation can however be helpful in narrowing the differential diagnosis; if in doubt, biopsy may be required.
- Early identification and diagnosis of invasive rhinosinusitis is essential for optimal early treatment; if clinically suspected, evaluate for early inflammatory changes outside the sinus or the MRI "black turbinate" sign.

# References

[1] Moore KL, Persaud TVN, Torchia MG. The Developing Human. 9th ed. Elsevier Inc; 2013
[2] Naidich TP, Blaser SI, Lien RJ, McLone DG, Fatterpekar GM, Bauer BS. Embryology and congenital lesions of the midface. In: Som PM, Curtin HD, eds. Head and Neck Imaging. 5th ed. St. Louis, MO: Mosby/Elsevier; 2011:3–97
[3] Harnsberger HR, Macdonald AJ. Diagnostic and Surgical Imaging Anatomy. Salt Lake City, UT: Amirsys; 2006
[4] Curtin HD, Hagiwara M. Embryology, anatomy, and imaging of the central skull base. In: Som PM, Curtin HD, eds. Head and Neck Imaging. 5th ed. St. Louis, MO: Mosby/Elsevier; 2011:928–946
[5] Belden CJ, Mancuso AA, Kotzur IM. The developing anterior skull base: CT appearance from birth to 2 years of age. AJNR Am J Neuroradiol. 1997; 18(5):811–818
[6] Som PM, Lawson W, Fatterpekar GM, Zinreich SJ, Shugar GM. Embryology, anatomy, physiology, and imaging of the sinonasal cavities. In: Som PM, Curtin HD, eds. Head and Neck Imaging. 5th ed. St. Louis, MO: Mosby/Elsevier; 2011:99–166
[7] Kilic C, Kamburoglu K, Yuksel SP, Ozen T. An assessment of the relationship between the maxillary sinus floor and the maxillary posterior teeth root tips using dental cone-beam computerized tomography. Eur J Dent. 2010; 4 (4):462–467

[8] Aoki S, Dillon WP, Barkovich AJ, Norman D. Marrow conversion before pneumatization of the sphenoid sinus: assessment with MR imaging. Radiology. 1989; 172(2):373–375

[9] Scuderi AJ, Harnsberger HR, Boyer RS. Pneumatization of the paranasal sinuses: normal features of importance to the accurate interpretation of CT scans and MR images. AJR Am J Roentgenol. 1993; 160(5):1101–1104

[10] Welker KM, DeLone DR, Lane JI, Gilbertson JR. Arrested pneumatization of the skull base: imaging characteristics. AJR Am J Roentgenol. 2008; 190(6):1691–1696

[11] Standring S. Gray's Anatomy: The Anatomical Basis of Clinical Practice. 41st ed. Philadelphia, PA: Elsevier Limited; 2016

[12] Basić N, Basić V, Jukić T, Basić M, Jelić M, Hat J. Computed tomographic imaging to determine the frequency of anatomical variations in pneumatization of the ethmoid bone. Eur Arch Otorhinolaryngol. 1999; 256(2):69–71

[13] Som PM, Park EE, Naidich TP, Lawson W. Crista galli pneumatization is an extension of the adjacent frontal sinuses. AJNR Am J Neuroradiol. 2009; 30(1):31–33

[14] Hajiioannou J, Owens D, Whittet HB. Evaluation of anatomical variation of the crista galli using computed tomography. Clin Anat. 2010; 23(4):370–373

[15] Socher JA, Santos PG, Correa VC, Silva LCBE. Endoscopic surgery in the treatment of crista galli pneumatization evolving with localized frontal headaches. Int Arch Otorhinolaryngol. 2013; 17(3):246–250

[16] Cervantes SS, Lal D. Crista galli mucocele: endoscopic marsupialization via frontoethmoid approach. Int Forum Allergy Rhinol. 2014; 4(7):598–602

[17] Thewissen JG. Mammalian frontal diploic vein and the human foramen caecum. Anat Rec. 1989; 223(2):242–244

[18] Tsutsumi S, Ono H, Yasumoto Y. A possible venous connection between the cranial and nasal cavity. Surg Radiol Anat. 2016; 38(8):911–916

[19] Gaffey MM, Friedel ME, Fatterpekar GM, Liu JK, Eloy JA. Spontaneous cerebrospinal fluid rhinorrhea of the foramen cecum in adulthood. Arch Otolaryngol Head Neck Surg. 2012; 138(1):79–82

[20] Hoang JK, Eastwood JD, Tebbit CL, Glastonbury CM. Multiplanar sinus CT: a systematic approach to imaging before functional endoscopic sinus surgery. AJR Am J Roentgenol. 2010; 194(6):W527–W536

[21] Solares CA, Lee WT, Batra PS, Citardi MJ. Lateral lamella of the cribriform plate: software-enabled computed tomographic analysis and its clinical relevance in skull base surgery. Arch Otolaryngol Head Neck Surg. 2008; 134(3):285–289

[22] Ohnishi T, Yanagisawa E. Lateral lamella of the cribriform plate–an important high-risk area in endoscopic sinus surgery. Ear Nose Throat J. 1995; 74(10):688–690

[23] Ohnishi T, Tachibana T, Kaneko Y, Esaki S. High-risk areas in endoscopic sinus surgery and prevention of complications. Laryngoscope. 1993; 103(10):1181–1185

[24] Gauba V, Saleh GM, Dua G, Agarwal S, Ell S, Vize C. Radiological classification of anterior skull base anatomy prior to performing medial orbital wall decompression. Orbit. 2006; 25(2):93–96

[25] Grevers G. Anterior skull base trauma during endoscopic sinus surgery for nasal polyposis preferred sites for iatrogenic injuries. Rhinology. 2001; 39(1):1–4

[26] Shin JH, Kang SG, Hong YK, et al. Role of the superior turbinate when performing endoscopic endonasal transsphenoidal approach. Folia Morphol (Warsz). 2014; 73(1):73–78

[27] Stammberger HR, Kennedy DW, Anatomic Terminology Group. Paranasal sinuses: anatomic terminology and nomenclature. Ann Otol Rhinol Laryngol Suppl. 1995; 167:7–16

[28] Daniels DL, Mafee MF, Smith MM, et al. The frontal sinus drainage pathway and related structures. AJNR Am J Neuroradiol. 2003; 24(8):1618–1627

[29] Bolger WE, Butzin CA, Parsons DS. Paranasal sinus bony anatomic variations and mucosal abnormalities: CT analysis for endoscopic sinus surgery. Laryngoscope. 1991; 101(1, Pt 1):56–64

[30] Calhoun KH, Waggenspack GA, Simpson CB, Hokanson JA, Bailey BJ. CT evaluation of the paranasal sinuses in symptomatic and asymptomatic populations. Otolaryngol Head Neck Surg. 1991; 104(4):480–483

[31] Braun H, Stammberger H. Pneumatization of turbinates. Laryngoscope. 2003; 113(4):668–672

[32] Som PM, Brandwein-Gensler MS. Lymph nodes of the neck. In: Som PM, Curtin HD, eds. Head and Neck Imaging. 5th ed. St. Louis, MO: Mosby/Elsevier; 2011:2287–2383

[33] Han MH, Chang KH, Min YG, Choi WS, Yeon KM, Han MC. Nontraumatic prolapse of the orbital contents into the ethmoid sinus: evaluation with screening sinus CT. Am J Otolaryngol. 1996; 17(3):184–189

[34] Huang BY, Lloyd KM, DelGaudio JM, Jablonowski E, Hudgins PA. Failed endoscopic sinus surgery: spectrum of CT findings in the frontal recess. Radiographics. 2009; 29(1):177–195

[35] Stallman JS, Lobo JN, Som PM. The incidence of concha bullosa and its relationship to nasal septal deviation and paranasal sinus disease. AJNR Am J Neuroradiol. 2004; 25(9):1613–1618

[36] Shpilberg KA, Daniel SC, Doshi AH, Lawson W, Som PM. CT of anatomic variants of the paranasal sinuses and nasal cavity: poor correlation with radiologically significant rhinosinusitis but importance in surgical planning. AJR Am J Roentgenol. 2015; 204(6):1255–1260

[37] Fadda GL, Rosso S, Aversa S, Petrelli A, Ondolo C, Succo G. Multiparametric statistical correlations between paranasal sinus anatomic variations and chronic rhinosinusitis. Acta Otorhinolaryngol Ital. 2012; 32(4):244–251

[38] Kim HJ, Jung Cho M, Lee J-W, et al. The relationship between anatomic variations of paranasal sinuses and chronic sinusitis in children. Acta Otolaryngol. 2006; 126(10):1067–1072

[39] Nouraei SA, Elisay AR, Dimarco A, et al. Variations in paranasal sinus anatomy: implications for the pathophysiology of chronic rhinosinusitis and safety of endoscopic sinus surgery. J Otolaryngol Head Neck Surg. 2009; 38(1):32–37

[40] Mathew R, Omami G, Hand A, Fellows D, Lurie A. Cone beam CT analysis of Haller cells: prevalence and clinical significance. Dentomaxillofac Radiol. 2013; 42(9):20130055

[41] Tomovic S, Esmaeili A, Chan NJ, et al. High-resolution computed tomography analysis of the prevalence of Onodi cells. Laryngoscope. 2012; 122(7):1470–1473

[42] Kantarci M, Karasen RM, Alper F, Onbas O, Okur A, Karaman A. Remarkable anatomic variations in paranasal sinus region and their clinical importance. Eur J Radiol. 2004; 50(3):296–302

[43] Dessi P, Moulin G, Triglia JM, Zanaret M, Cannoni M. Difference in the height of the right and left ethmoidal roofs: a possible risk factor for ethmoidal surgery. Prospective study of 150 CT scans. J Laryngol Otol. 1994; 108(3):261–262

[44] Lee JC, Song YJ, Chung Y-S, Lee B-J, Jang YJ. Height and shape of the skull base as risk factors for skull base penetration during endoscopic sinus surgery. Ann Otol Rhinol Laryngol. 2007; 116(3):199–205

[45] Souza SA, Souza MM, Gregório LC, Ajzen S. Anterior ethmoidal artery evaluation on coronal CT scans. Rev Bras Otorrinolaringol (Engl Ed). 2009; 75(1):101–106

[46] Prasanna LC, Mamatha H. The location of maxillary sinus ostium and its clinical application. Indian J Otolaryngol Head Neck Surg. 2010; 62(4):335–337

[47] Kimura Y, Hanazawa T, Sano T, Okano T. Lateral retropharyngeal node metastasis from carcinoma of the upper gingiva and maxillary sinus. AJNR Am J Neuroradiol. 1998; 19(7):1221–1224

[48] Tomovic S, Esmaeili A, Chan NJ, et al. High-resolution computed tomography analysis of variations of the sphenoid sinus. J Neurol Surg B Skull Base. 2013; 74(2):82–90

[49] DeLano MC, Fun FY, Zinreich SJ. Relationship of the optic nerve to the posterior paranasal sinuses: a CT anatomic study. AJNR Am J Neuroradiol. 1996; 17(4):669–675

[50] Hourany R, Aygun N, Della Santina CC, Zinreich SJ. Silent sinus syndrome: an acquired condition. AJNR Am J Neuroradiol. 2005; 26(9):2390–2392

[51] Daniels DL, Mark LP, Ulmer JL, et al. Osseous anatomy of the pterygopalatine fossa. AJNR Am J Neuroradiol. 1998; 19(8):1423–1432

[52] Chan LL, Chong J, Gillenwater AM, Ginsberg LE. The pterygopalatine fossa: postoperative MR imaging appearance. AJNR Am J Neuroradiol. 2000; 21(7):1315–1319

[53] Piagkou M, Xanthos T, Anagnostopoulou S, et al. Anatomical variation and morphology in the position of the palatine foramina in adult human skulls from Greece. J Craniomaxillofac Surg. 2012; 40(7):e206–e210

[54] Llorente JL, López F, Suárez C, Hermsen MA. Sinonasal carcinoma: clinical, pathological, genetic and therapeutic advances. Nat Rev Clin Oncol. 2014; 11(8):460–472

[55] Som PM, Brandwein-Gensler MS, Kassel EE, Genden SJ. Tumors and tumor-like conditions of the sinonasal cavities. In: Som PM, Curtin HD, eds. Head and Neck Imaging. 5th ed. St. Louis, MO: Mosby/Elsevier; 2011:253–410

[56] Barton RT. Nickel carcinogenesis of the respiratory tract. J Otolaryngol. 1977; 6(5):412–422

[57] d'Errico A, Pasian S, Baratti A, et al. A case-control study on occupational risk factors for sino-nasal cancer. Occup Environ Med. 2009; 66(7):448–455

[58] Perzin KH, Lefkowitch JH, Hui RM. Bilateral nasal squamous carcinoma arising in papillomatosis: report of a case developing after chemotherapy for leukemia. Cancer. 1981; 48(11):2375–2382

[59] Ganly I, Patel SG, Singh B, et al. Craniofacial resection for malignant paranasal sinus tumors: report of an international collaborative study. Head Neck. 2005; 27(7):575–584

[60] Singh N, Eskander A, Huang S-H, et al. Imaging and resectability issues of sinonasal tumors. Expert Rev Anticancer Ther. 2013; 13(3):297–312

[61] Eisen MD, Yousem DM, Montone KT, et al. Use of preoperative MR to predict dural, perineural, and venous sinus invasion of skull base tumors. AJNR Am J Neuroradiol. 1996; 17(10):1937–1945

[62] McIntyre JB, Perez C, Penta M, Tong L, Truelson J, Batra PS. Patterns of dural involvement in sinonasal tumors: prospective correlation of magnetic resonance imaging and histopathologic findings. Int Forum Allergy Rhinol. 2012; 2(4):336–341

[63] Raghavan P, Phillips CD. Magnetic resonance imaging of sinonasal malignancies. Top Magn Reson Imaging. 2007; 18(4):259–267

[64] Lund VJ, Stammberger H, Nicolai P, et al. European Rhinologic Society Advisory Board on Endoscopic Techniques in the Management of Nose, Paranasal Sinus and Skull Base Tumours. European position paper on endoscopic management of tumours of the nose, paranasal sinuses and skull base. Rhinol Suppl. 2010; 22:1–143

[65] Maroldi R, Nicolai P. Imaging in Treatment Planning for Sinonasal Diseases. Springer Science & Business Media Berlin, Heidelberg: Springer-Verlag; 2005

[66] Eisen MD, Yousem DM, Loevner LA, Thaler ER, Bilker WB, Goldberg AN. Preoperative imaging to predict orbital invasion by tumor. Head Neck. 2000; 22 (5):456–462

[67] Kim HJ, Lee TH, Lee H-S, Cho K-S, Roh H-J. Periorbita: computed tomography and magnetic resonance imaging findings. Am J Rhinol. 2006; 20(4):371–374

[68] Wong RJ. Current status of FDG-PET for head and neck cancer. J Surg Oncol. 2008; 97(8):649–652

[69] Compton CC, Byrd DR, Garcia-Aguilar J, Kurtzman SH, Olawaiye A, Washington MK. AJCC Cancer Staging Atlas: A Companion to the Seventh Editions of the AJCC Cancer Staging Manual and Handbook. New York, NY: Springer-Verlag; 2012

[70] Dulguerov P, Jacobsen MS, Allal AS, Lehmann W, Calcaterra T. Nasal and paranasal sinus carcinoma: are we making progress? A series of 220 patients and a systematic review. Cancer. 2001; 92(12):3012–3029

[71] Kida A, Endo S, Iida H, et al. Clinical assessment of squamous cell carcinoma of the nasal cavity proper. Auris Nasus Larynx. 1995; 22(3):172–177

[72] Lewis JS, Jr, Westra WH, Thompson LDR, et al. The sinonasal tract: another potential "hot spot" for carcinomas with transcriptionally-active human papillomavirus. Head Neck Pathol. 2014; 8(3):241–249

[73] Shah JP, Patel SG, Singh B. Jatin Shah's Head and Neck Surgery and Oncology. 4th ed. Philadelphia, PA: Elsevier; 2012

[74] de Almeida JR, Su SY, Koutourousiou M, et al. Endonasal endoscopic surgery for squamous cell carcinoma of the sinonasal cavities and skull base: oncologic outcomes based on treatment strategy and tumor etiology. Head Neck. 2015; 37(8):1163–1169

[75] Hoppe R, Phillips TL, Roach M. Leibel and Phillips Textbook of Radiation Oncology: Expert Consult. 3rd ed. Philadelphia, PA: Elsevier; 2010

[76] Banuchi V, Mallen J, Kraus D. Cancers of the nose, sinus, and skull base. Surg Oncol Clin N Am. 2015; 24(3):563–577

[77] Bachar G, Goldstein DP, Shah M, et al. Esthesioneuroblastoma: The Princess Margaret Hospital experience. Head Neck. 2008; 30(12):1607–1614

[78] 4. Definition of volumes. J ICRU. 2010; 10(1):41–53

[79] Chan AW, Liebsch NJ. Proton radiation therapy for head and neck cancer. J Surg Oncol. 2008; 97(8):697–700

[80] Turner JH, Reh DD. Incidence and survival in patients with sinonasal cancer: a historical analysis of population-based data. Head Neck. 2012; 34(6):877–885

[81] Leivo I. Update on sinonasal adenocarcinoma: classification and advances in immunophenotype and molecular genetic make-up. Head Neck Pathol. 2007; 1(1):38–43

[82] Moreau JJ, Bessede JP, Heurtebise F, et al. Adenocarcinoma of the ethmoid sinus in woodworkers. Retrospective study of 25 cases [in French]. Neurochirurgie. 1997; 43(2):111–117

[83] Bhayani MK, Yilmaz T, Sweeney A, et al. Sinonasal adenocarcinoma: a 16-year experience at a single institution. Head Neck. 2014; 36(10):1490–1496

[84] Reiersen DA, Pahilan ME, Devaiah AK. Meta-analysis of treatment outcomes for sinonasal undifferentiated carcinoma. Otolaryngol Head Neck Surg. 2012; 147(1):7–14

[85] Xu CC, Dziegielewski PT, McGaw WT, Seikaly H. Sinonasal undifferentiated carcinoma (SNUC): the Alberta experience and literature review. J Otolaryngol Head Neck Surg. 2013; 42:2

[86] Ejaz A, Wenig BM. Sinonasal undifferentiated carcinoma: clinical and pathologic features and a discussion on classification, cellular differentiation, and differential diagnosis. Adv Anat Pathol. 2005; 12(3):134–143

[87] Christopherson K, Werning JW, Malyapa RS, Morris CG, Mendenhall WM. Radiotherapy for sinonasal undifferentiated carcinoma. Am J Otolaryngol. 2014; 35(2):141–146

[88] Rischin D, Porceddu S, Peters L, Martin J, Corry J, Weih L. Promising results with chemoradiation in patients with sinonasal undifferentiated carcinoma. Head Neck. 2004; 26(5):435–441

[89] Lupinetti AD, Roberts DB, Williams MD, et al. Sinonasal adenoid cystic carcinoma: the M. D. Anderson Cancer Center experience. Cancer. 2007; 110(12): 2726–2731

[90] Eggesbø HB. Imaging of sinonasal tumours. Cancer Imaging. 2012; 12:136–152

[91] Hanna E, Vural E, Prokopakis E, Carrau R, Snyderman C, Weissman J. The sensitivity and specificity of high-resolution imaging in evaluating perineural spread of adenoid cystic carcinoma to the skull base. Arch Otolaryngol Head Neck Surg. 2007; 133(6):541–545

[92] Jeong H-S, Chung MK, Son Y-I, et al. Role of 18F-FDG PET/CT in management of high-grade salivary gland malignancies. J Nucl Med. 2007; 48(8):1237–1244

[93] Bjørndal K, Krogdahl A, Therkildsen MH, et al. Salivary adenoid cystic carcinoma in Denmark 1990–2005: outcome and independent prognostic factors including the benefit of radiotherapy. Results of the Danish Head and Neck Cancer Group (DAHANCA). Oral Oncol. 2015; 51(12):1138–1142

[94] Gondivkar SM, Gadbail AR, Chole R, Parikh RV. Adenoid cystic carcinoma: a rare clinical entity and literature review. Oral Oncol. 2011; 47 (4):231–236

[95] Wolfish EB, Nelson BL, Thompson LDR. Sinonasal tract mucoepidermoid carcinoma: a clinicopathologic and immunophenotypic study of 19 cases combined with a comprehensive review of the literature. Head Neck Pathol. 2012; 6(2):191–207

[96] Dulguerov P, Allal AS, Calcaterra TC. Esthesioneuroblastoma: a meta-analysis and review. Lancet Oncol. 2001; 2(11):683–690

[97] Petruzzelli GJ, Howell JB, Pederson A, et al. Multidisciplinary treatment of olfactory neuroblastoma: patterns of failure and management of recurrence. Am J Otolaryngol. 2015; 36(4):547–553

[98] Herrold KM. Induction of olfactory neuroepithelial tumors in Syrian hamsters by diethylnitrosamine. Cancer. 1964; 17:114–121

[99] Koike K, Jay G, Hartley JW, Schrenzel MD, Higgins RJ, Hinrichs SH. Activation of retrovirus in transgenic mice: association with development of olfactory neuroblastoma. J Virol. 1990; 64(8):3988–3991

[100] Dulguerov P, Calcaterra T. Esthesioneuroblastoma: the UCLA experience 1970–1990. Laryngoscope. 1992; 102(8):843–849

[101] Regenbogen VS, Zinreich SJ, Kim KS, et al. Hyperostotic esthesioneuroblastoma: CT and MR findings. J Comput Assist Tomogr. 1988; 12(1):52–56

[102] Howell MC, Branstetter BF, IV, Snyderman CH. Patterns of regional spread for esthesioneuroblastoma. AJNR Am J Neuroradiol. 2011; 32(5):929–933

[103] Som PM, Lidov M, Brandwein M, Catalano P, Biller HF. Sinonasal esthesioneuroblastoma with intracranial extension: marginal tumor cysts as a diagnostic MR finding. AJNR Am J Neuroradiol. 1994; 15(7):1259–1262

[104] Kadish S, Goodman M, Wang CC. Olfactory neuroblastoma. A clinical analysis of 17 cases. Cancer. 1976; 37(3):1571–1576

[105] Morita A, Ebersold MJ, Olsen KD, Foote RL, Lewis JE, Quast LM. Esthesioneuroblastoma: prognosis and management. Neurosurgery. 1993; 32(5):706–714, discussion 714–715

[106] Cunnane ME, Sepahdari A, Gardiner M, Mafee MF. Pathology of the eye and orbit. In: Som PM, Curtin HD, eds. Head and Neck Imaging. 5th ed. St. Louis, MO: Mosby/Elsevier; 2011:591–756

[107] O'Neill JP, Bilsky MH, Kraus D. Head and neck sarcomas: epidemiology, pathology, and management. Neurosurg Clin N Am. 2013; 24(1):67–78

[108] Reilly BK, Kim A, Peña MT, et al. Rhabdomyosarcoma of the head and neck in children: review and update. Int J Pediatr Otorhinolaryngol. 2015; 79(9): 1477–1483

[109] Crist WM, Anderson JR, Meza JL, et al. Intergroup rhabdomyosarcoma study-IV: results for patients with nonmetastatic disease. J Clin Oncol. 2001; 19 (12):3091–3102

[110] Mafee MF, Pai E, Philip B. Rhabdomyosarcoma of the orbit. Evaluation with MR imaging and CT. Radiol Clin North Am. 1998; 36(6):1215–1227, xii

[111] Raney RB, Maurer HM, Anderson JR, et al. The Intergroup Rhabdomyosarcoma Study Group (IRSG): major lessons from the IRS-I through IRS-IV studies as background for the current IRS-V treatment protocols. Sarcoma. 2001; 5(1):9–15

[112] Clifton N, Harrison L, Bradley PJ, Jones NS. Malignant melanoma of nasal cavity and paranasal sinuses: report of 24 patients and literature review. J Laryngol Otol. 2011; 125(5):479–485

[113] Haerle SK, Soyka MB, Fischer DR, et al. The value of 18F-FDG-PET/CT imaging for sinonasal malignant melanoma. Eur Arch Otorhinolaryngol. 2012; 269 (1):127–133

[114] Chang PC, Fischbein NJ, McCalmont TH, et al. Perineural spread of malignant melanoma of the head and neck: clinical and imaging features. AJNR Am J Neuroradiol. 2004; 25(1):5–11

[115] Melanoma Treatment. National Cancer Institute. https://www.cancer.gov/types/skin/hp/melanoma-treatment-pdq

[116] Dauer EH, Lewis JE, Rohlinger AL, Weaver AL, Olsen KD. Sinonasal melanoma: a clinicopathologic review of 61 cases. Otolaryngol Head Neck Surg. 2008; 138(3):347–352

[117] Cleary KR, Batsakis JG. Sinonasal lymphomas. Ann Otol Rhinol Laryngol. 1994; 103(11):911–914

[118] Li C-C, Tien H-F, Tang J-L, et al. Treatment outcome and pattern of failure in 77 patients with sinonasal natural killer/T-cell or T-cell lymphoma. Cancer. 2004; 100(2):366–375

[119] Peng KA, Kita AE, Suh JD, Bhuta SM, Wang MB. Sinonasal lymphoma: case series and review of the literature. Int Forum Allergy Rhinol. 2014; 4(8):670–674

[120] Ou C-H, Chen CC-C, Ling J-C, et al. Nasal NK/T-cell lymphoma: computed tomography and magnetic resonance imaging findings. J Chin Med Assoc. 2007; 70(5):207–212

[121] Ooi GC, Chim CS, Liang R, Tsang KW, Kwong YL. Nasal T-cell/natural killer cell lymphoma: CT and MR imaging features of a new clinicopathologic entity. AJR Am J Roentgenol. 2000; 174(4):1141–1145

[122] Kim SJ, Oh SY, Hong JY, et al. When do we need central nervous system prophylaxis in patients with extranodal NK/T-cell lymphoma, nasal type? Ann Oncol. 2010; 21(5):1058–1063

[123] Mendenhall WM, Fernandes R, Werning JW, Vaysberg M, Malyapa RS, Mendenhall NP. Head and neck osteosarcoma. Am J Otolaryngol. 2011; 32(6):597–600

[124] Guadagnolo BA, Zagars GK, Raymond AK, Benjamin RS, Sturgis EM. Osteosarcoma of the jaw/craniofacial region: outcomes after multimodality treatment. Cancer. 2009; 115(14):3262–3270

[125] Schwarz MB, Burgess LP, Fee WE, Jr, Donaldson SS. Postirradiation sarcoma in retinoblastoma. Induction or predisposition? Arch Otolaryngol Head Neck Surg. 1988; 114(6):640–644

[126] Huber GF, Dziegielewski P, Wayne Matthews T, Dort JC. Head and neck osteosarcoma in adults: the province of Alberta experience over 26 years. J Otolaryngol Head Neck Surg. 2008; 37(5):738–743

[127] Guo L, Liu J, Sun X, Wang D. Sinonasal tract chondrosarcoma: 18-year experience at a single institution. Auris Nasus Larynx. 2014; 41(3):290–293

[128] Khan MN, Husain Q, Kanumuri VV, et al. Management of sinonasal chondrosarcoma: a systematic review of 161 patients. Int Forum Allergy Rhinol. 2013; 3(8):670–677

[129] Rahal A, Durio JR, Hinni ML. Chondrosarcoma of the nasal septum. Ear Nose Throat J. 2009; 88(1):744–745

[130] Lawson W, Schlecht NF, Brandwein-Gensler M. The role of the human papillomavirus in the pathogenesis of Schneiderian inverted papillomas: an analytic overview of the evidence. Head Neck Pathol. 2008; 2(2):49–59

[131] Harrison LB, Sessions RB, Hong WK. Head and Neck Cancer: A Multidisciplinary Approach. 3rd ed. Philadelphia, PA: Lippincott Williams & Wilkins; 2009

[132] Szymańska A, Szymański M, Czekajska-Chehab E, Szczerbo-Trojanowska M. Invasive growth patterns of juvenile nasopharyngeal angiofibroma: radiological imaging and clinical implications. Acta Radiol. 2014; 55(6):725–731

[133] Som PM, Cohen BA, Sacher M, Choi IS, Bryan NR. The angiomatous polyp and the angiofibroma: two different lesions. Radiology. 1982; 144(2):329–334

[134] Apostol JV, Frazell EL. Juvenile nasopharyngeal angiofibroma. A clinical study. Cancer. 1965; 18:869–878

[135] Nicolai P, Schreiber A, Bolzoni Villaret A. Juvenile angiofibroma: evolution of management. Int J Pediatr. 2012; 2012:412545

[136] Radkowski D, McGill T, Healy GB, Ohlms L, Jones DT. Angiofibroma. Changes in staging and treatment. Arch Otolaryngol Head Neck Surg. 1996; 122(2):122–129

[137] Renkonen S, Hagström J, Vuola J, et al. The changing surgical management of juvenile nasopharyngeal angiofibroma. Eur Arch Otorhinolaryngol. 2011; 268(4):599–607

[138] Morales-Valero SF, Van Gompel JJ, Loumiotis I, Lanzino G. Craniotomy for anterior cranial fossa meningiomas: historical overview. Neurosurg Focus. 2014; 36(4):E14

[139] Rachinger W, Grau S, Tonn J-C. Different microsurgical approaches to meningiomas of the anterior cranial base. Acta Neurochir (Wien). 2010; 152(6):931–939

[140] Lopez DA, Silvers DN, Helwig EB. Cutaneous meningiomas–a clinicopathologic study. Cancer. 1974; 34(3):728–744

[141] Devi B, Bhat D, Madhusudhan H, Santhosh V, Shankar S. Primary intraosseous meningioma of orbit and anterior cranial fossa: a case report and literature review. Australas Radiol. 2001; 45(2):211–214

[142] Pieper DR, Al-Mefty O, Hanada Y, Buechner D. Hyperostosis associated with meningioma of the cranial base: secondary changes or tumor invasion. Neurosurgery. 1999; 44(4):742–746, discussion 746–747

[143] Biau J, Khalil T, Verrelle P, Lemaire JJ. Fractionated radiotherapy and radiosurgery of intracranial meningiomas. Neurochirurgie. 2015:[epub ahead of print]; pii: :S0028-3770(14)00283-5

[144] Komotar RJ, Starke RM, Raper DM, Anand VK, Schwartz TH. Endoscopic endonasal versus open transcranial resection of anterior midline skull base meningiomas. World Neurosurg. 2012; 77(5–6):713–724

[145] Kondziolka D, Mathieu D, Lunsford LD, et al. Radiosurgery as definitive management of intracranial meningiomas. Neurosurgery. 2008; 62(1):53–58, discussion 58–60

[146] Santacroce A, Walier M, Régis J, et al. Long-term tumor control of benign intracranial meningiomas after radiosurgery in a series of 4565 patients. Neurosurgery. 2012; 70(1):32–39, discussion 39

[147] Liu C-M, Hong C-Y, Shun C-T, et al. Inducible cyclooxygenase and interleukin 6 gene expressions in nasal polyp fibroblasts: possible implication in the pathogenesis of nasal polyposis. Arch Otolaryngol Head Neck Surg. 2002; 128(8):945–951

[148] Mafee MF, Tran BH, Chapa AR. Imaging of rhinosinusitis and its complications: plain film, CT, and MRI. Clin Rev Allergy Immunol. 2006; 30(3):165–186

[149] Encyclopedia of Otolaryngology, Head and Neck Surgery. Heidelberg, Germany: Springer; 2013

[150] Aferzon M, Millman B, O'Donnell TR, Gilroy PA. Cholesterol granuloma of the frontal bone. Otolaryngol Head Neck Surg. 2002; 127(6):578–581

[151] Capra GG, Carbone PN, Mullin DP. Paranasal sinus mucocele. Head Neck Pathol. 2012; 6(3):369–372

[152] Aribandi M, McCoy VA, Bazan C, III. Imaging features of invasive and noninvasive fungal sinusitis: a review. Radiographics. 2007; 27(5):1283–1296

[153] deShazo RD, Chapin K, Swain RE. Fungal sinusitis. N Engl J Med. 1997; 337 (4):254–259

[154] Schubert MS. Allergic fungal sinusitis. Otolaryngol Clin North Am. 2004; 37 (2):301–326

[155] deShazo RD, Swain RE. Diagnostic criteria for allergic fungal sinusitis. J Allergy Clin Immunol. 1995; 96(1):24–35

[156] Ryan MW. Allergic fungal rhinosinusitis. Otolaryngol Clin North Am. 2011; 44(3):697–710, ix–x

[157] Mukherji SK, Figueroa RE, Ginsberg LE, et al. Allergic fungal sinusitis: CT findings. Radiology. 1998; 207(2):417–422

[158] Manning SC, Merkel M, Kriesel K, Vuitch F, Marple B. Computed tomography and magnetic resonance diagnosis of allergic fungal sinusitis. Laryngoscope. 1997; 107(2):170–176

[159] DelGaudio JM, Swain RE, Jr, Kingdom TT, Muller S, Hudgins PA. Computed tomographic findings in patients with invasive fungal sinusitis. Arch Otolaryngol Head Neck Surg. 2003; 129(2):236–240

[160] Safder S, Carpenter JS, Roberts TD, Bailey N. The "Black Turbinate" sign: an early MR imaging finding of nasal mucormycosis. AJNR Am J Neuroradiol. 2010; 31(4):771–774

[161] Marple BF. Allergic fungal rhinosinusitis: current theories and management strategies. Laryngoscope. 2001; 111(6):1006–1019

[162] Gillespie MB, O'Malley BW, Jr, Francis HW. An approach to fulminant invasive fungal rhinosinusitis in the immunocompromised host. Arch Otolaryngol Head Neck Surg. 1998; 124(5):520–526

[163] Waitzman AA, Birt BD. Fungal sinusitis. J Otolaryngol. 1994; 23(4):244–249

[164] Parikh SL, Venkatraman G, DelGaudio JM. Invasive fungal sinusitis: a 15-year review from a single institution. Am J Rhinol. 2004; 18(2):75–81

[165] Schreiber A, Villaret AB, Maroldi R, Nicolai P. Fibrous dysplasia of the sinonasal tract and adjacent skull base. Curr Opin Otolaryngol Head Neck Surg. 2012; 20(1):45–52

[166] Sadeghi SM, Hosseini SN. Spontaneous conversion of fibrous dysplasia into osteosarcoma. J Craniofac Surg. 2011; 22(3):959–961

[167] Terkawi AS, Al-Qahtani KH, Baksh E, Soualmi L, Mohamed Ael-B, Sabbagh AJ. Fibrous dysplasia and aneurysmal bone cyst of the skull base presenting with blindness: a report of a rare locally aggressive example. Head Neck Oncol. 2011; 3:15

[168] Amit M, Collins MT, FitzGibbon EJ, Butman JA, Fliss DM, Gil Z. Surgery versus watchful waiting in patients with craniofacial fibrous dysplasia–a meta-analysis. PLoS One. 2011; 6(9):e25179

[169] Chapurlat RD, Orcel P. Fibrous dysplasia of bone and McCune-Albright syndrome. Best Pract Res Clin Rheumatol. 2008; 22(1):55–69

[170] DiCaprio MR, Enneking WF. Fibrous dysplasia. Pathophysiology, evaluation, and treatment. J Bone Joint Surg Am. 2005; 87(8):1848–1864

[171] Pakalniskis MG, Berg AD, Policeni BA, et al. The many faces of granulomatosis with polyangiitis: a review of the head and neck imaging manifestations. AJR Am J Roentgenol. 2015; 205(6):W619–W629

[172] Holle JU, Gross WL, Holl-Ulrich K, et al. Prospective long-term follow-up of patients with localised Wegener's granulomatosis: does it occur as persistent disease stage? Ann Rheum Dis. 2010; 69(11):1934–1939

[173] Tarabishy AB, Schulte M, Papaliodis GN, Hoffman GS. Wegener's granulomatosis: clinical manifestations, differential diagnosis, and management of ocular and systemic disease. Surv Ophthalmol. 2010; 55(5):429–444

[174] Lohrmann C, Uhl M, Warnatz K, Kotter E, Ghanem N, Langer M. Sinonasal computed tomography in patients with Wegener's granulomatosis. J Comput Assist Tomogr. 2006; 30(1):122–125

[175] Lloyd G, Lund VJ, Beale T, Howard D. Rhinologic changes in Wegener's granulomatosis. J Laryngol Otol. 2002; 116(7):565–569

[176] Schmidt J, Pulido JS, Matteson EL. Ocular manifestations of systemic disease: antineutrophil cytoplasmic antibody-associated vasculitis. Curr Opin Ophthalmol. 2011; 22(6):489–495

[177] Montecucco C, Caporali R, Pacchetti C, Turla M. Is Tolosa-Hunt syndrome a limited form of Wegener's granulomatosis? Report of two cases with anti-neutrophil cytoplasmic antibodies. Br J Rheumatol. 1993; 32(7):640–641

[178] Talar-Williams C, Sneller MC, Langford CA, Smith JA, Cox TA, Robinson MR. Orbital socket contracture: a complication of inflammatory orbital disease in patients with Wegener's granulomatosis. Br J Ophthalmol. 2005; 89(4): 493–497

[179] Nishino H, Rubino FA, DeRemee RA, Swanson JW, Parisi JE. Neurological involvement in Wegener's granulomatosis: an analysis of 324 consecutive patients at the Mayo Clinic. Ann Neurol. 1993; 33(1):4–9

[180] Foster WP, Greene JS, Millman B. Wegener's granulomatosis presenting as ophthalmoplegia and optic neuropathy. Otolaryngol Head Neck Surg. 1995; 112(6):758–762

[181] Murphy JM, Gomez-Anson B, Gillard JH, et al. Wegener granulomatosis: MR imaging findings in brain and meninges. Radiology. 1999; 213(3):794–799

[182] Finkielman JD, Lee AS, Hummel AM, et al. WGET Research Group. ANCA are detectable in nearly all patients with active severe Wegener's granulomatosis. Am J Med. 2007; 120(7):643.e9–643.e14

[183] Knopf A, Chaker A, Stark T, et al. Clinical aspects of granulomatosis with polyangiitis affecting the head and neck. Eur Arch Otorhinolaryngol. 2015; 272 (1):185–193

[184] Malm I-J, Mener DJ, Kim J, Seo P, Kim YJ. Otolaryngological progression of granulomatosis with polyangiitis after systemic treatment with rituximab. Otolaryngol Head Neck Surg. 2014; 150(1):68–72

[185] Charles P, Néel A, Tieulié N, et al. French Vasculitis Study Group. Rituximab for induction and maintenance treatment of ANCA-associated vasculitides: a multicentre retrospective study on 80 patients. Rheumatology (Oxford). 2014; 53(3):532–539

# 2 Sellar, Parasellar, and Clival Region

*Amy W. Lin, Walter Kucharczyk, Ehab Y. Hanna, Brian O'Sullivan, and Eugene Yu*

## 2.1 Embryological Development

The central skull base primarily develops from cartilage precursors, except for the most lateral portions of the greater wings of the sphenoid bone. Conversion of the mesenchyme into cartilage at the skull base begins around the 40th day of gestation. The various foramina of the skull base are present within this cartilaginous formation because the primitive nerves develop prior to chondrification and the cartilage develops around them.

During the 5th week of gestation, the notochord passes into the basiocciput from the upper cervical vertebral bodies. It then passes obliquely through the basiocciput, exiting ventrally to come in contact with the primitive pharynx, and then back into the basisphenoid and terminates just caudal to the pituitary fossa at the dural margin.[1] Chordomas and ecchordosis physaliphora are thought to arise from notochord remnants.

The Rathke's pouch, which gives rise to the anterior pituitary, arises from an invagination of the oral ectoderm from the roof of the stomodeum. It passes through the basal mesoderm just cephalad to the tip of the notochord to meet the precursor of the posterior pituitary, which forms from a diverticulum of the diencephalon.[2] This tract is usually obliterated by later ossification, but can rarely persist postnatally (termed the craniopharyngeal canal) and contain ectopic anterior pituitary tissue.[3]

The body of the sphenoid bone is formed from fusion of the two lateral hypophyseal cartilages containing and surrounding the developing pituitary gland. More rostrally, the paired presphenoid cartilages fuse to become the most anterior portion of the sphenoid bone. Laterally, there is fusion between precursors of the lesser (orbitosphenoid) and the greater (alisphenoid) wings.[1,2]

As ossification progresses, most of the cartilage is obliterated. However, remaining cartilage can be found in various synchondroses and persists into adult life, most commonly in the foramen lacerum and petroclival junction. Skull base chondrosarcomas are thought to mostly arise from remnants of embryonal cartilage.

## 2.2 Basic Anatomy Overview

Most of the central skull base is formed by the sphenoid bone. It is a structurally complex butterfly-shaped bone consisting of a central body (containing the sella turcica above and the sphenoid sinus below), two pairs of lateral extensions (greater and lesser wings), and one pair of inferior extensions (pterygoid processes; ▶ Fig. 2.1).

The sella turcica contains the pituitary gland and is a saddle-like bony formation on the upper surface of the sphenoid body (▶ Fig. 2.2). It is bounded anteriorly by the tuberculum sellae and posteriorly by the dorsum sellae. Anterior to the tuberculum sellae is the prechiasmatic sulcus and the planum sphenoidale. The sella turcica is surrounded by four bony projections, the anterior and posterior clinoid processes. The dorsum sellae is contiguous posteroinferiorly with the clivus through the spheno-occipital synchondrosis.

The sphenoid bone contains a number of important neurovascular canals (▶ Fig. 2.3). The superior orbital fissure is located between the greater and lesser wings, and transmits the superior ophthalmic vein and cranial nerves III, IV, VI, and V1. The optic canal is located above and is separated from the superior orbital fissure by the optic strut, and transmits the optic nerve and the ophthalmic artery. Other foramina near the junction between the sphenoid body and greater wing

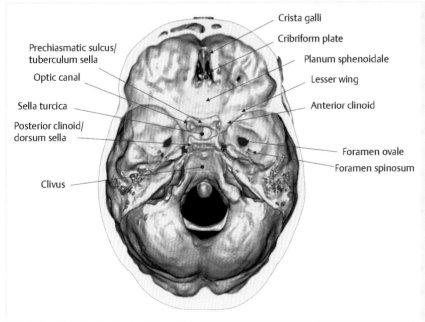

**Fig. 2.1** Bony anatomy of the skull base. The central skull base is shaded in yellow.

Crista galli
Cribriform plate
Planum sphenoidale
Lesser wing
Anterior clinoid
Foramen ovale
Foramen spinosum

Prechiasmatic sulcus/tuberculum sella
Optic canal
Sella turcica
Posterior clinoid/dorsum sella
Clivus

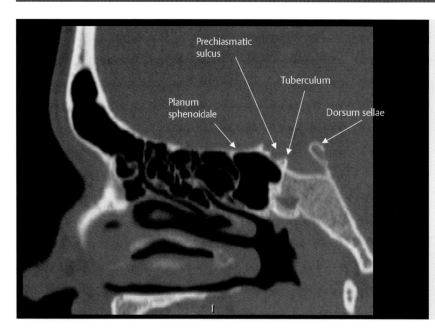

**Fig. 2.2** Sagittal midline anatomy.

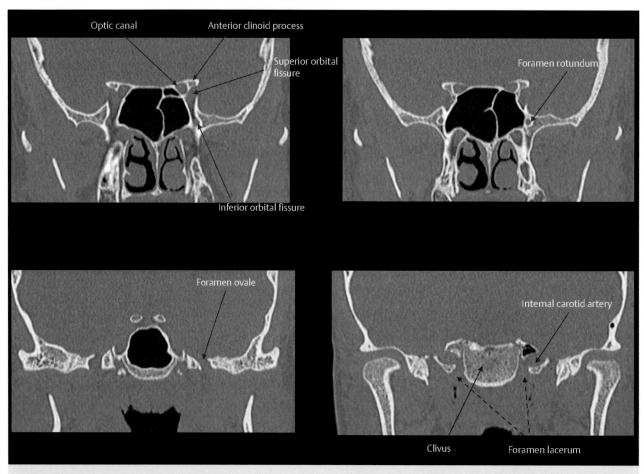

**Fig. 2.3** Coronal sections from anterior to posterior.

**Table 2.1** Sphenoid anatomy important for transsphenoidal surgery

Pneumatization pattern of the sphenoid sinus (sellar, presellar, conchal)

Lateral pneumatization for transpterygoid approaches

Presence of Onodi cell

Position of the intersphenoid septum relative to the internal carotid artery or optic nerve

Dehiscence of the bony covering around the internal carotid artery or optic nerve

Vascular variants (such as aberrant ICA or persistent trigeminal artery) and aneurysms

Presence of paranasal sinus inflammatory disease

Abbreviation: ICA, internal carotid artery.

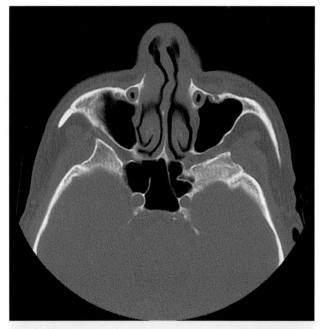

**Fig. 2.4** Sphenoid sinus septations attaching to the carotid artery canal. Care should be taken when surgically removing these septations to avoid carotid artery injury.

include the vidian/pterygoid canal (vidian artery and nerve), foramen rotundum (CN V2), foramen ovale (CN V3), and foramen spinosum (middle meningeal artery).

The sphenoid sinus is a variably pneumatized posterior extension of the paranasal sinuses. It is bordered by the ethmoid air cells anteriorly, clivus posteriorly, cavernous sinuses and cavernous internal carotid arteries laterally, sellae turcica and planum sphenoidale superiorly, and the nasopharynx inferiorly. There are several anatomic features related to the sphenoid that are important to assess when planning for surgery (▶ Table 2.1).

The sphenoid sinus is divided by complete and incomplete bony septations in various orientations. These septations may attach to the carotid canal, which is important because care must be taken to avoid carotid artery injury when removing these septations (▶ Fig. 2.4). It is also important to recognize the presence of any bony dehiscence of the carotid, as it protrudes centrally into the sphenoid (▶ Fig. 2.5). This would make the vessel more vulnerable to injury.

The Onodi cell is a posterior ethmoidal cell that pneumatizes and extends posterior and superior to the sphenoid sinus (▶ Fig. 2.6). This air cell is present in approximately 10% of the Western population. On coronal computed tomography (CT), a clue to the presence of the Onodi cell is visualization of a horizontal or cruciform septation, which represents the wall between the Onodi air cell superiorly and the sphenoid sinus inferiorly. As a result of its location, the optic nerve and/or the internal carotid artery (ICA) may be encompassed by it and be vulnerable to injury during surgery. The surgeon may also become disoriented with regard to the usual anatomy if this is not recognized.

Pneumatization of the sphenoid sinus is highly variable and can extend as far as the clivus and foramen magnum inferiorly, and the sphenoid wings laterally. The traditional classification by Hamberger et al[4] and Hammer and Radberg[5] describes three types of sphenoid pneumatization according to the proximity of the aerated cavity to the sellar floor: sellar (80%), presellar (17%), and conchal (3%) (▶ Fig. 2.7).[6] In the sellar type, the sphenoid sinus is pneumatized anterior and inferior to the sellar prominence. In the presellar type, the pneumatization is localized to the anterior sphenoid body and does not extend beyond the anterior sellar wall. A conchal sphenoid sinus has minimal to absent pneumatization. The sellar configuration is most favorable for transsphenoid surgery, whereas the conchal configuration is the most challenging anatomically. Lateral pneumatization into the sphenoid wing is most favorable for transpterygoid endoscopic approaches to the middle skull base.

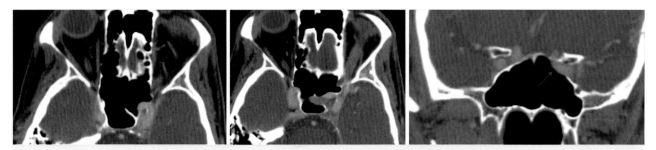

**Fig. 2.5** The left cavernous internal carotid artery is torturous with a dehiscent bony carotid canal (*arrow*), which makes it more vulnerable to injury during surgery.

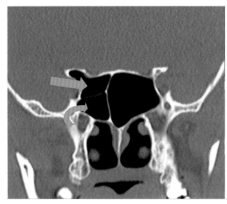
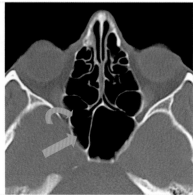

**Fig. 2.6** The Onodi cell (*arrow*) is a posterior ethmoid cell that pneumatizes posterior and superior to the sphenoid sinus (*curved arrow*). Note the presence of a horizontal septation which separates the Onodi cell superiorly and the sphenoid sinus inferiorly.

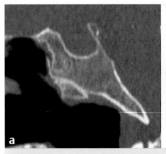
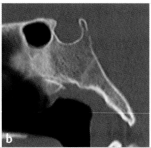
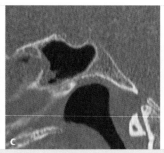
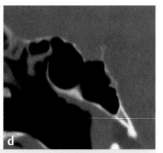

**Fig. 2.7** Variable pneumatization of the sphenoid sinus. In the conchal type (**a**), pneumatization does not extend into the sphenoid body. In the presellar type (**b**), pneumatization reaches but does not extend beyond the anterior sellar wall. In the sellar type (**c,d**), pneumatization extends posteriorly below the sella (incomplete sellar type, **c**), or all the way to the clival margin (complete sellar type, **d**). The sellar configuration is most favorable for transsphenoid surgery.

# 2.3 Tumors and Tumor-Like Conditions

One of the important roles of imaging in the evaluation of skull base neoplasia is to map the full extent of the disease. This is important in staging, which in turn will influence treatment approach and prognosis. Some imaging features important for surgical planning for central skull base tumors are listed in ► Table 2.2. Documentation of the presence of some of these may severely limit or preclude the complete surgical excision of disease.

## 2.3.1 Pituitary Adenoma

Pituitary adenomas are among the most common of all central nervous system (CNS) neoplasms. They are adenohypophysial tumors composed of secretory cells that produce pituitary hormones. The World Health Organization (WHO) classifies pituitary tumors as typical adenomas, atypical adenomas, and pituitary carcinomas. Pituitary adenomas are benign lesions, but both typical and atypical adenomas may have extensive invasion of the surrounding structures. Pituitary carcinomas are exceptionally rare and, by definition, have craniospinal dissemination or systematic metastases, although not all of them display classic cytological features of malignancy.[7]

Microadenomas are defined as those lesions 10 mm or less in diameter (► Fig. 2.8), whereas macroadenomas refer to those greater than 10 mm (► Fig. 2.9, ► Fig. 2.10, ► Fig. 2.11,

► Fig. 2.12). Most pituitary adenomas occur in adults (peak age of presentation between the fourth and seventh decades) and are sporadic. Approximately 5% of pituitary adenomas are familial and occur in patients with multiple endocrine neoplasia (MEN) type 1, Carney complex, McCune-Albright syndrome, and familial isolated pituitary adenoma syndrome.

Approximately 75% of pituitary adenomas are hormone secreting, and 25% are nonfunctional.[8] The clinical presentation of pituitary adenomas depends on the size of the lesion, hormonal activity, and the degree of extrasellar extension. Depending on the hormones being secreted, patients may present with amenorrhea, galactorrhea, hypogonadism, acromegaly, gigantism, Cushing's disease, or hyperthyroidism. Nonfunctional adenomas generally present due to mass effect, most commonly headache and visual disturbances. Rarely, a pituitary adenoma may present acutely with pituitary apoplexy due to intratumoral hemorrhage.

Prolactinoma is the most common type of pituitary adenoma in clinical series, making up about 50% of patients presenting with endocrine disturbance. However, elevated prolactin levels are not always due to a hormonally active adenoma. Any process that interferes with the production, release, or pituitary portal venous transport of prolactin-inhibiting factors from the hypothalamus can result in hyperprolactinemia because of the resulting disinhibition of normal prolactin cells. Nevertheless, serum prolactin levels greater than 150 ng/mL (normal is < 20 ng/mL) are almost always due to a prolactinoma. This is less certain in patients with elevated serum prolactin less than 150 ng/mL.[9]

**Table 2.2** Key imaging findings for surgical planning

1. Defining the epicenter and extent of tumor
   a) Intrasellar
   b) Suprasellar
   c) Clival

2. Displacement of the pituitary gland, infundibulum, and optic apparatus by tumor should be noted, as should the location of the diaphragma sellae

3. Describing the relationship to
   a) Internal carotid artery
   b) Optic nerve
   c) Optic chiasm
   d) Cavernous sinus

4. Extent of lateral extension into the orbit, including status of
   a) Lamina papyracea
   b) Periorbita
   c) Orbital fat
   d) Orbital muscles
   e) Orbital apex

5. Extent of intracranial extension
   a) Bony skull base erosion
   b) Dural involvement
   c) Intradural extension
   d) Relationship to ventricular system

6. Degree of lateral extension into skull base
   a) Pterygopalatine fossa
   b) Infratemporal fossa
   c) Pterygoid plates
   d) Petrous apex
   e) Foramen magnum
   f) Occipital condyle
   g) Hypoglossal canal

7. Presence and extent of perineural spread
   a) Vidian
   b) V1, 2, 3
   c) Superior and inferior orbital fissures

Clinically nonfunctional pituitary adenomas typically arise from gonadotroph cells. These cells make the alpha and beta subunits of the gonadotrophin hormones but not the intact molecule, and hence these lesions are not biologically active.

## Imaging

Dedicated magnetic resonance imaging (MRI) of the sella is the imaging modality of choice for assessing suspected pituitary abnormality. Although most adenomas are visible without intravenous contrast, several studies have shown improved visibility of small lesions with gadolinium.[10,11,12,13,14,15,16] Furthermore, dynamic contrast-enhanced MRI of the sella can be done to further increase detection sensitivity, taking advantage of the differential rates of contrast enhancement between adenomas and normal pituitary gland (▶ Fig. 2.13).[17,18,19,20] This increased sensitivity is most helpful in the detection and localization of adrenocorticotropic hormone (ACTH)-secreting adenomas in Cushing's disease because these tumors tend to be small. Accurate documentation of the presence and position of these adenomas is important because surgical removal is the most effective treatment.

A sellar or combined sellar and suprasellar mass that cannot be identified separately from the pituitary gland is the most characteristic imaging finding. An enlarged and remodeled sella turcia is commonly seen with macroadenomas. Inflammatory disorders (such as hypophysitis or sarcoidosis) can sometimes cause enlargement of the pituitary gland, which is often associated with enhancement of the adjacent meninges (a finding that is rare in adenomas).

Most pituitary adenomas are hypointense on T1-weighted images (T1WIs) and iso- to hyperintense on T2-weighted images (T2WIs) relative to normal pituitary tissue (▶ Fig. 2.8). Hemorrhagic and cystic areas may be present within the lesion.

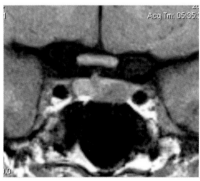
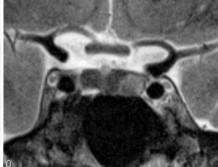

**Fig. 2.8** Pituitary microadenoma. Most pituitary adenomas are hypointense on T1-weighted images and iso- to hyperintense on T2-weighted images relative to normal pituitary tissue.

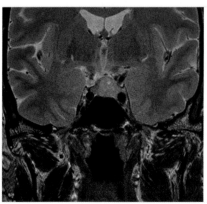
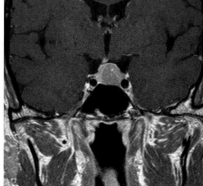

**Fig. 2.9** Pituitary macroadenoma. Cavernous sinus invasion is possible in this Knosp grade 2 lesion, which extends to the median intercarotid line on the left side. The normal pituitary gland is displaced to the right.

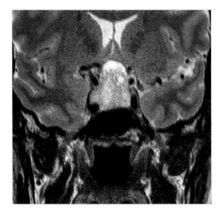
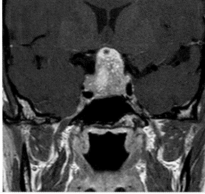

Fig. 2.10 Pituitary macroadenoma. Cavernous sinus invasion is likely in this Knosp grade 3 lesion, which extends beyond the lateral intercarotid line on the right side. The optic chiasm is elevated and compressed by the mass.

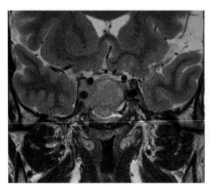
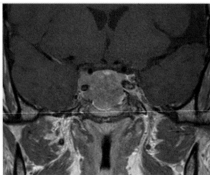

Fig. 2.11 Pituitary macroadenoma. The lesion completely encases the right cavernous internal carotid artery (Knosp grade 4) and invades the right cavernous sinus.

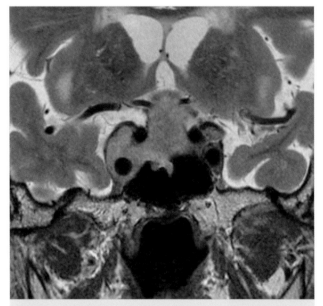

Fig. 2.12 Large pituitary macroadenoma with right cavernous sinus invasion, completely encasing the right cavernous internal carotid artery (Knosp grade 4). The lesion compresses and elevates the optic chiasm.

During dynamic imaging, pituitary adenomas tend to show slower enhancement than the rest of the gland.

No imaging feature definitively distinguishes between the various types of pituitary adenomas, although certain findings are more commonly seen with some. ACTH-secreting microadenomas are generally the smallest (mean size: 3 mm). Hormonally active adenomas have a certain topographic predilection within the gland that parallels the distribution of the normal secretory cells. Therefore, prolactin and growth hormone (GH) microadenomas tend to be lateral, whereas ACTH, thyroid-stimulating hormone (TSH), luteinizing hormone (LH), and follicle-stimulating hormone (FSH) microadenomas tend to be central in location. GH-secreting adenomas tend to show infrasellar rather than suprasellar extension. GH-secreting adenomas are also more commonly T2 hypointense, a finding predictive of a densely granulated appearance on histopathology (▶ Fig. 2.14).[21]

Lateral extension of the adenoma into the cavernous sinus impacts the surgeon's ability to completely resect the tumor. However, differentiation between compression and invasion of the cavernous sinus on MRI is not always easy because the medial wall is very thin. Various parameters have been described in an effort to predict cavernous sinus invasion. The Knosp-Steiner grade of parasellar extension is based on the

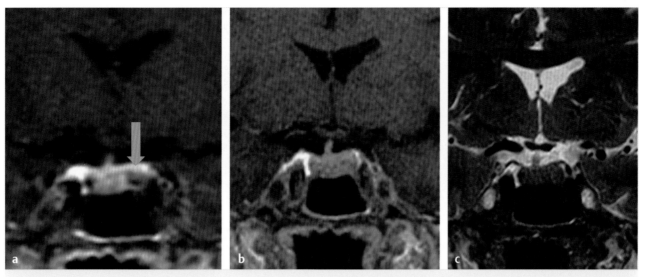

**Fig. 2.13** This pituitary microadenoma (*arrow*) is well seen on early dynamic contrast-enhanced image (**a**), but is difficult to appreciate on delayed contrast-enhanced (**b**) or T2-weighted images (**c**).

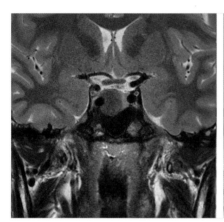
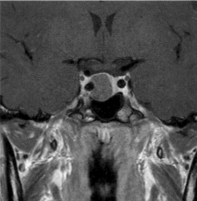

**Fig. 2.14** Growth hormone (GH)-secreting pituitary adenoma. Note this lesion is hypointense on T2-weighted images, which is a finding seen more commonly in GH-secreting adenomas, particularly those that are densely granulated.

relationship between the tumor and tangential lines drawn between the cavernous and supraclinoid internal carotid arteries on coronal MR images (▶ Fig. 2.15).[22] Knosp grades 3 and 4 (tumor extending beyond the lateral intercarotid line or totally encasing the cavernous carotid artery) are highly predictive of cavernous sinus invasion (▶ Fig. 2.10, ▶ Fig. 2.11, ▶ Fig. 2.12). Knosp grade 0 and 1 lesions do not invade the cavernous sinus. Knosp grade 2 lesions sometimes show invasion (▶ Fig. 2.9).

## Treatment

The initial treatment of pituitary adenomas varies depending on tumor type and configuration. Adenomas that produce prolactin, GH, ACTH, or TSH can be treated with different medications initially or after surgery. Dopamine agonists have become the initial treatment for most patients with prolactinoma. Surgery is usually the first-line treatment option for GH and ACTH-producing adenomas and nonfunctioning adenomas.[7]

Different surgical options include transcranial, microsurgical, transsphenoidal, or pure endoscopic procedures. In recent years, the transsphenoid route has become the standard approach for most intrasellar and some suprasellar tumors because of lower morbidity and mortality rates when compared with transcranial procedures.

Radiation is usually considered when initial treatment fails, when surgical excision is incomplete, or when there is tumor recurrence. The two major types of radiation therapy are stereotactic radiosurgery and fractionated radiation therapy. Stereotactic radiosurgery can be delivered as a single treatment and has the advantage of reduced radiation exposure to the brain, and is well suited for smaller adenomas less than 30 mm that do not abut the optic structures or infiltrate into the surrounding structures. Larger adenomas are more safely treated with fractionated radiation due to the mitigating effect of using smaller doses per fraction in damaging late responding normal tissues such as brain and optic nerves.[23]

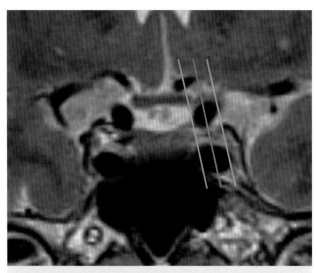

**Fig. 2.15** Knosp grading of parasellar extension, based on the relationship of the pituitary tumor and tangential lines drawn between the cavernous supraclinoid internal carotid arteries on coronal MRI images. *Blue line:* medial intercarotid line connecting the medial walls of the internal carotid arteries (ICAs). *Orange line:* median intercarotid line connecting the centers of the ICAs. *Green line:* lateral intercarotid line connecting the lateral walls of the ICAs. Knosp grade 0 (tumor medial to the medial line) and grade 1 (tumor reaching the median line but not extending beyond it) are unlikely to have cavernous sinus invasion. Knosp grade 2 (tumor extending between the median and the lateral line) lesions sometimes have cavernous sinus invasion. Knosp grades 3 and 4 (tumor extending beyond the lateral intercarotid line or totally encasing the cavernous carotid artery) are highly predictive of cavernous sinus invasion.

---

### Pituitary adenoma

Characteristic imaging features:
- Sellar or combined sellar and suprasellar mass that cannot be identified separately from the pituitary gland.
- Remodeling/enlargement of the sella turcica for macroadenomas.

Important imaging findings for treatment planning:
- Relationship to optic chiasm and optic nerves.
- Cavernous sinus extension.
- Internal carotid artery encasement.
- Effect on adjacent brain.
- Bony skull base invasion.

## 2.3.2 Craniopharyngioma

Craniopharyngiomas are rare and mostly benign tumors that arise from epithelial remnants of Rathke's pouch that occur exclusively in the region of the sella turcica and suprasellar cistern or in the third ventricle. There is a bimodal age distribution, with more than half occurring in children between 5 and 14 years of age, and a second smaller peak in adults between 50 and 75 years of age.[24]

Craniopharyngiomas primarily occur in the suprasellar cistern. Infrequently, the lesions may be completely intrasellar or located in the third ventricle. Secondary to their anatomic location, craniopharyngiomas may present with endocrine dysfunction (in 80–90%), visual disturbance, and signs of increased intracranial pressure.

Two histological subtypes exist—adamantinomatous (more common) and papillary (less common, usually in adults). In addition to being histologically disparate, the two subtypes have different molecular genetics and characteristic imaging features.

### Imaging

### Adamantinomatous craniopharyngioma

Adamantinomatous craniopharyngiomas are the more frequently encountered subtype, especially in the pediatric population. A partially calcified, mixed solid and cystic suprasellar lesion is the classic appearance (▶ Fig. 2.16). Approximately 90% contain calcification. Signal on MR varies with cyst content, and cyst signal can range from hypointense to hyperintense compared to brain on T1WI and T2WI.

T2 hyperintensity along the optic tracts is a common finding and usually represents edema rather than tumor invasion (▶ Fig. 2.17). This finding, rather than optic nerve signal abnormality, may suggest a craniopharyngioma over other parasellar lesions,[25] although it has reported in many other pathologies.[26,27]

Although craniopharyngiomas are grossly well circumscribed, microscopically the borders are frequently irregular and may be associated with gliosis in the adjacent brain tissue, which may be easily mistaken for glioma if biopsied.[28] This reactive gliosis also results in an indistinct and adherent interface between the craniopharyngioma and adjacent brain, often making identification and manipulation of surgical planes difficult.

### Papillary craniopharyngioma

Papillary craniopharyngiomas are usually found in adult patients. In distinction from their adamantinomatous counterpart, they are typically solid, without calcification, and are often found within the third ventricle (▶ Fig. 2.18). They have a nonspecific signal intensity pattern of a solid enhancing tumor. They are usually encapsulated and are readily separable from nearby structures, so recurrence rates are generally thought to be much less than within the adamantinomatous type.

### Treatment

Surgical resection is the primary treatment for craniopharyngiomas. For several decades, transcranial approaches have been used widely and successfully. In recent years, the evolution of endoscopic endonasal surgery has opened new surgical alternatives, with several authors showing safety and effectiveness of this approach, with arguably better surgical advantages and superior outcomes.[29]

Radiation therapy is indicated in patients with residual disease who have undergone a partial surgical resection or to treat disease that has recurred following initial gross total resection. It may also be used in patients who are not surgical candidates.

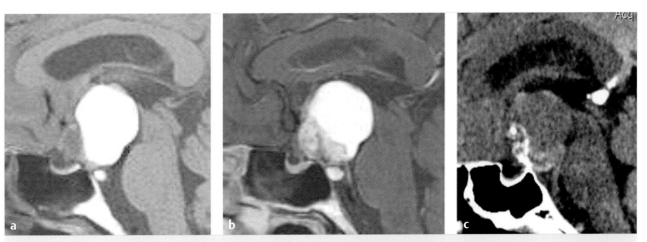

**Fig. 2.16** Adamantinomatous craniopharyngioma showing markedly heterogeneous composition, including a large cystic component containing intrinsically T1-hyperintense proteinatious material (**a,b**). (**b**) Enhancement of the solid component of the mass. (**c**) CT shows calcifications within the lesion.

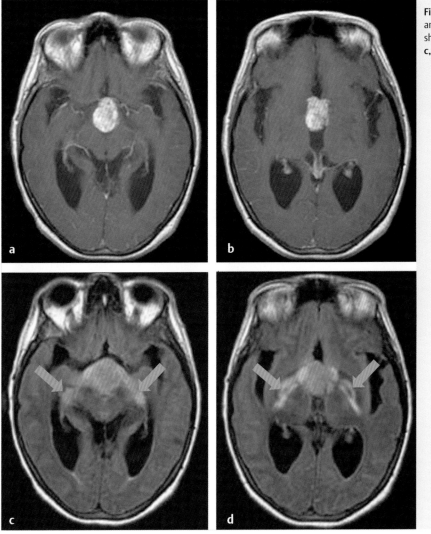

**Fig. 2.17** Axial postgadolinium T1-weighted (**a,b**) and FLAIR (**c,d**) images of a craniopharyngioma showing edema along the optic tracts (*arrows*; **c,d**).

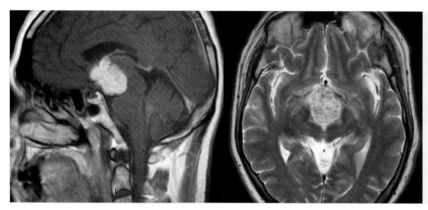

**Fig. 2.18** Papillary craniopharyngioma in a 58-year-old man. Large solid-enhancing mass centered in the suprasellar/hypothalamus region.

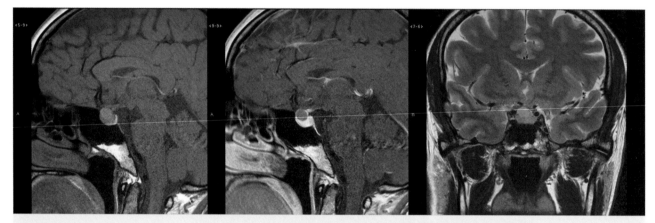

**Fig. 2.19** Rathke's cleft cyst. Cystic suprasellar mass with mild intrinsic T1 hyperintensity and mild peripheral enhancement.

Excellent long-term tumor control has been reported in radiotherapy series.

---

**Craniopharyngioma**

Characteristic imaging features:
- Multilobulated complex mass with cystic and solid components, usually centered in the suprasellar region.
- The adamantinomatous subtype is more common, especially in children.
- The papillary subtype is less common and is usually seen in adults, and is characteristically solid.
- T2 hyperintensity along the optic tracts is suggestive.
- Can be adherent to adjacent brain, which can show signal alteration due to secondary gliosis.

Important imaging findings for treatment planning:
- Relationship to the optic apparatus and adjacent arteries.
- Effect on adjacent brain.

---

## 2.3.3 Rathke's Cleft Cyst

Rathke's cleft cysts are thought to arise from remnants of the fetal Rathke's pouch. They are a common incidental finding at autopsy (about 11% in nonselected specimens).[30] They are predominantly intrasellar in location. Others may be centered in the suprasellar cistern, usually midline and just anterior to the pituitary stalk. Most Rathke's cleft cysts are small and asymptomatic, but symptoms can occur if it is large enough to compress the pituitary gland or optic chiasm, or in rare instances of hemorrhage. Most Rathke's cleft cysts remain stable or grow slowly over time.

### Imaging

Rathke's cleft cysts appear as a well-defined round or ovoid mass within or just above the sella turcica (▶ Fig. 2.19). The internal content varies from hypointense to hyperintense on T1WI, and is usually hyperintense on T2WI and fluid attenuation inversion recovery (FLAIR). An intracystic nodule can be present, which usually consists of mucin clump and is T1 hyperintense.[31,32] Calcification is uncommon. They do not typically enhance, although occasional thin marginal enhancement of the cyst wall has been observed.

### Treatment

No treatment is necessary for asymptomatic Rathke's cleft cysts. Partial resection or aspiration is usually sufficient for symptomatic lesions, usually via transsphenoidal surgery. Recurrence rates after surgery range between 16 and 18% in large series, with higher rates associated with suprasellar location, inflammation and reactive squamous metaplasia in the cyst wall, superinfection of the cyst, and placement of a fat graft into the cyst cavity.[33]

**Rathke's cleft cyst**

Characteristic imaging features:
- Well-defined round mass within or just above the sella turcica.
- T1 hyperintense intracystic nodule can be present and is suggestive.
- Lack of calcification may help distinguish from craniopharyngioma.

## 2.3.4 Meningioma

Approximately 10% of meningiomas occur in the parasellar region,[34] arising from a variety of locations including the tuberculum sellae, clinoid processes, medial sphenoid wing, and cavernous sinus. Meningiomas can also extend into the parasellar region from other sites, such as a planum sphenoidale meningioma extending posteriorly into the suprasellar cistern or sella turcica.

Meningiomas occur most frequently in the sixth decade of life and have a female predilection. Most are sporadic. Patients with neurofibromatosis type 2 and prior cranial radiation have an increased incidence. Meningiomas are usually slow-growing lesions that may be found incidentally or present because of compression, or less commonly invasion, of adjacent structures.

Most meningiomas are histologically typical (WHO grade 1), but about 4 to 8% are classified histologically as atypical menin-

giomas (WHO grade 2) and 1 to 3% are classified as malignant meningiomas (WHO grade 3).[35] The skull base is a relatively rare location for these more aggressive subtypes. In general, it can be difficult to determine the tumor grade based on imaging. Atypical and malignant meningiomas can have indistinct borders with the adjacent parenchymal cortex, and peritumoral edema is a common but nonspecific finding.

### Imaging

Most meningiomas are hyperdense compared to brain parenchyma on CT (▶ Fig. 2.20), and about 25% show calcification. On MR, they are usually hypointense to isointense relative to gray matter on T1WI, and isointense to moderately hyperintense on T2WI. Virtually all meningiomas enhance, usually strongly and homogenously. A dural tail is seen in the majority of meningiomas (▶ Fig. 2.21). Hyperostosis in the adjacent bone, best appreciated on CT, can be present and is a characteristic feature (▶ Fig. 2.20, ▶ Fig. 2.22). Necrosis, cyst, hemorrhage, or fat can be seen within meningiomas but are infrequently seen. Peritumoral cyst and edema within the adjacent brain are sometimes present (▶ Fig. 2.20).

Vascular encasement is not uncommon, particularly for tumors in the cavernous sinus. Meningiomas characteristically constrict the lumen of the encased vessel (▶ Fig. 2.23), in contrast with pituitary adenoma for which this is rare. However, luminal narrowing can be seen in other entities such as

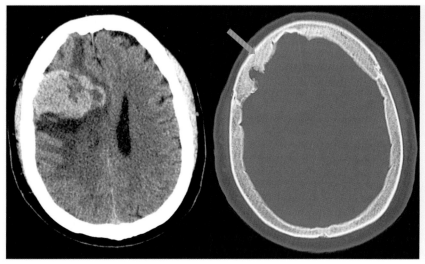

**Fig. 2.20** Meningiomas tend to be hyperintense relative to brain on CT. Hyperostosis in the adjacent bone (*arrow*) is another characteristic feature.

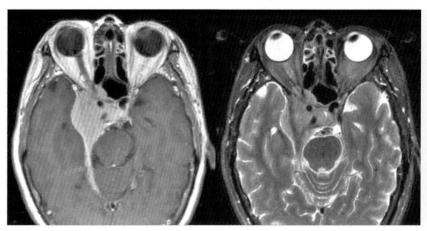

**Fig. 2.21** Meningioma centered in the right parasellar region extending into the right orbital apex and encasing the right internal carotid artery. Note the dural tail (*arrow*) and relatively low T2 signal.

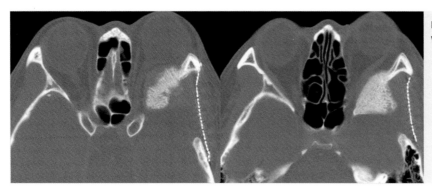

**Fig. 2.22** Meningioma along the lateral orbital wall with bone expansion and hyperostosis.

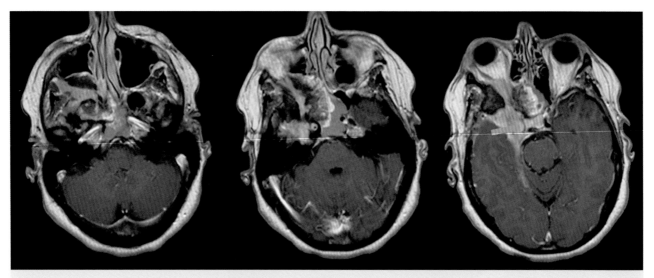

**Fig. 2.23** Extensive skull base meningioma involving the right middle cranial fossa and parasellar region, extending through multiple skull base foramen (superior orbital fissure, inferior orbital fissure, foramen rotundum), with tumor in the right orbital apex and retroantral space. The cavernous portion of the right internal carotid artery is encased by the tumor and markedly narrowed (*arrow*).

metastasis, chordoma, lymphoma, or Tolosa-Hunt. Some imaging features that are suggestive of atypical (WHO grade 2) and malignant (WHO grade 3) meningiomas include indistinct borders of the mass with the adjacent cortex, bony infiltration, and more pronounced peritumoral edema (▸ Fig. 2.24). WHO grade 2 and 3 meningiomas will also tend to show a greater degree of restricted diffusion which reflects their greater cellularity.

## Treatment

Elderly patients with small asymptomatic meningiomas may be observed and treatment initiated if and when there is progression. Surgery is most likely to achieve cure; however, the likelihood of accomplishing a complete resection is related to the location and extent of the tumor. Skull base meningiomas are particularly challenging because they often cannot be completely resected, and there may be significant surgical morbidity due to the complex anatomy with many nearby critical neural and vascular structures (▸ Fig. 2.25, ▸ Fig. 2.26). Radiotherapy and radiosurgery are alternative treatment methods with similar long-term local control and survival rates compared to surgery.[36] Radiation can be used primarily or adjunctive when resection is incomplete. In general, radiosurgery is

indicated if the lesion is small enough to be encompassed in the field, whereas larger, irregular tumors are treated with fractionated radiotherapy.

### Meningioma

Characteristic imaging features:
- Dural-based enhancing mass may contain calcification.
- Tends to narrow vessel when there is encasement.
- Atypical and malignant meningiomas are rare in the skull base. They tend to have an indistinct border with the adjacent cortex and peritumoral edema is more commonly seen.

Important imaging findings for treatment planning:
- Relationship with the optic apparatus, extension into the optic canal and orbital apex.
- Relationship with the adjacent arteries (displacement, encasement, and luminal narrowing).
- Relationship with cranial nerves and skull base foramina.
- Relationship with the pituitary gland and stalk.
- Relationship with the cavernous sinuses.
- Effect on adjacent brain.

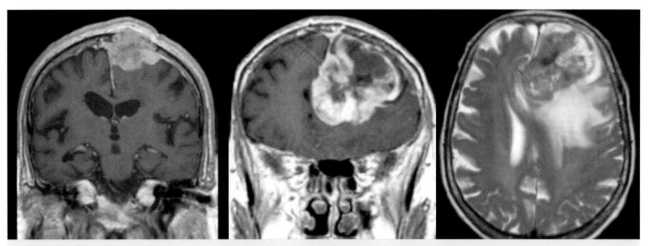

**Fig. 2.24** Atypical/malignant meningiomas are more likely to show bone erosion, are more commonly heterogeneous in signal and enhancement, and frequently show peritumoral edema, although these findings are nonspecific. These images are from different patients.

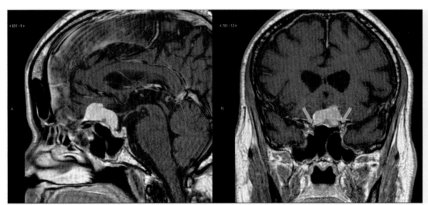

**Fig. 2.25** Meningioma centered in the planum sphenoidale region, with extension into the bilateral optic canals (*arrows*).

## 2.3.5 Germ Cell Tumors

Intracranial germ cell tumors (GCTs) are rare neoplasms that occur in children and young adults. The prevalence is higher in Asia compared to North America and Europe. The WHO classification system divides them into two basic groups—germinoma and nongerminomatous GCTs. The more common germinomas (60–65% of all intracranial GCTs) are similar to ovarian dysgerminoma and testicular seminoma on pathology. The less common nongerminomatous GCTs include embryonal carcinoma, endodermal sinus tumor, choriocarcinoma, teratoma, and mixed tumors with more than one element. Many intracranial GCTs secrete tumor makers such as alpha-fetoprotein and beta-human chorionic gonadotropin, and immunohistochemistry can be used to detect placental alkaline phosphatase and c-Kit on tumor cells. Therefore, cerebrospinal fluid (CSF) analysis and imaging evaluation are used to establish the diagnosis.

Intracranial GCTs arise almost exclusively from midline locations. The pineal region is the most common location. About 30 to 40% occur in the suprasellar region.[37,38] Pineal germinomas have a 10:1 male-to-female ratio, whereas suprasellar germinomas have no gender predilection. Suprasellar GCTs commonly present with hypothalamic and pituitary dysfunction, most frequently diabetes insipidus (polyuria, polydipsia). They can also cause decreased visual acuity or visual field defect due to chiasmic or optic nerve compression.

Some germinomas may be multiple, with the most frequent combination being a pineal and a suprasellar mass. Whether these are metastatic or synchronous is debatable.

### Imaging

Suprasellar germinomas are typically midline, centered at or just posterior to the pituitary infundibulum, which may be thickened. The normal pituitary posterior bright spot is absent in most.[39] They are predominantly solid tumors which are usually iso- to hypointense on T1WI and iso- to hyperintense on T2WI relative to gray matter, and enhance strongly and homogeneously (▶ Fig. 2.27). Variably sized intratumoral cysts are not uncommon, particularly in larger lesions. Calcification and hemorrhage are rare in germinomas but are more common in nongerminomatous GCTs.

Some suprasellar germinomas can present with diabetes insipidus before a mass is visible on MRI. Preceding the appearance of an obvious mass, a slight swelling of the infundibulum with loss of posterior pituitary hyperintensity can be seen.

CSF dissemination is common; therefore, the entire neuroaxis should be imaged in patients with suspected germinoma.

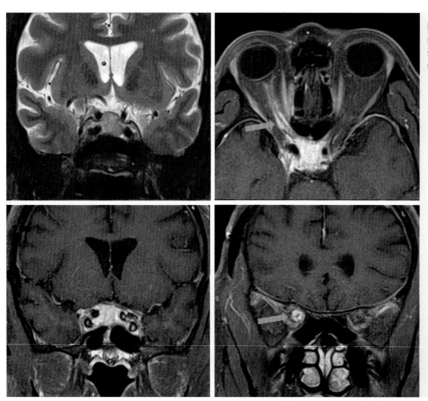

**Fig. 2.26** Sellar meningioma extending along the right optic nerve sheath (*arrow*). Optic nerve sheath extension makes this lesion surgically unresectable.

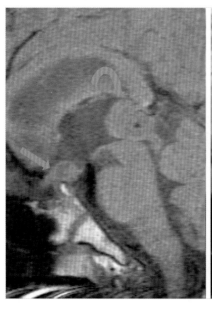 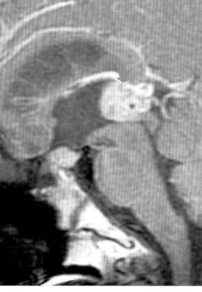

**Fig. 2.27** Synchronous germinomas in the suprasellar (*arrow*) and pineal (*curved arrow*) regions in a 10-year-old boy. Suprasellar germinomas are typically seen crawling along the floor of the third ventricle. There is homogeneous enhancement after contrast administration.

## Treatment

Surgical biopsy is done to establish a histologic diagnosis. Gross total resection at diagnosis is indicated only for patients with mature teratoma confirmed by histology and normal tumor markers. Germinomas are exquisitely sensitive to radiation therapy. Long-term, progression-free survival rate is greater than 90% with localized pure germinomas after radiation therapy. Cystic portions of the tumor tend to respond more slowly to radiation.[40]

### Germ cell tumors

Characteristic imaging features:
- Solid enhancing suprasellar mass centered at or just posterior to the pituitary infundibulum.
- Absent posterior pituitary bright spot.

Important imaging findings for treatment planning:
- Local extent.
- The presence of CSF dissemination throughout the neuroaxis.

## 2.3.6 Schwannoma

The many foramina in the central skull base transmit multiple major cranial nerves and smaller nerves. Schwannoma can arise from any of these nerves. The trigeminal nerve is most commonly involved in the central skull base and is the second most common site for intracranial schwannoma after vestibular schwannomas. They may involve any segment of the trigeminal nerve complex but mostly commonly arise from the gasserian ganglion in Meckel's cave. The usual presenting symptom is sensory impairment in one or more of the three divisions. Facial pain or weakness of the mastication muscles is less common.

Schwannomas can also arise from other cranial nerves in the cavernous sinus, particularly the oculomotor nerve.

### Imaging

The most characteristic feature of schwannomas is that they follow the course of the nerve from which they arise. They may cause expansion of the bony foramen with smooth margins, which is usually better appreciated on CT. Trigeminal schwannomas may be confined to Meckel's cave, or extend posteriorly into the prepontine cistern (giving the characteristic "dumbbell"

shape) or, less frequently, extend extracranially (▶ Fig. 2.28, ▶ Fig. 2.29).

Schwannomas are well-defined lesions that may be solid or have variable cystic or hemorrhagic components. Small lesions tend to be homogeneous, whereas larger ones are frequently heterogeneous. They are usually isointense to brain on T1WI and hyperintense on T2WI, and enhance intensely.

### Treatment

Treatment options vary. The advancement in skull base surgical techniques has greatly increased the total resection rate of these tumors with a significant decrease in morbidity.[41] Surgical approach selection depends on the anatomic extent of the tumor, and includes both transcranial and endonasal endoscopic techniques. Stereotactic radiosurgery is an effective management tool for small- to medium-sized tumors, and can be used as a primary treatment modality or for treating residual or recurrent tumor. Fractionated radiotherapy is an alternative option and commonly results in arrest of growth. Larger tumors and those with brainstem compression should not undergo primary radiosurgery due to potential swelling of the tumor. Schwannomas with cystic components tend to have poorer stereotactic radiosurgery results compared to solid ones.

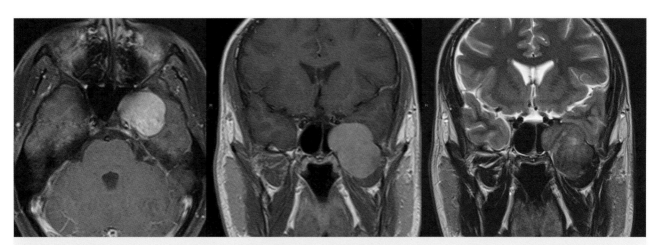

**Fig. 2.28** Trigeminal schwannoma. Large extra-axial mass extending from the left cavernous sinus region through the foramen ovale to the infratemporal fossa.

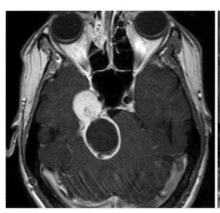
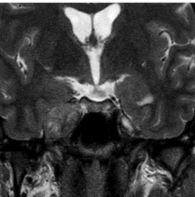

**Fig. 2.29** Partially solid, partially cystic dumbbell-shaped trigeminal schwannoma involving Meckel's cave and the prepontine cistern. The brainstem is compressed.

Characteristic imaging features:
- Well-defined enhancing mass following the course of the nerve from which they arise.
- Usually solid, but may have cystic or hemorrhagic components.
- May expand the bony foramen.

Important imaging findings for treatment planning:
- Location of the mass (intradural and extradural extension).
- Presence of cystic and hemorrhagic components.
- Brainstem compression.

## 2.3.7 Chordoma

Chordomas are rare, locally aggressive malignancies that are thought to arise from notochord remnants that have a predilection for the midline axial skeleton, with the most common sites being the sacrum, skull base, and spine. They are more common in men and have peak incidence between 50 and 60 years of age. Chordomas are slow growing and, therefore, are often clin-ically silent until the late stages of disease. Clival chordomas typically present with headaches and diplopia secondary to cranial nerve VI palsy. Larger lesions can cause multiple cranial neuropathies, endocrinopathy (due to sella involvement), visual disturbance, brainstem compression, and hydrocephalus.

Three histologic variants of chordoma are recognized: classical (conventional), chondroid, and dedifferentiated. Classical chordomas are soft, lobulated tumors that have an abundant, vacuo-lated cytoplasm described as physaliphorous (having bubbles or vacuoles).[42] Chondroid chordomas show histologic features of both chordoma and chondrosarcoma. Dedifferentiated chordomas are typically found in the sacrococcygeal region.

### Imaging

Chordomas are typically expansile, multilobulated, and well-circumscribed midline clival masses (▶ Fig. 2.30, ▶ Fig. 2.31, ▶ Fig. 2.32). They are usually very hyperintense on T2WI, reflecting high fluid content within the physaliphorous cells. CT shows a moderately hyperdense mass that sometimes contain intratumoral calcification (generally representing sequestrations from destroyed bone). Moderate to marked heterogeneous enhancement is typically seen after contrast administration.

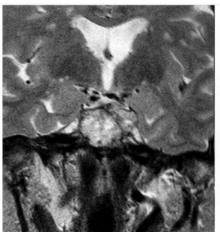
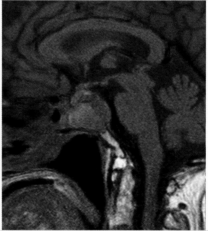
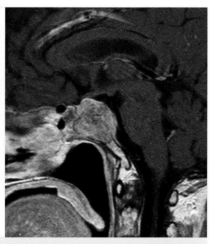

Fig. 2.30 Chordoma, seen as an expansile T2 hyperintense mass in the clivus. Note the areas of high signal on T1-weighted images representing intratumoral hemorrhage, calcification, or mucinous material.

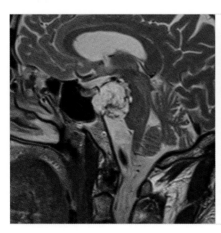
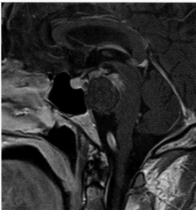

Fig. 2.31 Chordoma, seen as a multilobulated, markedly T2 hyperintense mass extending from the clivus to the prepontine cistern, indenting the brainstem. Although chordoma classically shows significant enhancement, mild enhancement can also be seen, as the tumor does centrally in the cases. More avid enhancement is seen peripherally in this tumor.

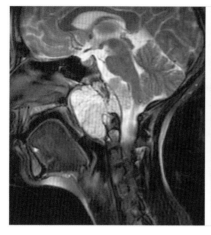 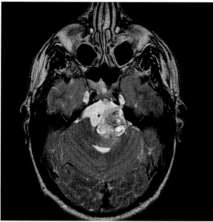

**Fig. 2.32** Large multilobulated chordoma centered in the clivus extending into the prepontine cistern and the nasopharynx. Note that the basilar artery (*arrow*) is encased by the mass.

MRI is the imaging modality of choice for delineating the full extent of the tumor and its relationship to the adjacent neurovascular structures. Vessel encasement and displacement is common (▶ Fig. 2.32), but arterial luminal narrowing is infrequent. While most chordomas stay extradural, some are more invasive and extend intradurally which is an important consideration in surgical planning for resection and reconstruction.

Clival chordomas can be difficult to differentiate from chondrosarcoma, as they have similar signal characteristics on MRI. Skull base chondrosarcomas, however, are usually located more laterally along the petrooccipital fissure and tend to show finer chondroid ("rings and arcs") calcifications on CT.

Another major differential diagnosis for clival chordoma is invasive pituitary macroadenoma. The pituitary gland can typically be identified separate from the clival chordoma, whereas the gland cannot be separated from macroadenoma.

## Treatment

The general paradigm for treatment of clival chordomas is maximally safe aggressive resection on presentation with an emphasis on neurological preservation, followed by radiation therapy.[43] Complete surgical resection is often not feasible because of anatomic constraints to surgical access and proximity to critical structures. Adjuvant radiation therapy is generally advocated for chordomas because of the poor prognosis in those who recur. It is difficult to administer adequately high doses of radiation with conventional two- or three-dimensional techniques; however, newer high-dose focused radiation delivery techniques with particles (primarily protons) or photons (stereotactic radiosurgery, stereotactic radiation therapy, and image-guided intensity-modulated radiation therapy) have allowed for administration of a higher dose to the tumor while sparing the surrounding structures.[43,44,45]

### Chordoma

Characteristic imaging features:
- Expansile, multilobulated, well-circumscribed midline clival mass.
- Markedly hyperintense on T2WI.
- May contain calcifications.
- Moderate to marked heterogeneous enhancement.
- Indents ("thumb") the anterior pons.

Important imaging findings for treatment planning:
- Relationship to adjacent neurovascular structures (basilar artery, internal carotid arteries, and cranial nerves).
- Effect on adjacent brainstem.

## 2.3.8 Epidermoid and Dermoid

Intracranial epidermoid and dermoid cysts are inclusion cysts that arise from epithelial cells that are retained during the closure of neural tube. Epidermoid cysts are lined by stratified squamous epithelium and contain keratinaceous debris and crystalline cholesterol from desquamation of the lining epithelium. Dermoid cysts contain elements of retained hair, sweat, and sebaceous glands in addition to squamous epithelium. Both of these lesions will slowly expand over time. Malignant transformation into squamous cell carcinoma has been described but is exceedingly rare.

Intracranial epidermoid cysts are usually off midline and have a predilection for the basal cisterns. The cerebellopontine angle cistern is the most common location, followed by the parasellar and middle cranial fossa (Sylvian fissure) locations. They usually present in adulthood owing to slow growth causing compression of neural or vascular structures.

Intracranial dermoid cysts are at least four times less common than epidermoid cysts and are most often midline in

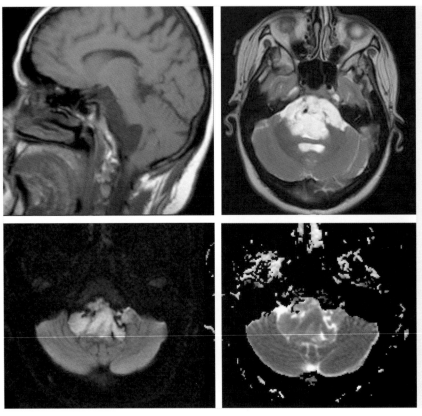

**Fig. 2.33** Large epidermoid centered in the prepontine cistern. Note the insinuating growth pattern with encasement of the basilar artery. It is hyperintense in diffusion-weighted images but has similar ADC value compared to brain parenchyma.

location. The most common site is the suprasellar cistern, followed by the posterior fossa and frontonasal region. They present at significantly younger ages (peaking in the second to third decades) compared to epidermoid cysts. They typically present with symptoms caused by local mass effect. Spontaneous rupture of dermoid cysts is rare but can be fatal.

### Imaging

Epidermoid cysts characteristically have irregular frondlike excrescences and an insinuating growth pattern, wrapping around vessels and cranial nerves in cisterns. They resemble CSF on nonenhanced CT scan, and T1WI and T2WI on MRI. Calcification (usually peripheral) can be seen in about 20%. On FLAIR imaging, they do not suppress in signal at all or will suppress incompletely. They are characteristically hyperintense on diffusion-weighted images (due to a combination of true restricted diffusion and T2 shine-through; ▶ Fig. 2.33, ▶ Fig. 2.34). Enhancement is usually absent, but mild peripheral enhancement is possible.

A "white" epidermoid is a rare type of epidermoid cyst which has high protein content and is hyperintense on T1WI and hypointense on T2WI.

Dermoid cysts appear as a well-circumscribed fat-containing mass (▶ Fig. 2.35, ▶ Fig. 2.36). Capsular calcification (▶ Fig. 2.35) is seen in about 20% of cases. The fat content shows characteristic low density on CT and hyperintensity on T1-weighted MRI. Fat suppression sequence and presence of chemical shift artifact can be seen. Lesions do not enhance centrally, although mild marginal enhancement can be present. With dermoid rupture, fat droplets can disseminate in the CSF in cisterns and ventricles,

and could cause chemical meningitis with resulting vasospasm and leptomeningeal enhancement (▶ Fig. 2.37).

### Treatment

Treatment for symptomatic epidermoid and dermoid cysts is surgical resection. The insinuating growth pattern for epidermoid cysts can make gross total resection impossible. Incompletely resected epidermoid and dermoid cysts may gradually recur.

| Epidermoid and dermoid |
| --- |
| Characteristic imaging features: <br>• Epidermoid: insinuating mass that is hyperintense on diffusion weighted imaging. <br>• Dermoid: fat-containing mass; CSF dissemination of fat droplets if ruptured. |

### 2.3.9 Arachnoid Cyst

Arachnoid cysts are frequent incidental findings on cranial MR and are most common in the anterior one-third of the temporal fossa. They are collections of CSF-like fluid within layers of the arachnoid membrane, which may or may not communicate with the subarachnoid space. Approximately 15% are in the juxtasellar region.[46] Most are asymptomatic and found incidentally, but some suprasellar arachnoid cysts become very large and cause obstructive hydrocephalus. Arachnoid cysts are usually stable over time, but may very gradually enlarge

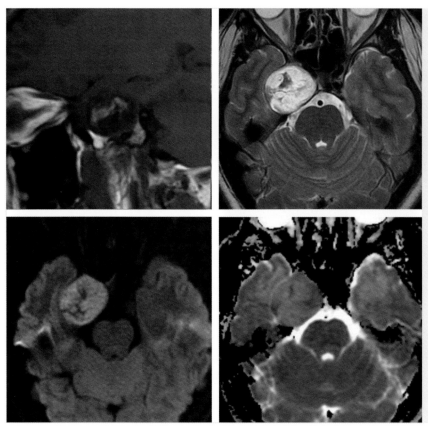

**Fig. 2.34** Epidermoid in cavernous sinus region with characteristic hyperintensity on DWI. ADC value is similar to brain parenchyma. Also note small T1 hyperintense areas with the lesion, which is likely due to high triglycerides and unsaturated fatty acids that can sometimes be seen in epidermoids.

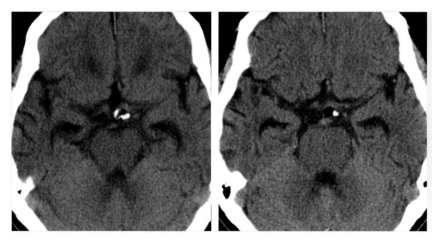

**Fig. 2.35** Suprasellar dermoid with fat and capsular calcification.

(particularly in very young children). Hemorrhage into an arachnoid cyst is rare but can cause sudden enlargement.

## Imaging

Uncomplicated arachnoid cysts are sharply demarcated ovoid extra-axial lesions that have the exactly same appearance as CSF on CT and MR (▶ Fig. 2.38, ▶ Fig. 2.39). Larger lesions can cause pressure on remodeling of the adjacent bone. MR cisternography sequences (CISS, FIESTA) can be used to delineate the cyst wall and therefore help distinguish an arachnoid cyst from an enlarged subarachnoid space. CSF flow imaging such as 2D cine phase contrast may be used to look for communication between the lesion and the adjacent subarachnoid space (▶ Fig. 2.40).[47]

## Treatment

Asymptomatic arachnoid cysts do not require any treatment. For symptomatic arachnoid cysts, treatment options include endoscopic or open resection or fenestration, or cystoperitoneal shunting.

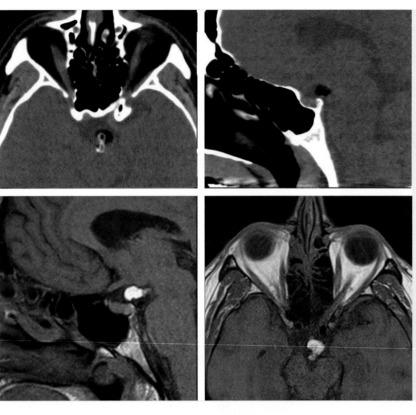

Fig. 2.36 Suprasellar dermoid containing fat and calcification. T1 hyperintensity within the lesion on MRI corresponding to the low attenuation fat content on CT.

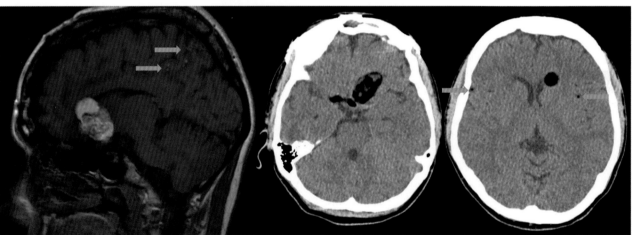

Fig. 2.37 This dermoid centered in the left suprasellar region has ruptured. Note the fat droplets scattered in the subarachnoid space (*arrows*).

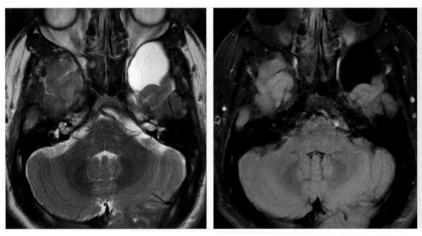

Fig. 2.38 Arachnoid cyst in the left middle cranial fossa. It has the same signal as cerebrospinal fluid (hyperintense on T2-weighted images and suppresses in signal on fluid attenuation inversion recovery).

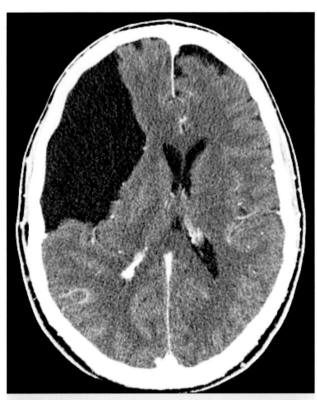

Fig. 2.39 Arachnoid cyst with mass effect on the brain and causing midline shift to the left, and displacing the cortical vessels around it. It has the same attenuation as cerebrospinal fluid.

**Arachnoid cyst**

Characteristic imaging features:
- Follows CSF signal on all sequences.
- May remodel adjacent bone.

## 2.3.10 Ecchordosis Physaliphora

Ecchordosis physaliphora is a benign lesion arising from an ectopic notochordal remnant that is typically located along the clivus in the prepontine cistern. They can also be found elsewhere along the craniospinal axis, reflecting the course of the embryonic notochord. Autopsy series shows them to be present in 2% of individuals. They are generally asymptomatic and usually found incidentally on imaging. They are similar to chordoma on histology, but are more hypocellular with absent mitoses.

### Imaging

Ecchordosis physaliphora appears as a small gelatinous nodule that is attached to the clivus by a small stalk or bony protuberance (▶ Fig. 2.41). CT may show a well-defined small lesion in the clivus with sclerotic margins. A small bony stalk may be evident. On MRI, the lesion is usually similar to CSF in signal. No enhancement is seen postcontrast, which is helpful for differentiating ecchordosis physaliphora from chordoma.

## Treatment

No treatment is necessary for this benign lesion unless significant brainstem compression or symptoms are present. Symptomatic lesions can be surgically resected.

**Ecchordosis physaliphora**

Characteristic imaging features:
- Small T2 hyperintense mass in the prepontine cistern connected to the clivus by an osseous stalk.
- Part of the lesion may be in the clivus and show well-defined sclerotic margins on CT.

## 2.3.11 Nasopharyngeal Carcinoma

Nasopharyngeal carcinoma arises from the nasopharyngeal epithelium, frequently originating from the fossa of Rosenmuller. It differs from other head and neck squamous cell carcinomas in epidemiology, histology, natural history, and response to treatment. The incidence of nasopharyngeal carcinoma in endemic areas in Southeast Asia is at least 10 times that in North America and Western Europe. It is two to three times more common in males than in females, with a peak incidence between 40 and 60 years of age.

Clinical presentation includes headaches, conductive hearing loss secondary to middle ear obstruction, epistaxis, cranial nerve neuropathies, and neck mass due to cervical node metastases. However, many patients remain asymptomatic for a prolonged period. The majority of patients present with locally and/or regionally advanced disease.

The WHO classifies nasopharyngeal carcinoma into keratinizing, nonkeratinizing, and basaloid squamous cell carcinoma types. The nonkeratinizing type is the most common (particularly in endemic areas where it constitutes > 95% cases), is most strongly associated with Epstein-Barr virus (EBV), and has a more favorable prognosis than the other types. For nasopharyngeal carcinoma associated with EBV, tumor immunostaining for EBV-encoded RNA (EBER) is a typical diagnostic criterion, and plasma levels of EBV copy number can be used to monitor the course of the disease, including following the completion of treatment.

### Imaging

Imaging is vital for accurate staging of tumor according to the UICC/AJCC classification, most recently updated in 2016 (▶ Table 2.3) and with additional proposed changes planned for the upcoming TNM eighth edition.[48] MR is the recommended modality for the assessment of local extent, as it is the most sensitive means to evaluate skull base and intracranial tumor spread. Nasopharyngeal carcinoma usually appears as a poorly marginated mucosal mass with epicenter in the fossa of Rosenmuller at the superolateral aspect of the nasopharynx. It is usually hypo- to isointense on T1WI, moderately hyperintense on T2WI compared to muscle, and shows mild homogenous enhancement postcontrast. The borders of the tumor are usually best delineated on T2-weighted and T1 postcontrast fat-suppressed images.

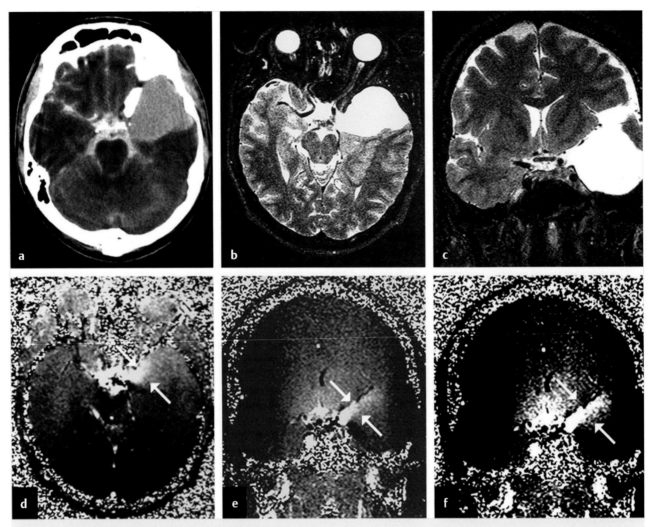

**Fig. 2.40** Phase contrast cine MR showing left middle cranial fossa arachnoid cyst communicating with adjacent subarachnoid space. (**a**) CT cisternography shows homogeneous contrast enhancement in the cyst. Transverse (**b**) and coronal (**c**) T2-weighted images obtained before PC cine MR imaging helps in proper section orientation. Transverse (**d**) and coronal (**e**) PC cine MR images show hyperintensity (*arrows*) arising from left chiasmatic cistern, which represents communication with the subarachnoid space. (**f**) Adjusting the windowing makes the flow jet (*arrows*) more clear. (Used with permission from Yildiz H, Erdogan C, Yalcin R, et al. Evaluation of communication between intracranial arachnoid cysts and cisterns with phase-contrast cine MR imaging. Am J Neuroradiol. 2005; 26(1):145–151.)

The tumor can extend anteriorly into the nasal cavity, pterygoid fossa, and maxillary sinuses; laterally beyond the pharyngobasilar fascia into the parapharyngeal and masticator spaces; and posteriorly and superiorly into the skull base, clivus, and intracranial compartment. When the tumor is small, its lateral extent is often limited by the pharyngobasilar fascia and the cartilaginous portion of the Eustachian tube. However, once these barriers are breached, the tumor can extend into the parapharyngeal and masticator space, the latter of which can lead to perineural spread along V3 intracranially through the foramen ovale (▶ Fig. 2.42). Superior extension may also occur through direct transgression via the petroclival fissure, foramen lacerum, Eustachian tube, sphenoid sinus, or clivus (▶ Fig. 2.43, ▶ Fig. 2.44).

Nasopharyngeal carcinoma tends to have earlier cervical lymph node involvement compared to other head and neck primary malignancies, and has a propensity for bilateral involvement. Retropharyngeal and level 2 nodes are typically involved first. Nodal disease in the lower neck does not typically occur in the absence of disease in the upper nodal stations.[49]

PET/CT is more sensitive and accurate compared to other modalities in the detection of nodal and distant metastasis, and therefore is often obtained for more advanced stage disease.

## Treatment

Radiotherapy is the primary treatment modality for nasopharyngeal carcinoma. Intensity-modulated radiation therapy (IMRT) is preferred where it is available. Surgery at the primary site is not used as a first-line therapy due to the deep anatomical location of the nasopharynx, close proximity to crucial neurovascular structures, and relative radiosensitivity of these tumors. Concurrent chemoradiotherapy is used for all but the most localized tumors with minimal regional nodal disease because of the risk of distant metastases. Contemporary treatments have almost completely eradicated locoregional failure, but distant metastasis remains the main form of failure and is seen in approximately 30% of patients, most typically those with advanced primaries and extensive neck disease.

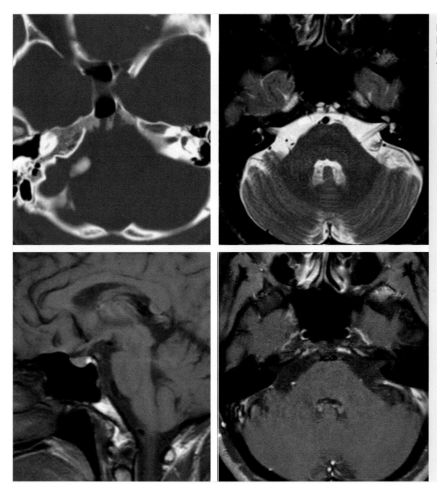

**Fig. 2.41** Ecchordosis physaliphora. Small lytic lesion in the clivus with well-marginated borders is seen on CT, corresponding to a lobulated T2-hyperintense nonenhancing lesion on MRI.

**Table 2.3** Classification criteria and stage grouping according to the 8th edition of the American Joint Committee on Cancer/International Union against Cancer staging system

**T category**

T1. Nasopharynx, oropharynx, nasal fossa

T2. Parapharyngeal extension, adjacent soft tissue involvement (medial pterygoid, lateral pterygoid, prevertebral muscles)

T3. Bony structure (skull base, cervical vertebra), paranasal sinuses

T4. Intracranial extension, cranial nerve, hypopharynx, orbit, extensive soft tissue involvement (beyond the lateral surface of the lateral pterygoid muscle, parotid gland)

**N Category**

N0. None

N1. Retropharyngeal (regardless of laterality); Cervical: unilateral, ≤ 6 cm, and above caudal border of cricoid cartilage

N2. Cervical: bilateral, ≤ 6 cm, and above caudal border of cricoid cartilage

N3. > 6 cm and/or below caudal border of cricoid cartilage (regardless of laterality)

Note: The nodal size is based on the maximum dimension in any direction.

Source: Adapted for Pan et al.[48]

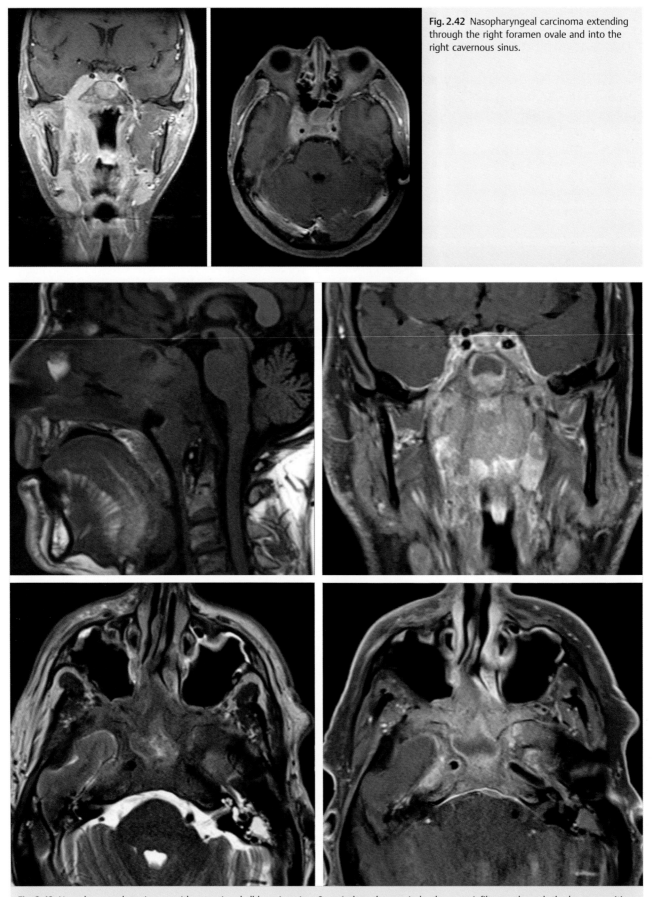

Fig. 2.42 Nasopharyngeal carcinoma extending through the right foramen ovale and into the right cavernous sinus.

Fig. 2.43 Nasopharyngeal carcinoma with extensive skull base invasion. Superiorly and posteriorly, the mass infiltrates through the longus capitis muscles to involve the entire clivus, anterior occipital bone, and occipital condyles. Intracranially, the tumor infiltrates the bilateral cavernous sinuses with dural thickening and enhancement along the medial walls and floors of middle cranial fossae. Posteriorly, there is retroclival soft-tissue tumor extension with dural enhancement.

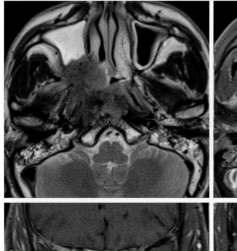
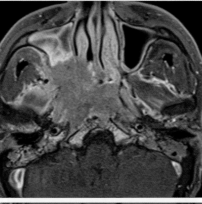
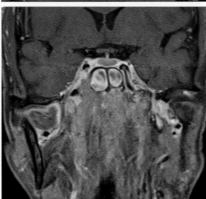

**Fig. 2.44** Nasopharyngeal carcinoma centered in the right nasopharynx. Anteriorly, the tumor extends to the back of the right nasal cavity, with involvement of the nasal septum, and through the right pterygopalatine fossa to the ipsilateral maxillary sinus. Laterally, the tumor extends into the right parapharyngeal space, with no definite involvement of the right masticator space. Medially, the tumor extends across midline to the left lateral wall of the nasopharynx. Posteriorly, there is involvement of the prevertebral muscles and diffuse involvement of the clivus, bilateral jugular tubercles, and right occipital condyle. Superiorly, there is tumor extending through the floor of the sphenoid sinus. The bilateral pterygoid processes and plates are involved with tumor. There is extension into the right cavernous sinus with cuffing of the petrous portion of the right carotid artery, as well as extension into the right infraorbital fissure and right foramen rotundum.

---

### Nasopharyngeal carcinoma

Characteristic imaging features:
- Infiltrative mass centered in the lateral pharyngeal recess.
- May infiltrate the adjacent soft tissue and skull base, and extend intracranially via direct spread or via skull base foramina.
- May have perineural tumor spread (most commonly V2 and V3).

Important imaging findings for treatment planning:
- Local tumor extent (see UICC/AJCC staging criteria).
- Nodal status.
- Perineural tumor spread.

## 2.3.12 Perineural Tumor Spread

Perineural tumor spread refers to the continuous neoplastic extension along a nerve which is associated with significantly increased locoregional recurrence rate and decreased 5-year survival rate. Up to 30 to 45% of patients with perineural spread may be asymptomatic; therefore, imaging assessment for this plays an important role.[50,51] Adenoid cystic carcinoma and the desmoplastic variant of melanoma are well known for their propensity for perineural spread. However, other malignancies such as squamous cell carcinoma, lymphoma, melanoma, basal cell carcinoma, and sarcoma can also show extension along nerves. In practice, most cases of perineural invasion occur in squamous cell carcinoma because it has the highest incidence among all head and neck cancers.

Any nerve may serve as a conduit for perineural spread, but the phenomenon is most commonly seen along the maxillary and mandibular divisions of the trigeminal nerve, and the facial nerve. The maxillary nerve innervates many areas in the face, oropharynx, and paranasal sinuses, and may therefore serve as a conduit for many tumors in these areas. It can also be involved by any tumor that invades the pterygopalatine fossa. Mandibular nerve involvement is often seen in masticator space malignancies and nasopharyngeal carcinoma. Perineural spread along the maxillary and mandibular nerves can extend intracranial through the foramen rotundum and foramen ovale (▶ Fig. 2.45, ▶ Fig. 2.46, ▶ Fig. 2.47), involving the Meckel's cave and cavernous sinus, and even extending to the brainstem. Malignant tumors in the parotid space can extend to the central skull base through involvement of the auriculotemporal nerve which connects with the mandibular nerve (▶ Fig. 2.48),[52] or along the greater superficial petrosal nerve to the vidian nerve.[53]

### Imaging

Perineural tumor spread is best assessed with contrast-enhanced MRI using multiple planes. It is important to follow the affected nerve in both the antegrade and retrograde directions. T1 images without fat saturation can be used to assess for obliteration of the perineural fat tissue at foraminal openings or in the pterygopalatine fossa. Enhancement and enlargement of the involved nerve can be assessed using T1 postgadolinium images either with or without fat suppression. Pathological enhancement is more conspicuous when imaged with fat suppression; however, susceptibility artifact may be an issue for

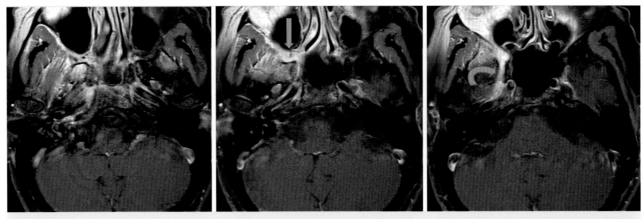

**Fig. 2.45** Perineural spread from the pterygopalatine fossa (*arrow*) along the right maxillary nerve in the foramen rotundum (*curved arrow*) by adenoid cystic carcinoma.

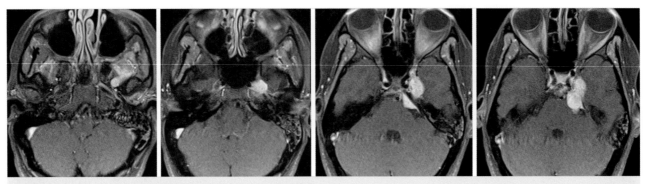

**Fig. 2.46** Angiosarcoma with perineural spread along the left mandibular nerve through the foramen ovale into the cavernous sinus and prepontine cistern.

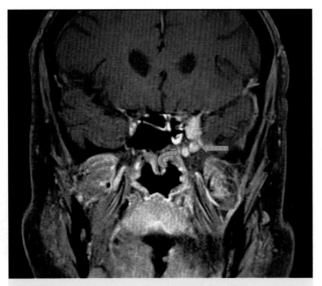

**Fig. 2.47** Perineural spread along the left maxillary nerve (*arrow*) and vidian nerve (*curved arrow*) from maxillary sinus squamous cell carcinoma.

frequency-selection fat suppression techniques in areas adjacent to an aerated sphenoid sinus and result in obscuration of the nearby foramen rotundum, vidian canal, and foramen ovale.[54]

Findings of muscle denervation can be seen as a result of nerve dysfunction due to perineural tumor spread (► Fig. 2.49). This can be seen in the masticator muscles and hemitongue when the mandibular nerve and the hypoglossal nerves are involved. MRI shows hyperintensity on T2WIs in the acute to subacute phase due to an increase in extracellular water, and muscle atrophy and fatty replacement in the chronic phase.[55]

## Treatment

Treatment strategies depend on the histologic subtype and staging. For squamous cell carcinoma, presence of perineural spread may be an indication for a more aggressive therapeutic approach that includes neck dissection, adjuvant therapy, or a larger radiation target volume.[56]

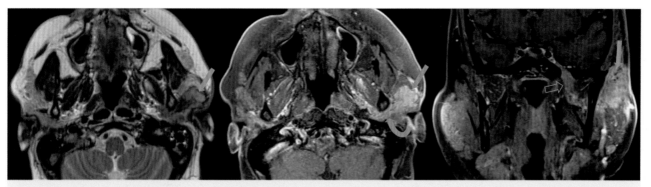

Fig. 2.48 Parotid mass (*arrow*) with perineural spread along the auriculotemporal nerve (*curved arrow*) to the mandibular nerve (*open arrow*).

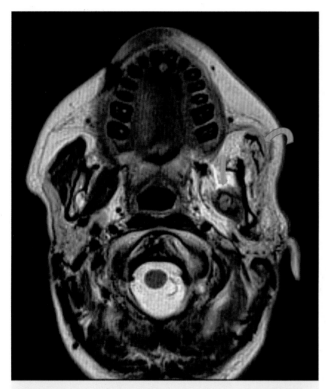

Fig. 2.49 Perineural spread along the left mandibular nerve (*arrow*), with resulting denervation and atrophy of the muscles of mastication on the left (*curved arrow*).

## 2.4 Tumor Mimics

### 2.4.1 Cephalocele

A cephalocele is a protrusion of intracranial contents through a defect in the skull. When the herniation contains only meninges and CSF, it is termed a meningocele. If the herniation also involves the brain then it is termed an encephalocele. These can be congenital or acquired lesions.

Congenital skull base cephaloceles are related to mesodermal defects and usually occur at the site of cranial sutures (▶ Fig. 2.50). The lesions involving the central skull base are termed basal cephaloceles and can be subdivided into transsphenoidal, sphenoethmoidal, transethmoidal, and sphenoorbi-

tal types based on location.[57] Many congenital cephaloceles are associated with other malformations and are recognized early in life; however, some skull base cephaloceles may remain undiagnosed and present later in life with recurrent meningitis, CSF leak, nasal mass, dysfunction of the herniated or adjacent tissue (such as the pituitary gland or optic chiasm), or seizures.

The majority of skull-base defects and cephaloceles in adults are acquired secondary to trauma (▶ Fig. 2.51) or iatrogenic defects or, more rarely, tumors and infections. Skull-base surgery may be complicated by CSF leaks and cephaloceles (▶ Fig. 2.52). Pseudomeningoceles at the surgical site may be clinically inconsequential if small, but need to be surgically corrected if large.

Cephaloceles and CSF leak can also develop spontaneously. This is seen more commonly in patients with clinical symptoms and radiologic signs of elevated intracranial pressure. They can occur anywhere in the skull base, but is most common at the cribriform plate, tegmen tympani (▶ Fig. 2.53), and sphenoid sinus (perisellar and lateral recess regions). A cephalocele discovered during investigation of a spontaneous CSF leak is usually small and appears as a pouch of CSF with a few strands of soft tissue on MRI.[58]

CT and MR are complimentary in the assessment of cephaloceles. Modern thin-slice CT is able to demonstrate osseous defects with high sensitivity. MR (including MR cisternography) is best for assessing content in the protruding pouch. CT cisternography and nuclear cisternography are also sometimes used in the workup of CSF leaks.

## 2.4.2 Cavernous Carotid Aneurysm and Fistula

Vascular abnormalities such as aneurysms or cavernous carotid fistulas (CCFs) should always be kept in mind whenever assessing any type of mass lesion in the skull base.

### Cavernous Carotid Artery Aneurysm

Cavernous carotid artery aneurysms have a strong female predilection and can be found incidentally or present with ophthalmoplegia or facial pain due to compression of the nerves in the cavernous sinus. If they rupture, patients can develop carotid cavernous fistula or occasionally subarachnoid hemorrhage. They have a significantly lower rate of rupture and mortality

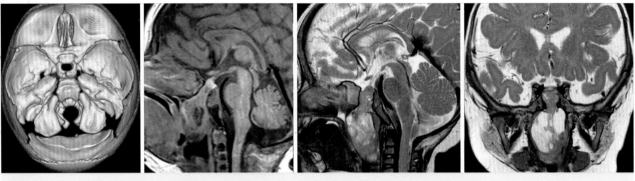

**Fig. 2.50** Teratoma within a persistent craniopharyngeal canal.

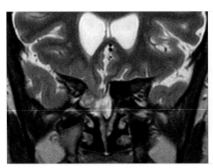

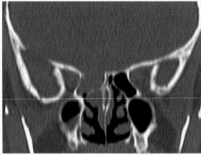

**Fig. 2.51** Traumatic encephalocele involving the right sphenoid sinus and posterior ethmoid air cells due to large defect in the planum sphenoidale and cribriform plate.

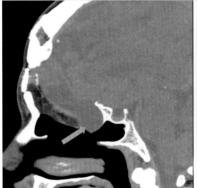

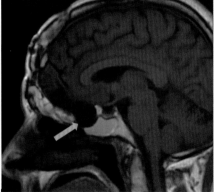

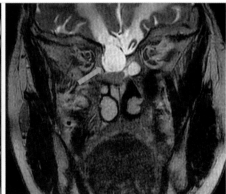

**Fig. 2.52** Postsurgical encephalocele (*arrow*) in a patient with previous olfactory groove meningioma resection, along a defect in the anterior cranial floor reconstruction.

compared to aneurysms located in the subarachnoid compartment, and therefore asymptomatic unruptured ones are not usually treated. Cavernous carotid artery aneurysms in patients with progressive neurologic symptoms can be treated with a variety of endovascular strategies, including coiling, stent-assisted coiling, parent vessel occlusion, and flow-diverting stents.[59]

The imaging appearance of aneurysm can vary depending on patency of the lumen and presence of thrombosis. Patent aneurysm lumens are well demonstrated with CTA, MRA, or cerebral angiography (► Fig. 2.54). Thrombosed portions of the aneurysm are better seen with cross-sectional imaging and can have a variable MR signal (► Fig. 2.55). Aneurysm walls may calcify.

## Cavernous Carotid Fistula

Cavernous carotid fistulas (CCF) are abnormal vascular shunts that allow blood to flow either directly or indirectly from the carotid artery into the cavernous sinus. Direct/high-flow CCFs result from a direct connection between the cavernous ICA and the surrounding cavernous sinus, and may be secondary to trauma or rupture of a cavernous carotid artery aneurysm. Indirect/low-flow CCFs are a subtype of dural arteriovenous (AV) fistula that result from communication between the cavernous sinus and branches of the internal or external artery in the adjacent dura. Treatment depends on the type of CCF and its angioarchitecture, and includes transarterial embolization, transvenous embolization, ICA occlusion, and covered stent placement.

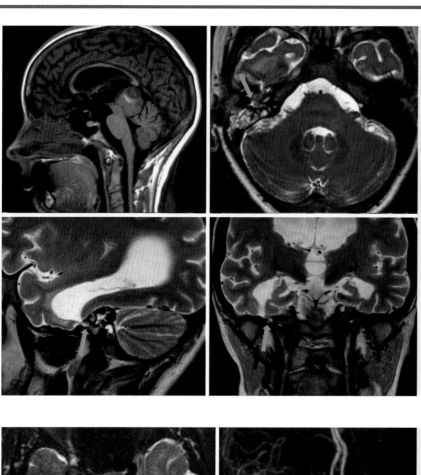

**Fig. 2.53** Patient with hydrocephalus secondary to obstruction of the cerebral aqueduct due to tectal tumor, presenting with otorrhea and bacterial meningitis. The patient was found to have an encephalocele (*arrow*) through the tegmen tympani, presumably secondary to increased intracranial pressure.

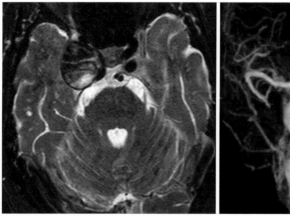
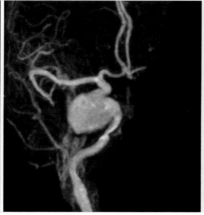

**Fig. 2.54** Large right cavernous carotid artery aneurysm.

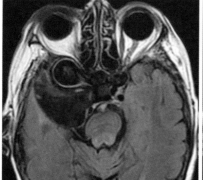
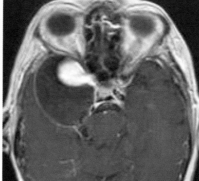
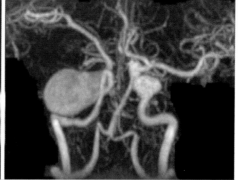

**Fig. 2.55** Bilateral cavernous carotid artery aneurysms. The giant right cavernous carotid artery aneurysm is partially thrombosed. Images are courtesy of Dr. Karel terBrugge.

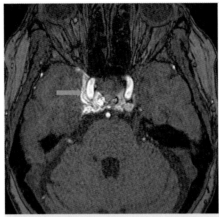
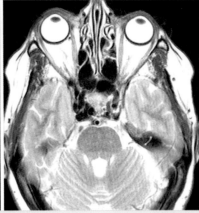
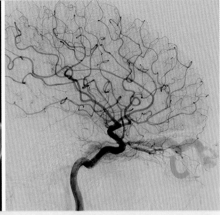

**Fig. 2.56** Right cavernous carotid fistula (indirect type). Time-of-flight MRA source images show abnormal opacification of the right cavernous sinus (*arrow*). T2WI shows asymmetric prominent flow voids in the right cavernous sinus. Lateral digital subtraction angiography (DSA) of selective injection of right internal carotid artery shows early opacification of the right cavernous sinus and the right superior ophthalmic vein (*curved arrow*).

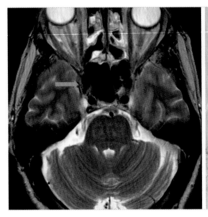
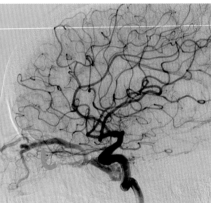

**Fig. 2.57** Another case of indirect-type right cavernous carotid fistula. T2-weighted image shows asymmetric small flow voids in the right cavernous sinus (*arrow*). Lateral DSA of selective injection of right internal carotid artery shows early opacification of the right cavernous sinus and the right superior ophthalmic vein (*curved arrow*).

Imaging findings suggestive of CCFs include a dilated superior ophthalmic vein(s) and the cavernous sinus, proptosis, and extraocular muscle enlargement (▶ Fig. 2.56, ▶ Fig. 2.57). However, venous drainage patterns may be variable and some CCFs drain predominantly into the inferior and superior petrosal sinuses and/or cortical veins. Lesions that show cortical vein reflux or directly drain into a cortical vein are at increased risk of hemorrhage. CTA and MRA may show early enhancement of the cavernous sinus and superior ophthalmic vein (▶ Fig. 2.56). Time-resolved MRA can be useful for demonstrating arteriovenous shunting, although it has lower spatial resolution than conventional CTA or MRA. Digital subtraction cerebral angiography is the gold standard of diagnosis.

### 2.4.3 Hypophysitis

Several forms of hypophysitis are recognized histologically, including lymphocytic, granulomatous, plasmacytic, and xanthomatous.[60] Clinical presentation usually consists of headache and multiple endocrine deficiencies. Lymphocytic hypophysitis is the most common form and often occurs in late pregnancy or the postpartum period. Its etiology is uncertain but may be autoimmune (▶ Fig. 2.58). Granulomatous hypophysitis is characterized histologically by infiltration of histiocytes and giant cells and sometimes accompanies a known granulomatous condition such as granulomatosis with polyangiitis (Wegener's granulomatosis) and tuberculosis. Plasmacytic hypophysitis is characterized by infiltration of plasma cells, which produce IgG4, and can be associated with IgG4-related disease in other organs (▶ Fig. 2.59). Xanthomatous hypophysitis is rare and is characterized histologically by infiltration by foamy histiocytes.[60]

Ipilimumab-induced hypophysitis is a recently observed entity associated with the immunotherapeutic agent ipilimumab which is used most commonly to treat unresectable or metastatic melanoma, with reported incidence of up to 13% in clinical trials.[61] Clinical, endocrine, and imaging features are similar to other forms of hypophysitis (▶ Fig. 2.60).[62,63]

Imaging appearances of the various types of hypophysitis are similar. There is usually a thick nontapering pituitary stalk with diffuse enlargement of the pituitary gland and loss of the normal T1 bright spot in the posterior pituitary. Enhancement is typically uniform but can be heterogeneous. Thickening of the adjacent dura can be seen.

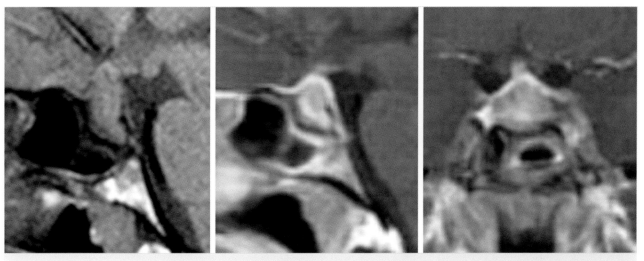

**Fig. 2.58** Biopsy-proven lymphocytic hypophysitis in a 45-year-old woman with polyuria and headache. There is enlargement of the pituitary stalk and pituitary gland, and loss of the normal posterior pituitary T1 bright spot.

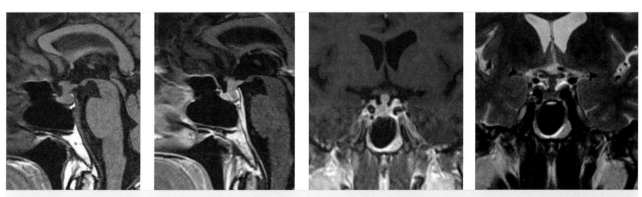

**Fig. 2.59** IgG4 disease–related hypophysitis. This is a 44-year-old man with past history of submandibular sialadenitis and pancreatitis presenting with polyuria and polydipsia.

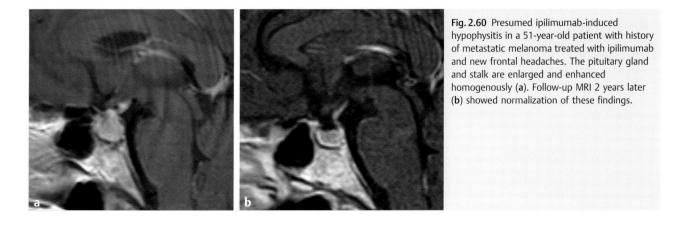

**Fig. 2.60** Presumed ipilimumab-induced hypophysitis in a 51-year-old patient with history of metastatic melanoma treated with ipilimumab and new frontal headaches. The pituitary gland and stalk are enlarged and enhanced homogenously (**a**). Follow-up MRI 2 years later (**b**) showed normalization of these findings.

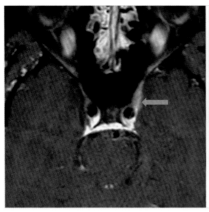
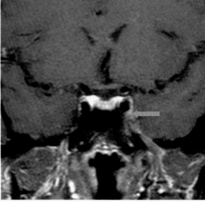

Fig. 2.61 Mild asymmetric enlargement and enhancement of the left cavernous sinus (*arrow*) in a patient with Tolosa-Hunt syndrome.

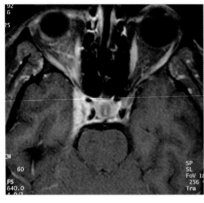
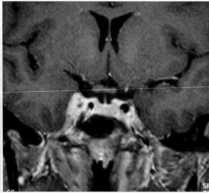

Fig. 2.62 Asymmetric enlargement and enhancement of the right cavernous sinus in a patient with Tolosa-Hunt syndrome.

## 2.4.4 Tolosa-Hunt Syndrome

Tolosa-Hunt syndrome is a rare syndrome of painful ophthalmoplegia caused by an idiopathic granulomatous inflammation of the cavernous sinus. This entity likely represents the same disease process as orbital pseudotumor, distinguished only by anatomic location. The diagnosis of Tolosa-Hunt syndrome is based on clinical presentation, neuroimaging finding, clinical response to corticosteroids, and exclusion of an alternative diagnosis.

MRI shows fullness and enhancement of the cavernous sinus and the superior orbital fissure (▶ Fig. 2.61, ▶ Fig. 2.62). The abnormal soft tissue is usually relatively hypointense on T2WIs, reflecting a very cellular infiltrate and fibrosis. The cavernous ICA may be narrowed. These MR findings are not specific to Tolosa-Hunt and can be seen in other entities such as lymphoma and sarcoidosis.

## 2.4.5 Neurosarcoidosis

Sarcoidosis is a chronic multisystem inflammatory disorder of unknown etiology that is characterized by noncaseating granulomas. The hilar lymph nodes and the lungs are the most common organs involved. The CNS is involved in approximately 5% of cases, usually in combination with disease elsewhere, but can rarely be the only site of involvement. Neurosarcoidosis can involve any part of the nervous system or meninges. The most common location is the leptomeninges at the base of the brain (▶ Fig. 2.63, ▶ Fig. 2.64). The hypothalamic–pituitary axis is another favored site. The most common finding on MRI is nod-ular or diffuse leptomeningeal thickening. However, sarcoidosis is a great mimicker of many other diseases and many imaging appearances are possible, including dural-based masses, diffuse perivascular infiltrates, multifocal small enhancing parenchymal lesions, and large tumefactive parenchymal masses.

## 2.4.6 Central Skull Base Infection

Sphenoid sinusitis is the most common inflammatory process in the central skull base. The imaging appearance of uncomplicated sphenoid sinus infection is similar to infection in other sinuses. However, because of its location, aggressive sphenoid sinus infections can spread to the cavernous sinus and cause cavernous sinus thrombosis. Infections from other areas in the face or orbit can also spread to the cavernous sinuses through their connections with the facial veins and pterygoid plexus via the inferior and superior ophthalmic veins. The organisms associated with septic cavernous sinus thrombosis reflect the primary sites of infection, with bacteria (most commonly *Staphylococcus aureus*) accounting for most infections and fungal pathogens being less common.[64,65] Diagnosis can be made on contrast-enhanced CT or MR imaging by identifying filling defects within the normally enhancing cavernous sinus (▶ Fig. 2.65), bulging of the lateral wall, increased enhancement along the lateral wall, or indirect signs relating to venous obstruction (such as dilatation of the superior ophthalmic vein).[66,67,68] Cavernous sinus thrombosis can be complicated by carotid artery narrowing and thrombosis, which can be assessed by CTA or MRA.

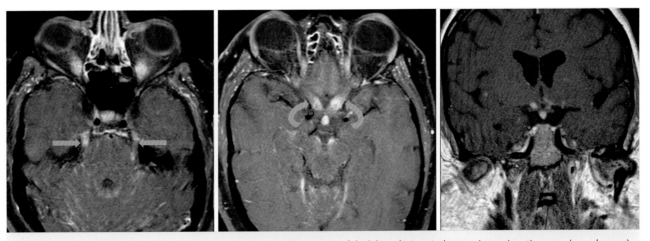

**Fig. 2.63** Patient with neurosarcoidosis. There is thickening and enhancement of the bilateral trigeminal nerves (*arrows*), optic nerves (*curved arrows*), and pituitary stalk; leptomeningeal enhancement around the basal cisterns and along the cerebellar folia; and patchy parenchymal enhancement.

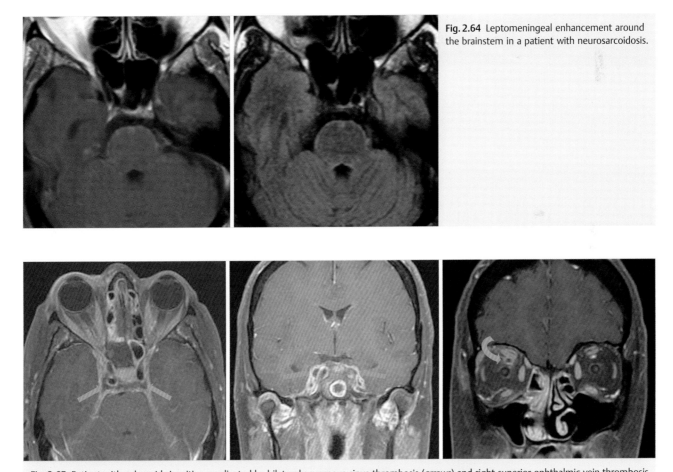

**Fig. 2.64** Leptomeningeal enhancement around the brainstem in a patient with neurosarcoidosis.

**Fig. 2.65** Patient with sphenoid sinusitis complicated by bilateral cavernous sinus thrombosis (*arrows*) and right superior ophthalmic vein thrombosis (*curved arrow*).

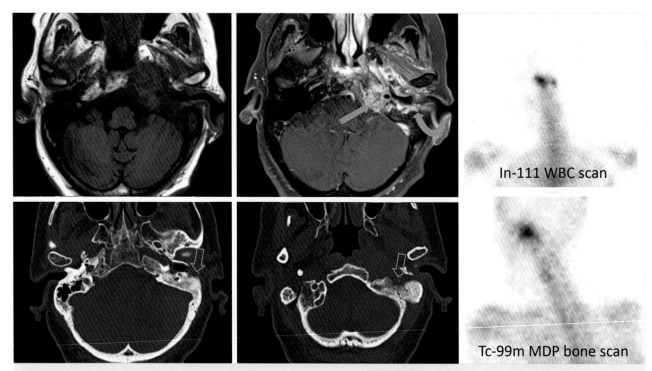

**Fig. 2.66** Skull base osteomyelitis secondary to necrotizing otitis externa. There is abnormal enhancement involving the left petrous apex and the left aspect of the clivus (*arrow*), and the left pre-vertebral soft tissue. Note also the enhancement around the left external auditory canal (*curved arrow*). Bony erosive changes (*open arrow*) are better seen on CT. Indium-111-labeled WBC scan shows increased WBC accumulation at the left skull base, corresponding to the area of increased scintigraphic activity on bone scan. MDP, methylene diphosphonate; WBC, white blood cell.

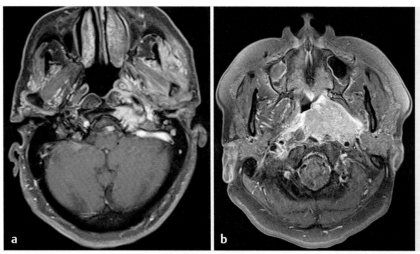

**Fig. 2.67** Postcontrast T1 images in a patient with skull base osteomyelitis (**a**) and in a patient with nasopharyngeal carcinoma (**b**). Note that the tissue planes appear relatively preserved in the patient with osteomyelitis, whereas nasopharyngeal carcinoma (NPC) obliterates the tissue planes.

Skull base osteomyelitis is a rare entity that most frequently results as a complication of otitis externa in patients with diabetes, usually caused by pseudomonas infection (▶ Fig. 2.66). Central skull base osteomyelitis unrelated to an otogenic source has also been reported, again mostly seen in patients with diabetes.[69] Imaging findings include soft-tissue infiltration and bone erosion. MR is better for assessing bone marrow signal change and subtle dural enhancement, whereas CT is better for the evaluation of bone erosion.[70] Clinical and imaging features of central skull base osteomyelitis may mimic malignancy. One study suggests that at presentation, MR shows greater extent of bone involvement than CT for osteomyelitis, whereas the extent of involvement is more similar on CT and MR for malignancy.[71] The tissue planes usually appear relatively preserved on T1 postcontrast images in cases of osteomyelitis, which is not seen in malignancy (▶ Fig. 2.67).[71] Various nuclear medicine imaging techniques, such as indium-111 white blood cell scans (▶ Fig. 2.66, ▶ Fig. 2.68) and technetium-99 methylene diphosphonate bone scans, can be used in the assessment of suspected skull base osteomyelitis, particularly in the postoperative setting where changes on CT/MRI may be more difficult to interpret, and in follow-up of patients being treated for osteomyelitis.[72]

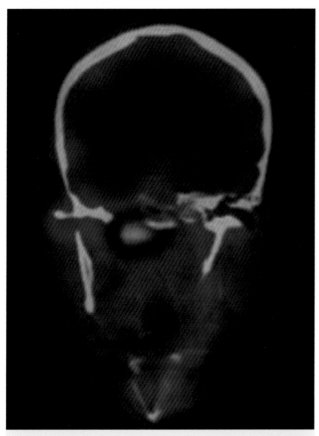

Fig. 2.68 Indium-111 white blood cell scan showing abnormal localization of tracer in the right skull base in this patient with osteomyelitis.

Tuberculous meningitis has a predilection for the meninges around the basal cisterns (▶ Fig. 2.69). MR is more sensitive than CT, and shows signal abnormality within the cisterns and marked smooth or nodular meningeal enhancement. Tuberculomas, which are usually parenchymal, can also be seen. Arteries within the basal cisterns can be directly involved by exudate or indirectly by reactive arteritis, and can result in infarcts typically involving perforator territories.

## 2.5 Conclusion

A variety of disease processes can involve the central skull base. This chapter has reviewed in depth the most common neoplasms that can occur in the region. The key distinguishing radiologic and clinical features have been discussed for each entity. In addition, highly relevant anatomical features that need to be closely scrutinized on cross-sectional imaging have also been highlighted. Such radiologic features are important in helping determine potential resectability of tumors and, as a consequence, will affect patient staging and influence treatment options and prognosis. The most common and relevant nonneoplastic entities that can arise in the central skull base have also been discussed. Such lesions can be very challenging to diagnose and manage. The clinical and distinguishing imaging features of these diseases have also been reviewed.

## 2.6 High Yield Summary

- For those lesions that arise in the sella or suprasellar region, the identification of the normal pituitary gland can help distinguish pituitary micro/macroademnomas from non–pituitary-based lesions.

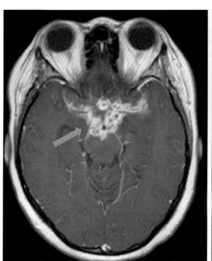
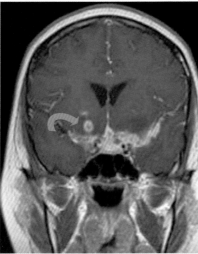

Fig. 2.69 Tuberculous meningitis with marked thickening and enhancement of the meninges in the basal cisterns (*arrow*). A small developing tuberculous abscess (*curved arrow*) is also noted.

- Key upstaging features that determine resectability in the central skull base include involvement of the optic nerves, cavernous sinus, carotid artery, and the extent of bony and intracranial invasion.
- The presence of perineural tumor spread can also make certain neoplasms unresectable.
- Skull base soft-tissue infection and/or osteomyelitis can mimic tumors both clinically and radiologically by giving rise to an enhancing infiltrative and aggressive-appearing mass.
- Aneurysms arising in the central skull base can also provide a diagnostic dilemma if the clinician or radiologist is unaware or not suspicious as to their possible existence; inadvertent biopsy or inappropriate surgical manipulation can lead to catastrophic outcomes.
- During the interpretation of central skull base imaging studies, it is also important to report on the presence of any anatomical variants that can lead to a higher risk of perioperative morbidity or mortality or potentially influence the difficulty of access; such features to note include the presence of Onodi air cells, the degree of sphenoid sinus pneumatization, and dehiscent cavernous carotid arteries.

# References

[1] Laine FJ, Nadel L, Braun IFCT. CT and MR imaging of the central skull base. Part 2. Pathologic spectrum. Radiographics. 1990; 10(5):797–821

[2] Curtin HD, Hagiwara M. Embryology, anatomy, and imaging of the central skull base. In: Som PM, Curtin HD, eds. Head and Neck Imaging. 5th ed. St. Louis, MO: Mosby Elsevier; 2011

[3] Abele TA, Salzman KL, Harnsberger HR, Glastonbury CM. Craniopharyngeal canal and its spectrum of pathology. AJNR Am J Neuroradiol. 2014; 35(4): 772–777

[4] Hamberger CA, Hammer G, Norlen G, Sjogren B. Transantrosphenoidal hypophysectomy. Arch Otolaryngol 1961; 74: 28.

[5] Hammer G, Radberg C. The sphenoidal sinus: an anatomical and roentgenologic study with reference to transsphenoid hypophysectomy. Acta Radiol 1961; 56(6): 401422.

[6] Singh A, Roth J, Anand VK, Schwartz TH. Anatomy of the pituitary gland and paraseller areas. In: Schwartz TH, Anand VK, eds. Endoscopic Pituitary Surgery—A Comprehensive Guide. 1st ed. New York, NY: Thieme; 2011:384

[7] Di Ieva A, Rotondo F, Syro LV, Cusimano MD, Kovacs K. Aggressive pituitary adenomas–diagnosis and emerging treatments. Nat Rev Endocrinol. 2014; 10 (7):423–435

[8] Katznelson L, Alexander JM, Klibanski A. Clinical review 45: Clinically nonfunctioning pituitary adenomas. J Clin Endocrinol Metab. 1993; 76(5):1089–1094

[9] Symons SP, Montanera WJ, Aviv RI, Kucharczyk W. Magnetic resonance imaging of the brain and spine. In: Atlas SW, ed. Magnetic Resonance Imaging of the Brain and Spine. 3rd ed. Philadelphia, PA: Lippincott Williams & Wilkins; 2008

[10] Davis PC, Hoffman JC, Jr, Malko JA, et al. Gadolinium-DTPA and MR imaging of pituitary adenoma: a preliminary report. AJNR Am J Neuroradiol. 1987; 8(5): 817–823

[11] Doppman JL, Frank JA, Dwyer AJ, et al. Gadolinium DTPA enhanced MR imaging of ACTH-secreting microadenomas of the pituitary gland. J Comput Assist Tomogr. 1988; 12(5):728–735

[12] Dwyer AJ, Frank JA, Doppman JL, et al. Pituitary adenomas in patients with Cushing disease: initial experience with Gd-DTPA-enhanced MR imaging. Radiology. 1987; 163(2):421–426

[13] Nakamura T, Schörner W, Bittner RC, Felix R. The value of paramagnetic contrast agent gadolinium-DTPA in the diagnosis of pituitary adenomas. Neuroradiology. 1988; 30(6):481–486

[14] Newton DR, Dillon WP, Norman D, Newton TH, Wilson CB. Gd-DTPA-enhanced MR imaging of pituitary adenomas. AJNR Am J Neuroradiol. 1989; 10(5):949–954

[15] Steiner E, Imhof H, Knosp E. Gd-DTPA enhanced high resolution MR imaging of pituitary adenomas. Radiographics. 1989; 9(4):587–598

[16] Bartynski WS, Lin L. Dynamic and conventional spin-echo MR of pituitary microlesions. AJNR Am J Neuroradiol. 1997; 18(5):965–972

[17] Miki Y, Matsuo M, Nishizawa S, et al. Pituitary adenomas and normal pituitary tissue: enhancement patterns on gadopentetate-enhanced MR imaging. Radiology. 1990; 177(1):35–38

[18] Sakamoto Y, Takahashi M, Korogi Y, Bussaka H, Ushio Y. Normal and abnormal pituitary glands: gadopentetate dimeglumine-enhanced MR imaging. Radiology. 1991; 178(2):441–445

[19] Gao R, Isoda H, Tanaka T, et al. Dynamic gadolinium-enhanced MR imaging of pituitary adenomas: usefulness of sequential sagittal and coronal plane images. Eur J Radiol. 2001; 39(3):139–146

[20] Suzuki M, Matsui O, Ueda F, et al. Dynamic MR imaging for diagnosis of lesions adjacent to pituitary gland. Eur J Radiol. 2005; 53(2):159–167

[21] Hagiwara A, Inoue Y, Wakasa K, Haba T, Tashiro T, Miyamoto T. Comparison of growth hormone-producing and non-growth hormone-producing pituitary adenomas: imaging characteristics and pathologic correlation. Radiology. 2003; 228(2):533–538

[22] Knosp E, Steiner E, Kitz K, Matula C. Pituitary adenomas with invasion of the cavernous sinus space: a magnetic resonance imaging classification compared with surgical findings. Neurosurgery. 1993; 33(4):610–617, discussion 617–618

[23] Loeffler JS, Shih HA. Radiation therapy of pituitary adenomas. In: Post TW, ed. UpToDate. Waltham, MA: 2015

[24] Bunin GR, Surawicz TS, Witman PA, Preston-Martin S, Davis F, Bruner JM. The descriptive epidemiology of craniopharyngioma. J Neurosurg. 1998; 89(4): 547–551

[25] Hirunpat S, Tanomkiat W, Sriprung H, Chetpaophan J. Optic tract edema: a highly specific magnetic resonance imaging finding for the diagnosis of craniopharyngiomas. Acta Radiol. 2005; 46(4):419–423

[26] Saeki N, Uchino Y, Murai H, et al. MR imaging study of edema-like change along the optic tract in patients with pituitary region tumors. AJNR Am J Neuroradiol. 2003; 24(3):336–342

[27] Asaeda M, Kurosaki M, Kambe A, et al. MR imaging study of edema along the optic tract in patient with Rathke's cleft cyst [in Japanese]. No To Shinkei. 2004; 56(3):243–246

[28] Kawamata T, Kubo O, Hori T. Histological findings at the boundary of craniopharyngiomas. Brain Tumor Pathol. 2005; 22(2):75–78

[29] Fernandez-Miranda JC, Gardner PA, Snyderman CH, et al. Craniopharyngioma: a pathologic, clinical, and surgical review. Head Neck. 2012; 34(7): 1036–1044

[30] Teramoto A, Hirakawa K, Sanno N, Osamura Y. Incidental pituitary lesions in 1,000 unselected autopsy specimens. Radiology. 1994; 193(1):161–164

[31] Byun WM, Kim OL, Kim D. MR imaging findings of Rathke's cleft cysts: significance of intracystic nodules. AJNR Am J Neuroradiol. 2000; 21(3):485–488

[32] Binning MJ, Gottfried ON, Osborn AG, Couldwell WT. Rathke cleft cyst intracystic nodule: a characteristic magnetic resonance imaging finding. J Neurosurg. 2005; 103(5):837–840

[33] Han SJ, Rolston JD, Jahangiri A, Aghi MK. Rathke's cleft cysts: review of natural history and surgical outcomes. J Neurooncol. 2014; 117(2):197–203

[34] Russell DS, Rubinstein LJ. Pathology of Tumors of the Nervous System. 5th ed. Baltimore, MD: Lippincott Williams & Wilkins; 1989

[35] Osborn AG. Osborn's Brain: Imaging, Pathology, and Anatomy. 1st ed. Salt Lake City, UT: Amirsys Pub; 2013

[36] Mendenhall WM, Friedman WA, Amdur RJ, Foote KD. Management of benign skull base meningiomas: a review. Skull Base. 2004; 14(1):53–60, discussion 61

[37] Jennings MT, Gelman R, Hochberg F. Intracranial germ-cell tumors: natural history and pathogenesis. J Neurosurg. 1985; 63(2):155–167

[38] Hoffman HJ, Otsubo H, Hendrick EB, et al. Intracranial germ-cell tumors in children. J Neurosurg. 1991; 74(4):545–551

[39] Kanagaki M, Miki Y, Takahashi JA, et al. MRI and CT findings of neurohypophyseal germinoma. Eur J Radiol. 2004; 49(3):204–211

[40] Moon WK, Chang KH, Han MH, Kim IO. Intracranial germinomas: correlation of imaging findings with tumor response to radiation therapy. AJR Am J Roentgenol. 1999; 172(3):713–716

[41] MacNally SP, Rutherford SA, Ramsden RT, Evans DG, King AT. Trigeminal schwannomas. Br J Neurosurg. 2008; 22(6):729–738

[42] Chugh R, Tawbi H, Lucas DR, Biermann JS, Schuetze SM, Baker LH. Chordoma: the nonsarcoma primary bone tumor. Oncologist. 2007; 12(11): 1344–1350

[43] Walcott BP, Nahed BV, Mohyeldin A, Coumans JV, Kahle KT, Ferreira MJ. Chordoma: current concepts, management, and future directions. Lancet Oncol. 2012; 13(2):e69–e76

[44] Snyderman C, Lin D. Chordoma and chondrosarcoma of the skull base. In: Post TW, ed. UpToDate. Waltham, MA: 2015

[45] Sahgal A, Chan MW, Atenafu EG, et al. Image-guided, intensity-modulated radiation therapy (IG-IMRT) for skull base chordoma and chondrosarcoma: preliminary outcomes. Neuro-oncol. 2015; 17(6):889–894

[46] Wiener SN, Pearlstein AE, Eiber A. MR imaging of intracranial arachnoid cysts. J Comput Assist Tomogr. 1987; 11(2):236–241

[47] Yildiz H, Erdogan C, Yalcin R, et al. Evaluation of communication between intracranial arachnoid cysts and cisterns with phase-contrast cine MR imaging. AJNR Am J Neuroradiol. 2005; 26(1):145–151

[48] Pan JJ, Ng WT, Zong JF, et al. Proposal for the 8th edition of the AJCC/UICC staging system for nasopharyngeal cancer in the era of intensity-modulated radiotherapy. Cancer. 2016; 122(4):546–558

[49] Tang L, Mao Y, Liu L, et al. The volume to be irradiated during selective neck irradiation in nasopharyngeal carcinoma: analysis of the spread patterns in lymph nodes by magnetic resonance imaging. Cancer. 2009; 115(3):680–688

[50] Warden KF, Parmar H, Trobe JD. Perineural spread of cancer along the three trigeminal divisions. J Neuroophthalmol. 2009; 29(4):300–307

[51] Mendenhall WM, Parsons JT, Mendenhall NP, et al. Carcinoma of the skin of the head and neck with perineural invasion. Head Neck. 1989; 11(4):301–308

[52] Schmalfuss IM, Tart RP, Mukherji S, Mancuso AA. Perineural tumor spread along the auriculotemporal nerve. AJNR Am J Neuroradiol. 2002; 23(2):303–311

[53] Ginsberg LE, De Monte F, Gillenwater AM. Greater superficial petrosal nerve: anatomy and MR findings in perineural tumor spread. AJNR Am J Neuroradiol. 1996; 17(2):389–393

[54] Curtin HD. Detection of perineural spread: fat suppression versus no fat suppression. AJNR Am J Neuroradiol. 2004; 25(1):1–3

[55] Ong CK, Chong VF. Imaging of perineural spread in head and neck tumours. Cancer Imaging. 2010; 10(1A):S92–S98

[56] Paes FM, Singer AD, Checkver AN, Palmquist RA, De La Vega G, Sidani C. Perineural spread in head and neck malignancies: clinical significance and evaluation with 18F-FDG PET/CT. Radiographics. 2013; 33(6):1717–1736

[57] Tomita T, Ogiwara H. Primary (congenital) encephalocele. In: Post TW, ed. UpToDate. Waltham, MA: 2015

[58] Connor SE. Imaging of skull-base cephalocoeles and cerebrospinal fluid leaks. Clin Radiol. 2010; 65(10):832–841

[59] ter Brugge KG. Cavernous sinus segment internal carotid artery aneurysms: whether and how to treat. AJNR Am J Neuroradiol. 2012; 33(2):327–328

[60] Synder PJ. Causes of hypopituitarism. In: Post TW, ed. UpToDate. Waltham, MA: 2015

[61] Bertrand A, Kostine M, Barnetche T, Truchetet ME, Schaeverbeke T. Immune related adverse events associated with anti-CTLA-4 antibodies: systematic review and meta-analysis. BMC Med. 2015; 13:211

[62] Carpenter KJ, Murtagh RD, Lilienfeld H, Weber J, Murtagh FR. Ipilimumab-induced hypophysitis: MR imaging findings. AJNR Am J Neuroradiol. 2009; 30(9):1751–1753

[63] Faje AT, Sullivan R, Lawrence D, et al. Ipilimumab-induced hypophysitis: a detailed longitudinal analysis in a large cohort of patients with metastatic melanoma. J Clin Endocrinol Metab. 2014; 99(11):4078–4085

[64] Ebright JR, Pace MT, Niazi AF. Septic thrombosis of the cavernous sinuses. Arch Intern Med. 2001; 161(22):2671–2676

[65] Southwick FS. Septic dural sinus thrombosis. In: Post TW, ed. UpToDate. Waltham, MA: 2015

[66] Schuknecht B, Simmen D, Yüksel C, Valavanis A. Tributary venosinus occlusion and septic cavernous sinus thrombosis: CT and MR findings. AJNR Am J Neuroradiol. 1998; 19(4):617–626

[67] Ellie E, Houang B, Louail C, et al. CT and high-field MRI in septic thrombosis of the cavernous sinuses. Neuroradiology. 1992; 34(1):22–24

[68] Lee JH, Lee HK, Park JK, Choi CG, Suh DC. Cavernous sinus syndrome: clinical features and differential diagnosis with MR imaging. AJR Am J Roentgenol. 2003; 181(2):583–590

[69] Johnson AK, Batra PS. Central skull base osteomyelitis: an emerging clinical entity. Laryngoscope. 2014; 124(5):1083–1087

[70] Adams A, Offiah C. Central skull base osteomyelitis as a complication of necrotizing otitis externa: Imaging findings, complications, and challenges of diagnosis. Clin Radiol. 2012; 67(10):e7–e16

[71] Lesser FD, Derbyshire SG, Lewis-Jones H. Can computed tomography and magnetic resonance imaging differentiate between malignant pathology and osteomyelitis in the central skull base? J Laryngol Otol. 2015; 129(9):852–859

[72] Seabold JE, Simonson TM, Weber PC, et al. Cranial osteomyelitis: diagnosis and follow-up with In-111 white blood cell and Tc-99m methylene diphosphonate bone SPECT, CT, and MR imaging. Radiology. 1995; 196(3):779–788

# 3 Cerebellopontine Angle and Jugular Fossa

*Laila S. Alshafai, Chris Heyn, John A. Rutka, Arjun Sahgal, Vincent Lin, Michael D. Cusimano, Sean Symons, Nabeel S. Alshafai, and Peter Som*

## 3.1 Basic Anatomy Overview

### 3.1.1 Cerebellopontine Angle Cistern

The cerebellopontine angle (CPA) cisterns are paired lateral infratentorial cerebrospinal fluid (CSF)-filled spaces bound by the pons, cerebellum, and petrous temporal bones. On axial images, they are triangular in shape. Although they communicate with other cisterns, they are also compartmentalized by porous trabeculated walls (▶ Fig. 3.1). These walls may be deficient either as a normal variant or as part of a pathological process. Under normal circumstances, there is continuous exchange of CSF from one compartment to another through these openings which can be obstructed by certain conditions (e.g., subarachnoid hemorrhage, pus, and protein).[1,2,3]

### Contents

The literature of the CPA cistern can be confusing because it has been subdivided by some researchers into a superior compartment (this corresponds to what is generally regarded by most as the "CPA cistern") and an inferior compartment (which is called the "lateral cerebellomedullary cistern"). The contents are shown in ▶ Fig. 3.2. To avoid confusion, we will discuss only the superior compartment of the CPA cistern.

### Boundaries

The boundaries of the CPA cistern are as follows:
- *Posteriorly*: The posterior quadrangular and superior semilunar lobulus of the anterior cerebellar hemisphere.

- *Posteromedially*: The pontomedullary sulcus, the flocculus of the cerebellum.
- *Medially*: The lateral portion of pons. It is continuous with the prepontine cistern superiorly and premedullary cistern inferiorly.
- *Superiorly*: The ambient cistern just below the tentorial hiatus. The CPA roof is limited by the tentorium and its attachment to the petrous bone.
- *Inferiorly*: The lateral cerebellomedullary cistern. The lateral outlet of the fourth ventricle, the foramen of Luschka, marks the boundary with the lateral cerebellomedullary cistern.
- *Laterally*: The posterior petrous segment of the temporal bone, internal auditory meatus, and Meckel's cave. The CPA cistern extends into the internal auditory canal (IAC) around the cranial nerves (CNs) VII and VIII.

The normal orientation of the CNs at the IAC porus acusticus is as follows: The facial nerve is anterosuperior, the cochlear nerve is anteroinferior, the superior vestibular nerve is posterosuperior, and the inferior vestibular nerve is anteroinferior. "Seven-up, Coke down" is an easy way to remember their location (▶ Fig. 3.3).[1,2,3]

### 3.1.2 Jugular Fossa

The jugular bulb is the junction between the lower sigmoid sinus and the internal jugular vein (IJV). It is situated between the occipital bone and the mastoid portion of the temporal bone. The lateral bony wall of the intraosseous jugular bulb is adjacent to the hypotympanum and, when dehiscent, can cause pulsatile tinnitus. An alternate name for the jugular bulb is the

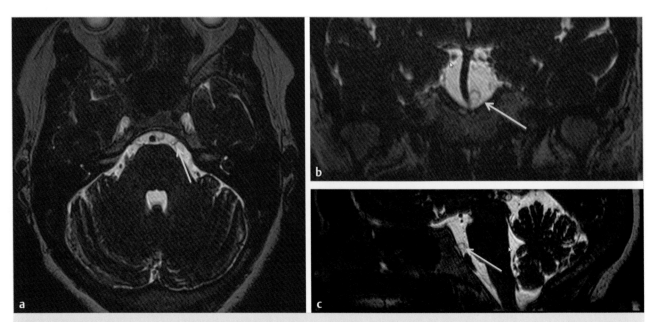

**Fig. 3.1** High-resolution T2-weighted sequence in the posterior fossa in axial (**a**), coronal (**b**), and sagittal (**c**) sequences. There is demonstration of normal membrane or porous trabeculations (*arrows*) within the prepontine cistern. These can also be seen in the cerebellopontine angle cistern.

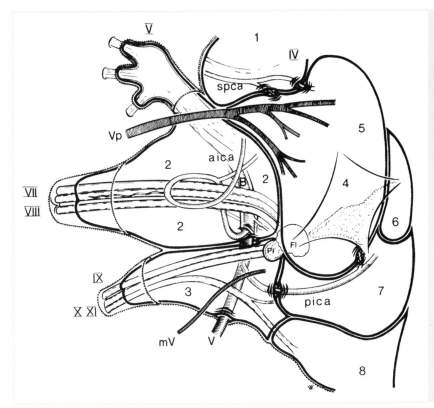

**Fig. 3.2** Schematic diagram showing the position and contents of the superior and inferior cerebellopontine cisterns. The inferior cerebellopontine angle cistern is also known as the lateral cerebellomedullary cistern. (Used with permission from Yasargil MG, ed. *Microneurosurgery Vol. 1*. New York, NY: Thieme; 1984:49.)

jugular fossa (JF). When the top of the jugular bulb extends cranial to the plane of the lateral semicircular canal, it is referred to as a high-riding jugular bulb. The right jugular bulb is larger than the left bulb in approximately 80% of people, as the primary drainage of blood from the brain is on the right side. The JF courses anteriorly, laterally, and inferiorly and is divided by a fibrous or a bony septum into two compartments, the larger posterolateral pars vascularis and the smaller anteromedial pars nervosa (▶ Fig. 3.4).

The pars vascularis contains the jugular bulb, part of the sigmoid sinus, CN 11, and CN 10 with its auricular branch (nerve of Arnold). The latter can be seen on thin section computed tomography (CT) traversing through the mastoid canaliculus on the lateral wall of the JF adjacent to the mastoid segment of the CN 7 (▶ Fig. 3.5). The pars nervosa contains the inferior petrosal sinus and CN 9 with its tympanic branch (nerve of Jacobson). The latter can be occasionally seen on CT within the inferior tympanic canaliculus (which also contains the inferior tympanic artery) at the level of the caroticojugular spine (▶ Fig. 3.6).[4]

# 3.2 Lesions of the Cerebellopontine Angle

The four most common CPA cistern lesions are the vestibular schwannoma (VS), meningioma, epidermoid cyst, and nonvestibular posterior fossa schwannoma. Together, they account for 75 to 98% of CPA cistern mass lesions.[5]

## 3.2.1 Vestibular Schwannoma

The VS is a benign slow-growing primary nerve sheath neoplasm that arises from the Schwann cells which wrap around CN 8 in the IAC. This tumor has no malignant potential. VS involves the superior vestibular division of CN 8 far more commonly than the cochlear division, and hence the name VS, which was officially recommended by the National Institutes of Health Consensus Developmental Panel in 1991.[6,7] Less favored terms are acoustic schwannoma or neurinoma.

VS accounts for 8 to 10% of all intracranial neoplasms and it is the most common CPA cistern mass accounting for 85 to 90% of the cases. It is also the second most common extra-axial mass in adults. Sporadic VS is the most commonly (> 90%) found lesion in patients with unilateral sensorineural hearing loss (SNHL). The incidence of sporadic VS is 0.2% across all imaging scans in asymptomatic patients. Mutations of the neurofibromatosis 2 (NF2) tumor suppressor gene is present in 60% of sporadic VS.

There is a female predominance of up to 2:1, especially for larger and more vascular tumors and pregnancy can potentially accelerate the clinical course. It has also been reported that purely intracanalicular tumors are more common in males.

The most common age of presentation is in the fourth to fifth decades of life and VSs more commonly affect Caucasians. When VS is present in young adults or children, or is associated with other lesions, a careful evaluation for other features of neurofibromatosis should be performed.

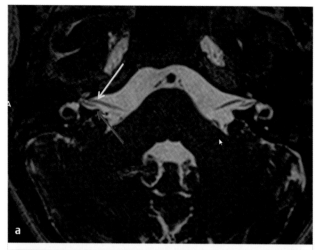

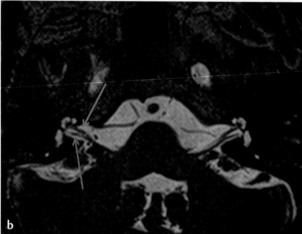

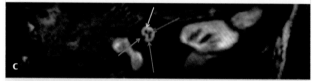

Fig. 3.3 High-resolution T2-weighted series through the cerebello-pontine angle. (a) Axial image shows the facial nerve (*yellow arrow*) situated anteriorly and superiorly. Adjacent to it is the superior division of the vestibular nerve (*red arrow*). (b) Axial slice at the level of the inferior internal auditory canal (IAC) showing the cochlear nerve (*green arrow*) anteriorly positioned and the inferior vestibular nerve (*blue arrow*) posteriorly positioned. (c) Sagittal reformat at the level of the IAC showing the relationship of the four nerves.

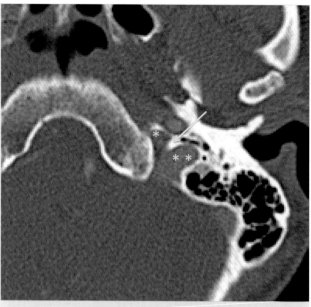

Fig. 3.4 High-resolution unenhanced axial CT image at the level of the jugular foramen. The jugular fossa is divided by a bony septum (*arrow*) into two compartments, the larger posterolateral pars vascularis (**) and the smaller anteromedially situated pars nervosa (*).

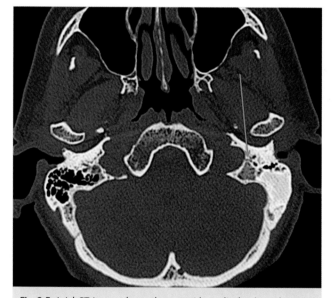

Fig. 3.5 Axial CT image shows the mastoid canaliculus (*arrow*) connecting the jugular fossa to the facial nerve canal.

The vestibular nerve has a transitional zone from oligoden-drocytes to Schwann cells at the porus acusticus. Therefore, most VSs arise inside the IAC, or near its opening, but they can then secondarily grow into the CPA cistern. Small VSs are usually entirely contained within the IAC.

The most common presenting symptom is a slowly progressive SNHL mainly affecting the perception of high-frequency sounds. Vertigo, tinnitus, and balance issues are uncommon (< 10%). Other symptoms can arise secondary to mass effect on the facial and trigeminal nerves, the brain stem, cerebellum, or fourth ventricle (obstructive hydrocephalus). Rarely, large lesions can present with subarachnoid hemorrhage. Brain stem–evoked response audiometry (BERA) is considered a sensitive preimaging test for diagnosis.[3,5,8,9]

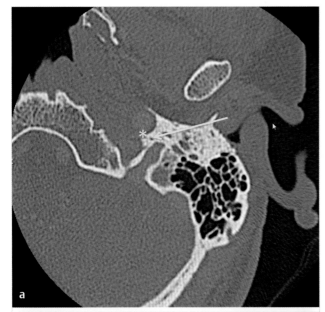

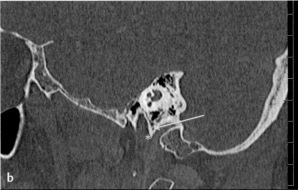

**Fig. 3.6** (**a,b**) High-resolution axial CT of the left temporal bone at the level of the jugular fossa. The tympanic branch of the glossopharyngeal nerve (nerve of Jacobson) travels within the inferior tympanic canaliculus (*arrow*). The inferior tympanic artery also travels within this canal. The caroticojugular spine is delineated by the *asterisk*.

## Imaging

There is no consensus on a size grading scale for VS, but some have adopted the following[10]:

- *Small VS*: Limited to the IAC with less than 1 cm extension into the CPA cistern.
- *Medium VS*: 1 to 2 cm sized cisternal component.
- *Large VS*: 2 to 4 cm sized cisternal component.
- *Giant VS*: Greater than 4 cm sized cisternal component.

Small VS or those that are completely intracanalicular can easily be missed on routine CT and magnetic resonance imaging (MRI) of the brain. When VS is suspected, a high-resolution temporal bone CT or, more preferably, a MRI that includes focused high-resolution imaging of the IAC and posterior fossa should be performed preferably with contrast enhancement.

The imaging features of VS reflect the presence of the two types of cellular regions present within schwannomas. Antoni A regions are the highly cellular dense regions which forms palisades histologically. This is reflected on imaging as a solid and homogenously enhancing tumor. The Antoni B regions are hypocellular with cells separated in a reticulated myxoid matrix. On imaging, this gives rise to areas of cystic change in the VS.

CT features of VS are variable. Small intracanalicular lesions may not be visible unless they expand or remodel the bony margins of the IAC. Larger lesions may be visible once they extend into the CPA cistern and cause mass effect upon the adjacent brain (▶ Fig. 3.7). Valvassori observed an abnormal IAC on CT in 78% of pathologically proven VS. The difference between the abnormal and the normal IAC was found to be a canal height disparity (>2 mm on the affected side), a shorter posterior wall of the canal (>3 mm on the affected side), and a downward displacement of the crista falciformis.[11]

Erosion and enlargement/flaring of the porous acusticus can be seen to occur in 70 to 90% of VS with or without a CPA cisternal soft-tissue component.[12]

MRI is generally the best imaging test for the assessment of VS. A high-resolution T2-weighted sequence can detect lesions as small as 0.06 cm.[13] Small VSs appear as a round or funnel-shaped

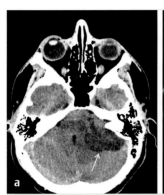
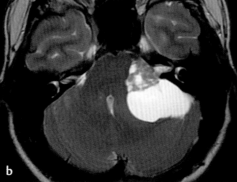
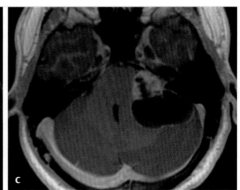

**Fig. 3.7** (**a**) Contrast CT demonstrates a heterogeneous mass in the left cerebellopontine angle (CPA; *arrow*) that is causing mass effect on the adjacent brain parenchyma. (**b**) Axial T2-weighted MRI demonstrates a mixed solid and cystic left cerebellopontine angle mass with extension into the internal auditory canal (IAC). (**c**) Axial T1-weighted postgadolinium image demonstrates enhancement of the solid component and extension into the left IAC.

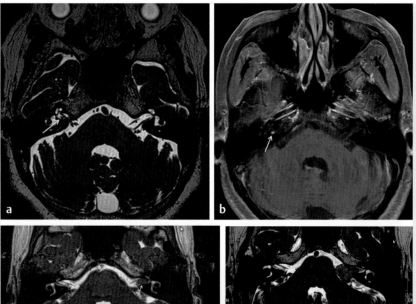

**Fig. 3.8** (a) Axial high-resolution T2-weighted MRI shows a 1- to 2-mm rounded lesion (*arrow*) in the right internal auditory canal (IAC) compatible with a small VS. (b) Fat-saturated axial T1-weighted postgadolinium demonstrates nodular enhancement of the lesion (*arrow*). (c) High-resolution MRI T2-weighted image of a larger 8-mm elongated lesion filling left IAC in keeping with a VS (*arrow*). (d) Axial high-resolution MRI T2-weighted image sequence of the same patient as in (c). This scan was taken 6 years later showing interval growth and the extension of the lesion into the cerebellopontine angle cistern with secondary mass effect on the left pons/middle cerebellar peduncle.

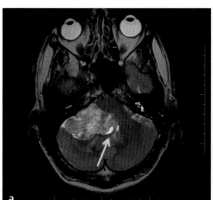
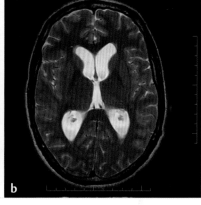

**Fig. 3.9** (a) Axial T2-weighted image of a very large VS (*arrow*) causing mass effect upon the adjacent cerebellum. There is marked compression of the fourth ventricle. The mass also forms acute angles to the posterior cisternal face of the petrous bone. (b) Axial image at a level more superiorly demonstrates secondary obstructive hydrocephalous as a result of the fourth ventricular compression.

mass centered in the long axis of the IAC. Larger VSs are seen as a well-marginated spherical, ovoid, or lobulated CPA cistern mass with a convex medial margin and extension into a widened porous (▶ Fig. 3.8). Giant VS may not have an intracanalicular component. The cisternal component of larger VS typically forms an acute angle with the petrous bone in 85% of cases (▶ Fig. 3.9).

On T1-weighted images, VSs are isointense to gray matter. On T2-weighted images, VSs are usually hyperintense. An arachnoid cyst or trapped CSF can be associated with 0.5% of cases. A potential explanation for this is the trabeculae in the CPA cistern that may thicken and entrap CSF or accumulate hypertonic fluid rich in protein that is excreted from the surface of the tumor.[2,14]

Use of contrast enhancement on MRI can help the detection of VS approach 100% sensitivity.[15] This is best accomplished with the use of T1-weighted, fat-suppressed sequences. Small lesions will homogeneously enhance, while larger VSs appear heterogeneous, and demonstrate degenerative changes with

cystic regions (15%) and occasional hemorrhage (0.5%), thrombosis, and rarely fatty degeneration.

With larger VS, it is important to assess the degree of mass effect on the brain stem and cerebellar peduncle, the presence of perilesional edema, and the development of obstructive hydrocephalus secondary to compression on the fourth ventricle (▶ Fig. 3.9). Such findings are features that help identify patients who should be directed toward surgical decompression. When contrast MRI is used, a noncontrast (precontrast) fat-suppressed sequence should be routinely obtained to assess for areas of high signal intensity that reflect the presence of tumoral fat or hemorrhage. Such an inherent high T1 signal can also falsely mimic enhancement on the postcontrast sequences.

There are certain MRI features that are important to note on follow-up studies as they may predict a higher risk for hearing loss:

- A growth rate more than 2.5 mm/year is associated with a doubling of the risk of hearing loss.[16]

- Initial size has no bearing on the development of hearing loss. Size does not correlate with symptomatology and does not predict growth rate.
- The presence of blood or fibrosis in the tumor may lead to vestibulocochlear damage and hearing loss. This is best evaluated on a T2* gradient sequence which will show marked reduction in signal intensity or "blooming."[16]
- Impaction of tumor at the cochlear aperture.[8] Tumors that fill the IAC have a worse prognosis for hearing preservation with surgery or stereotactic radiosurgery (SRS)/radiotherapy.

## Imaging of VS post–radiation therapy

Radiation therapy is one potential treatment option for VS. In a series of 86 patients by Nakamura,[17] three patterns of contrast change were observed:

1. Transient loss of contrast, 84%.
2. Continuous increase in enhancement, 5%.
3. No change in the pattern of enhancement, 11%.

There was no significant correlation between change in tumor volume and the degree of enhancement. An increase in T2 signal intensity in the adjacent brain stem and cerebellum was noted, reflecting the presence of edema. No correlation between radiation dose, tumor size, and the T2 signal changes was found.

In another series of 89 patients by Norén et al,[18] with 12 months of follow-up after radiosurgery, size changes were noted as follows; 73% remained stable, 22% shrunk, and 3% grew. Seventy-nine percent of patients lost their central enhancement 5 to 15 months post–radiation therapy and some regained central enhancement after a period of time. Enhancement in the adjacent parenchyma was also noted to occur. Nine percent had an increase in T2 signal in the adjacent parenchyma which did not correspond with focal neurological deficits. Delayed trigeminal enhancement was also noted.

It should also be noted that for some partially resected or radiated VSs, such procedures can lead to a shedding of proteins from the tumor, which can result in communicating hydrocephalus in about 4% of cases.

For follow-up, an annual CT or MR is often performed to monitor tumor growth. There is no relation between the initial VS size and subsequent growth rate. If there is a family history of NF2, screening with MRI of family members is recommended.[2,3,5,8,9]

Some important findings to assess on imaging include the following:

- Size—especially, the volume of tumor.
- Location—intracanalicular, CPA cistern, extension to tentorial hiatus, the jugular foramen or beyond.
- Local mass effect—cerebellar, brain stem, edema, CNs, arteries, and veins.
- Location of the jugular bulb.
- Dominance of the transverse sigmoid sinuses.
- Presence or absence of hydrocephalus.
- Degree on tumor extension into the IAC.
- Presence of enhancement along the facial nerve canal or the geniculate ganglion as this would suggest the presence of a facial nerve schwannoma rather than a VS.

The size of the CPA component of VS is especially important as it will affect the method of treatment—namely, surgery versus radiation treatment. Surgery is usually preferred if the tumor is larger than 2.5 to 3.0 cm within the CPA, or if there is compression on the brainstem, brainstem edema, or obstructive hydrocephalus. Lesions that do not extend to the distal end of the IAC have a better prognosis for hearing preservation at surgery. This is primarily because there is a better chance that the blood supply, which is end-organ arterial (labyrinthine and cochlear arteries), can be preserved during surgery. Also, tumors that do not extend to the very distal end of the IAC will help limit the degree of dissection required for tumor exposure and removal.

Before deciding upon a translabyrinthine versus retrosigmoid (suboccipital) approach, it is important to know the status of the sigmoid sinus and jugular bulb. Surgeons want an unencumbered and thus easier route of access to the region. The decision on preferred surgical approach is more often surgeon related than related to patient or tumor factors. However, if the jugular bulb is particularly high and the sigmoid on the ipsilateral side is dominant, this may limit the transtemporal approaches and favor a retrosigmoid route. On the other hand, larger lesions may also require more bone exposure to access the superior and inferior extensions of the lesion, something that is less limited via the retrosigmoid access.

## Prognosis and Treatment

Seventy-five percent of VSs grow slowly, 10% grow rapidly (≥ 1 cm/year), and 15% grow very slowly. If left untreated, hearing loss followed by symptoms related to local mass effect will progress slowly over time. If hydrocephalus or intratumoral hemorrhage occurs, clinical deterioration can be rapid. Sudden irreversible, hearing loss can occur even in patients with small tumors. Patients with NF2 typically have worse outcomes.

Treatment options include monitored observation, surgery, stereotactic single fraction radiosurgery (SRS), and fractionated stereotactic radiotherapy (SRT). The size of the lesion, age of the patient, comorbidities, and whether hearing is considered serviceable are the main patient-related factors affecting the choice of treatment.

In a study by Hajioff et al[19] that followed 72 patients for a minimum of 10-year follow-up, it was noted that when a tumor reaches the CPA a growth rate of approximately 1 to 2 mm/year in cross-sectional diameter was observed. Within the IAC, growth rates are generally less at 0.5 mm/year. Tumor growth rate in a subset of 19 patients with intracanalicular tumor was 0 mm/year. In the group with CPA extension less than 2 cm, the growth rate was 1 to 2 mm/year. About 15% of patients had some regression in the size of their tumor over this time frame. Most experts agree that watching a tumor until it reaches a size of approximately 2 cm within the CPA is reasonable. Once greater than 2 cm, some active treatment option could be considered (either microsurgical removal or SRS). However, others suggest intervention when growth is observed on at least on two serial scans. Maximal tumor dimension is an important consideration for surgery, given that the incidence of facial nerve paralysis at surgery increases from 5%, if the tumor is less than 2 cm, to 10 to 15% if larger than 2 cm but still less than 3 cm if total tumor removal is performed.

Tumor size is also important in radiation decision making. The decision for SRS versus fractionated radiosurgery is largely dependent on tumor maximal diameter. Typically for tumors less than 2 to 3 cm, single fraction SRS can be delivered and most often with a total dose of 12- to 13-Gy depending on the histology of the tumor and anatomic proximity to critical organs-at-risk. For larger tumors, fractionated SRT is delivered with a total dose of 45 to 54 Gy in 1.8 to 2.0 Gy per day fractions over 5 to 6 weeks. This approach maximizes safety while being efficacious in terms of long-term local tumor control. With either modality, the long-term local control rates do not significantly differ and range from 80 to 90% at 10 years. For larger tumors, fractionated stereotactic radiation is safer. More recently, hypofractionated SRS delivering typically 25 Gy in five fractions is emerging as a means to treat larger tumors (3–4 cm). This requires a week of treatment as opposed to 5 to 6 weeks which is much more convenient for patients. For tumors larger than 4 cm, 5 to 6 weeks of fractionated SRT is recommended.

A hybrid approach is increasingly being practiced for large tumors needing surgery. The surgical aim is to debulk the tumor and decompress the brainstem and brain parenchyma with a planned tumor residual being left in vicinity of the facial nerve. This residual can then be observed and/or treated upfront postoperatively with radiation. The aim of this approach is to minimize the chance of facial nerve damage that can be debilitating to patients.

For those patients in whom surgery is being contemplated, the degree of hearing loss and the full extent of VS are important factors. If hearing preservation is of the utmost importance, a middle cranial fossa (only for intracanalicular tumors) or retrosigmoid/suboccipital approach is favored. The middle cranial fossa approach is best for intracanalicular VS situated more laterally in the IAC. A retrosigmoid approach is considered when there is a significant cisternal or medial IAC component. The translabyrinthine approach is used when there is already poor hearing or the mass is considered so large that hearing sacrifice is unavoidable.

Specific to radiosurgery, positive predictors for hearing and facial nerve preservation post-SRS include tumor size (< 5 cm³), younger than 60 years, radiation dose less than 13 Gy, and dose to the cochlea (radiation plans that expose the cochlea to mean doses below 4–8 Gy have higher rates of hearing preservation). There is debate in the radiation treatment for patients with baseline hearing. The decision centers on whether hearing can be preserved maximally with fractionated SRT versus SRS due to the benefits of fractionation. This is because of the long-term late effects of radiation such as hearing damage, which are influenced by the dose per fraction. Currently, there are no conclusive data on this subject and future clinical trials will be needed to resolve these issues.

## 3.2.2 Facial Nerve Schwannoma

Facial nerve schwannomas can involve any or multiple segments of the facial nerve. This is a rare tumor and can be associated with NF2. There is no gender predilection and the age of presentation is usually in the fifth decade of life.

The geniculate ganglion is the most commonly affected site followed by the labyrinthine and then the CPA–IAC portion of the nerve. Involvement of the intraparotid segment is rare. Multisegment involvement is common.

Fifty percent of the facial nerve schwannomas are asymptomatic. In the other 50% of the cases, the most common presentation is facial nerve paralysis which usually takes years to develop. This is likely related to the fact that schwannomas compress and do not invade the nerve. Symptoms will also depend on the segment involved. When the tumor is situated in the IAC or CPA, SNHL can be the presenting symptom due to secondary mass effect on the thinly myelinated sensory fibers of CN 8 which are more vulnerable to compression compared to the more thickly myelinated motor fibers of CN 7.

Tumors involving the geniculate ganglion are often clinically silent. However, with continued growth, the mass can bulge into the middle cranial fossa and cause local mass effect upon the brain; it can also involve the greater superficial petrosal nerve resulting in a loss of lacrimation. These tumors may also cause hyperacusis due to involvement of the stapedial nerve and paralysis of the stapedius muscle. Tumors involving the tympanic segment of the nerve can give rise to conductive hearing loss due to interference with the ossicular chain. Facial schwannomas that arise in the mastoid segment are likely to cause facial palsy as the canal is a small, limited, and of fixed volume. Other symptoms include vertigo and hemifacial spasm. On occasion, large tumors involving the stylomastoid foramen can present as painless neck mass.[2,5]

As a facial nerve schwannoma can give rise to facial paralysis, it is important to differentiate it from idiopathic facial nerve palsy (Bell's palsy). Patients with a Bell's palsy typically have an acute onset and symptoms resolve within approximately 2 months. In those patients with history of progressive facial nerve paralysis beyond 3 weeks, absence of recovery after 6 months, or ipsilateral recurrence, a facial nerve schwannoma would be a consideration. Differentiation of other lesions affecting the facial nerve, such as autoimmune or viral diseases, is also necessary and this is most often investigated with imaging studies.

## Imaging

A classic appearance on CT is an IAC mass with associated widening of the canal, thus mimicking a VS. However, careful assessment will show enlargement of the labyrinthine portion of the facial nerve as the schwannoma follows the natural course of the facial nerve through the fallopian canal. Enlargement of the geniculate ganglion may also be seen (▶ Fig. 3.10). MRI features will parallel those on CT, such as, enlargement and enhancement of the facial nerve and geniculate ganglion (▶ Fig. 3.11).

Facial schwannoma can also present as a posterior middle cranial fossa mass and the imaging clue would be the presence of contiguous extension toward the geniculate ganglion and or other segments of the facial nerve (▶ Fig. 3.12).

Care must be taken when assessing the facial nerve for enhancement as normal physiologic enhancement can be present along portions of the nerve. The normal facial nerve can demonstrate some enhancement on MRI in up to 76% of examinations, and in 69% of cases this can be asymmetric. This has been attributed to the presence of the normal circumneural facial arteriovenous plexus. Enhancement can be present in all

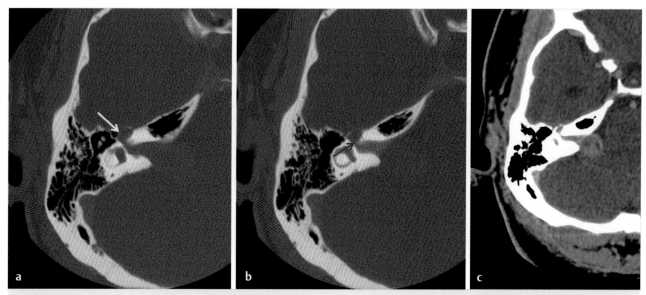

**Fig. 3.10** Axial high-resolution enhanced CT of the right temporal bones (**a**), in bone window (**b**), and in soft-tissue window (**c**) showing a widening of the right geniculate ganglion (*yellow arrow*; **a**) and labyrinthine (*red arrow*; **b**) portion of the facial nerve. (**c**) An enhancing mass widens the internal auditory canal and bulges into the cerebellopontine angle cistern.

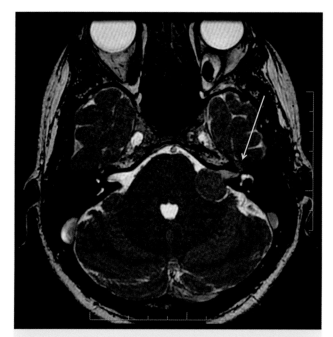

**Fig. 3.11** Axial T2 high-resolution FIESTA sequence shows a large cerebellopontine angle mass that extends into the internal auditory canal. The enlargement of the geniculate ganglion (*arrow*) is compatible with this mass being a facial schwannoma.

segments except the cisternal, canalicular (IAC) portions and extracranial segment beyond the stylomastoid foramen.[4,20] These latter portions normally do not enhance.

Some pathology that can mimic a facial nerve schwannoma includes a persistent stapedial artery which will enlarge the facial tympanic canal and an arachnoid diverticulum which may enlarge the geniculate ganglion.

Critical imaging features to assess and report are the portion(s) of the facial nerve that are involved, whether the tumor extends into the IAC, and if there is any involvement of the inner ear.

## Prognosis and Treatment

Watchful waiting is one approach as some facial nerve schwannomas may not grow. Intervention is considered once there is facial nerve paresis or other symptoms. Radiosurgery or fractionated radiotherapy will have a good chance of preserving facial nerve function.

Since surgery requires facial nerve grafting, the best result obtainable would result in a House-Brackmann (HB) grade 3 score (moderate dysfunction, noticeable asymmetry at rest, and complete eye closure with effort). This degree of facial nerve outcome is often of significant concern to the patient.

The surgical goal is complete tumor resection with preservation of hearing and restoration of facial nerve function by restoring the continuity of the nerve by either end-to-end anastomosis or cable grafting. Since surgery may actually worsen the symptoms,[2,5,8] consideration must be given to all potential treatment modalities and in particular radiation therapy.

If a patient develops an acute facial paralysis that does not improve over 6 months and the tumor is located within the horizontal or vertical segments of the facial nerve in the middle ear/mastoid segments, respectively, this may make surgical treatment more urgent. If, on clinical follow-up, the facial function deteriorates to a greater than House Brackmann grade 3/6 appearance, then surgery would more than likely be suggested. This is on the basis that a facial hypoglossal nerve anastomosis would at best provide a grade 3/6 appearance to facial function. The issue for the surgeon to consider is whether surgical decompression therapy would be a reasonable approach to alleviate pressure from the facial nerve and allow the tumor to expand.

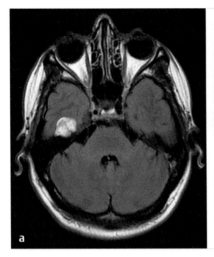 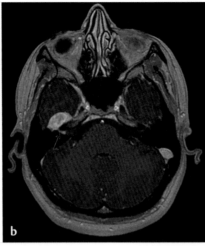

**Fig. 3.12** (a) Axial FLAIR sequence shows a hyperintense extra-axial mass in the right posterior middle cranial fossa. (b) Axial postgadolinium T1-weighted sequence shows enhancement of the mass and contiguous enhancement and labyrinthine segment (*arrow*) of the facial nerve. The large lobulated mass is the epicenter of the facial schwannoma within the geniculate ganglion.

The main reasons to avoid surgical resection are the presence of significant medical comorbidities, or the fact that a resection will definitely result in permanent total facial nerve paralysis (HB grade 6/6). This latter outcome may cause many patients to elect to avoid surgery.

SRS, and more often fractionated SRT (45–54 Gy over 5–6 weeks), is a treatment option for these patients. Although limited literature exists, it does not have the adverse event profile of permanent facial nerve palsy and this treatment can result in long-term local tumor control.

### 3.2.3 Schwannomas along the Carotid Sheath

Schwannomas can arise within the carotid sheath (CS) anywhere from the level of the skull base to above the aortic arch. CNs that can be involved include CNs 9, 10, and 11. Medial to the CS and in front of flexure muscles of the cervical spine are the sympathetic chain and superior sympathetic ganglion. The proximity to the CS structures warrants their inclusion in this discussion.

Schwannomas usually arise in otherwise healthy individuals. The literature is confusing as some authors mention a male predominance,[9] while others do not describe any such gender predilection.[21] The affected age range can be broad ranging from 18 to 63 years. CS schwannomas can also be associated with NF2.

The suprahyoid location of these tumors is much more common than an infrahyoid location. Seventeen percent to 25% of the lesions occur in the retrostyloid parapharyngeal space (PPS) with the most common nerves of origin in descending order being the vagus > glossopharyngeal > superior sympathetic chain.

Small lesions are rarely symptomatic. Larger lesions typically present as a painless palpable neck mass or posterolateral pharyngeal wall mass at the level of the naso- or oropharynx. The infrahyoid lesions can present as an anterolateral neck mass. Large lesions can also have mass effect and result in dysphagia, IJV occlusion, Horner's syndrome, sleep apnea, or a sore throat.

Specific nerve palsies or deficits can occur and be a clue to the nerve of origin:

- *Vagal schwannomas*: Hoarseness from vocal cord paralysis and pain radiating to the ear and eye, angle of mandible and tonsillar region.
- *Glossopharyngeal schwannomas*: Paralysis of the ipsilateral stylopharyngeus muscle (this muscle helps elevate the larynx and expand the pharynx during swallowing) which can lead to some impairment of swallowing and speech, loss of taste in the posterior one-third of tongue, loss of temperature, touch and deep sensation of the base of tongue, Eustachian tube, pharynx and tonsil, and abnormal gag reflexes.
- *Accessory nerve schwannomas*: Downward and lateral rotation of the scapula and shoulder droop from atrophy of the trapezius and sternocleidomastoid muscles with compensatory hypertrophy of the ipsilateral levator scapulae muscle in chronic cases. This is similar to the shoulder drop syndrome that can follow a radical neck dissection.

### Imaging

Schwannomas arising within the CS appear as ellipsoid, smoothly marginated masses with either uniform enhancement or cystic areas. Imaging features are similar to all other schwannomas. When they arise within the JF, the margins of the surrounding bone are smoothly widened.

The internal carotid artery (ICA) and IJV can be displaced by the schwannoma and the direction of carotid displacement may also help predict the likely nerve of origin. As the vagus nerve is posterior to the ICA within the CS, vagal schwannomas will displace the ICA anteriorly and usually medially while displacing the IJV posteriorly and laterally (splay common carotid artery or ICA away from IJV; ▶ Fig. 3.13, ▶ Fig. 3.14).

Alternatively, since the superior sympathetic chain is situated medial to the CS, sympathetic chain schwannomas will typically displace all the vessels together anterolaterally. Such sympathetic schwannomas can also slip between the CS and pharyngeal wall and result in posterior displacement of the ICA (▶ Fig. 3.15). With the latter form of displacement, the appearance could mimic that of a salivary gland tumor arising either from the deep parotid lobe or originating primarily

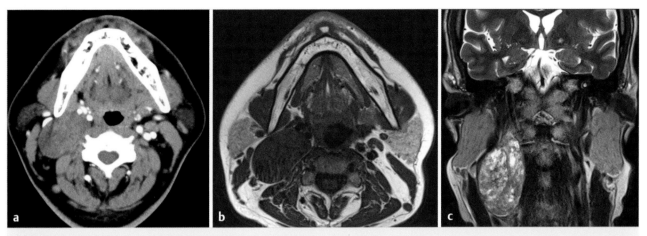

Fig. 3.13 (a) Axial enhanced CT, (b) axial T1-weighted image, and (c) coronal T2-weighted image demonstrating a fusiform minimally enhancing vagal schwannoma located in the right carotid space (poststyloid parapharyngeal space). There is displacement of the internal carotid artery anteriorly and medially and of the IJV laterally.

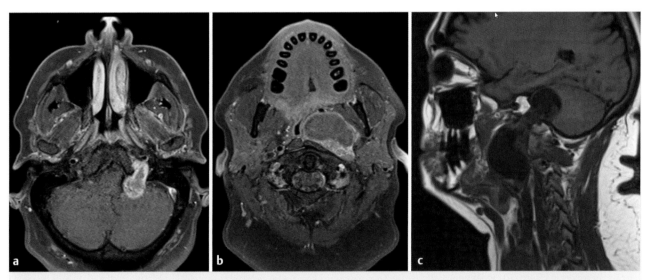

Fig. 3.14 (a,b) Contrast-enhanced T1-weighted images demonstrate a left vagal schwannoma in the left carotid space that displaces the left internal carotid artery anteriorly and medially. The mass demonstrates intracranial extension through the jugular foramen. (c) Sagittal T1-weighted image shows the mass to be both cystic and solid with protrusion through the jugular foramen into the posterior fossa.

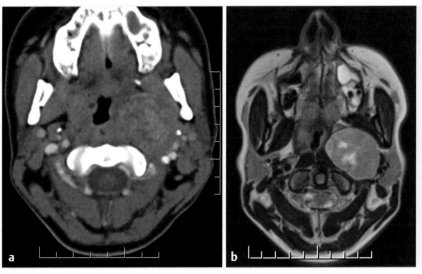

Fig. 3.15 Contrast-enhanced axial CT (a) and axial T2-weighted (b) images of a sympathetic chain schwannoma. This well-marginated minimally enhancing lesion is displacing the carotid and jugular vessels posteriorly.

within the prestyloid PPS from extraparotid minor salivary cells.[2,5,9]

Important imaging findings to communicate to the clinician include whether the schwannoma is in intimate contact with the carotid artery and the rate of growth of the tumor over serial scans. Tumor intimacy with the common or ICAs is important as surgery may result in arterial injury and potential dissection and secondary ischemic/thromboembolic events. The degree of intracranial extension though the jugular foramen is also important to note if surgery is contemplated. Typically, lesions with more than 1.5 cm of intracranial extension may necessitate a neurosurgical approach from above to gain superior access and control of the lesion.

## Prognosis and Treatment

A watch-and-wait approach is a consideration with CS schwannomas.

Ultimately, experienced head and neck surgeons would resect a vagal schwannoma if there is 30 to 40% growth in size over 3 to 4 years, if there is compression on other CNs with progressive neurological symptoms, or if there is evidence of malignant transformation. Removal of a nerve sheath tumor generally causes a nerve palsy of the involved nerve if it has not occurred already from the tumor. The worst feared intraoperative complications are stroke related to injury of the carotid arteries and associated lower CN palsies that could result in significant comorbidities such as chronic aspiration and hoarseness.

Fractionated SRT is a treatment option for these patients. Although limited literature is available, it does not have the adverse event profile of surgery and can yield long-term local tumor control.

# 3.2.4 Paraganglioma (Glomus): Glomus Jugulare and Vagale

Paragangliomas are benign, slow growing, highly vascularized lesions originating from paraganglionic tissue of the extra-adrenal nonchromaffin chemotactic cells which are distributed around the tympanic portion of the facial nerve, the jugular foramen, within the parapharyngeal portion of the vagus nerve and in the carotid body. These latter tumors are in an intimate relationship to the vagus nerve. Other names for these lesions include chemodectoma and glomus tumor. However, according to Glenner and Grimley,[22] paraganglioma is the most appropriate name for these lesions. Paragangliomas have the potential for local invasion and can frequently invade the skull base with resulting intracranial extradural extension. These tumors rarely metastasize.

Paragangliomas in the neck are named according to their site of origin:

- *Glomus jugulare*: Situated at the level of the jugular bulb and skull base, arising from the tympanic branch of the glossopharyngeal nerve (nerve of Jacobson), or the auricular branch of the vagus nerve (nerve of Arnold).
- *Glomus tympanicum*: Situated in the tympanic cavity and mastoid, along the course of Jacobson's nerve.
- *Glomus jugulotympanicum*: Those lesions span both the middle ear and jugular foramen.
- *Glomus vagale*: From the intravagal paraganglia at or below the skull base level and primarily parapharyngeal in location.

- *Carotid body tumor*: Arising from the carotid body at the carotid bifurcation.

In this section, the glomus jugulare/jugulotympanicum and vagale tumors will be discussed.

The incidence of paragangliomas is 1 per 1.3 million people per year and they are significantly more common in females with a male-to-female ratio of 3–4:1. Two-thirds of patients at the time of presentation are in their fourth to sixth decades of life. These lesions can be bilateral (2%) or multifocal (10%), with the most common association being a jugulare/jugulotympanicum paraganglioma and an ipsilateral carotid body tumor. Paragangliomas can also be familial, with a nearly 30% incidence of multiple lesions. The glomus jugulare/jugulotympanicum is the second most common tumor involving the temporal bone after VS. Ten percent of cases are associated with other entities such as medullary thyroid carcinoma, islet cell, or nonendocrine tumors of mesodermal origin, such as pulmonary chondroma and gastric leiomyosarcoma.[23]

The average time from symptom onset to diagnosis is 3 to 6 years. Glomus jugulare and tympanicum/jugulotympanicum are usually initially asymptomatic. When symptomatic, the presenting symptom depends on the location and extent of the tumor and the compression of surrounding neural structures. Very rarely, large paragangliomas can secrete norepinephrine or, less often, adrenocorticotropic hormone, serotonin, calcitonin, or dopamine. However, only 1 to 3% of these secreting paragangliomas present with clinical symptoms because the majority secrete low levels of hormones.[2,23]

Glomus jugulotympanicum can grow laterally to produce otologic symptoms (conductive hearing loss, pulsatile tinnitus, or retrotympanic mass) or can grow medially and extend further into the jugular foramen and cause jugular foramen syndrome (Vernet's syndrome) consisting of CNs 9 to 11 deficits. The incidence of lower CN palsies is 35% with CN 10 palsy being the most common (61%)—CN 7 (45%), CN 11 (52%), CN 9 (48%)—and CN 12 being the least common. Compression of CN 12 will give rise to Collet-Sicard syndrome, which consists of unilateral CN 9, 10, 11, and 12 palsies. It is distinguished from Villaret's syndrome by lack of sympathetic involvement.[24,25]

Involvement of CN 7 in the mastoid portion of the temporal bone can give rise to a facial palsy. Sympathetic chain involvement in the carotid canal can result in a Horner's syndrome. Cavernous sinus extension will result in a cavernous sinus syndromes including ophthalmoplegia, diplopia (which could be acute or slowly progressive in onset and can be painful), and exophthalmos.[26,27]

Paragangliomas can also extend into the posterior fossa resulting in mass effect upon the brain stem/cerebellum and result in obstructive hydrocephalus.

## Imaging

On CT, a glomus jugulare is usually seen as an enhancing mass centered in the JF that can cause irregular demineralization (moth-eaten appearance) and expansion of the margins of the JF and caroticojugular spine (▶ Fig. 3.16). Actual vessels can occasionally be seen within the tumor. This is in contrast to schwannomas which are well-circumscribed lesions, less vascular, and frequently demonstrate cystic degeneration without

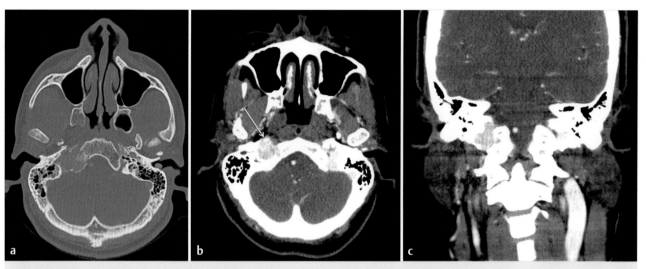

Fig. 3.16 Axial CT bone window (a) image of a right glomus jugulare tumor. There is expansion and permeative erosion of the jugular foramen. Axial (b) and coronal (c) soft-tissue window images of another patient with a right glomus jugulare tumor. The lesion shows avid enhancement. The axial image (b) also shows intimate contact with the right internal carotid artery (arrow).

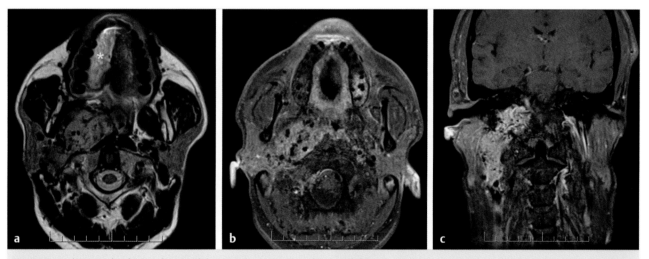

Fig. 3.17 Axial T2-weighted (a) and postgadolinium-enhanced T1-weighted axial (b) and coronal (c) images of a right glomus vagale tumor. The prominent flow voids are noted throughout the lesion. This tumor extends up into the jugular fossa. Note the presence of ipsilateral tongue fatty atrophy (asterisk; a) secondary to mass effect upon the hypoglossal nerve.

bone destruction. A glomus vagale tumor will also appear as a vascular mass but will be positioned primarily in the poststyloid PPS, below the skull base. A glomus vagale tumor, however, can also grow to extend up into the JF (▶ Fig. 3.17).

Glomus tympanicum tumors classically appears as a well-defined enhancing soft-tissue mass situated over the cochlear promontory along the course of Jacobson's nerve (▶ Fig. 3.18). By definition, they are confined to the middle ear cavity.

A glomus jugulotympanicum is a glomus jugulare that has extended into the middle ear cavity (▶ Fig. 3.19, ▶ Fig. 3.20). These lesions tend to grow along the planes of least resistance (fissures, air cell tracts, vascular channels, and foramina). The most common location of soft-tissue extension is along the Jacobson' and Arnold's nerves (in the adventitia of the jugular bulb, the inferior tympanic canaliculus, cochlear promontory, mastoid canaliculus, and the mastoid facial nerve canal). When

large, these lesions can also descend intraluminally through the jugular vein or along the CS.

MRI of paragangliomas reveals an avidly enhancing lesion that may demonstrate a classic salt-and-pepper appearance on T1-weighted imaging (▶ Fig. 3.21). The high-signal "salt" foci correspond to foci of subacute hemorrhage and the dark "pepper" foci represent vascular flow voids. However, the microvascular variety of these tumors may not always demonstrate vascular flow voids and thus can have a tumor imaging morphology similar to a vagal schwannoma.

On catheter angiogram, paragangliomas are characteristically hypervascular with a tumor blush which is coarser than a meningioma but less than that of an AVM. The most common feeders are branches of the ascending pharyngeal artery. The larger the tumor, the more arterial recruitment from the external or ICAs is likely to arise.

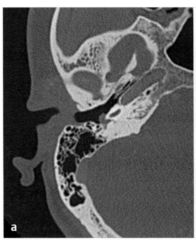
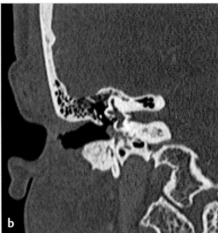

**Fig. 3.18** Axial (**a**) and coronal (**b**) CT images of a right glomus tympanicum. The lesion appears as a lobulated mass centered on the cochlear promontory.

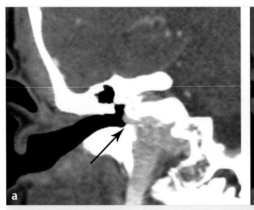
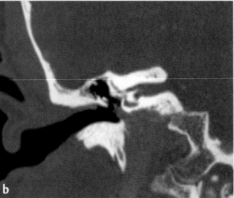
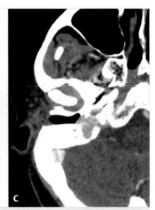

**Fig. 3.19** Contrast-enhanced coronal soft-tissue (**a**), bone window (**b**), and axial (**c**) CT images of a right glomus jugulotympanicum tumor. The lesion is primarily situated in the jugular fossa which has subtle bony erosion and expansion. The enhancing mass (*arrow*; **a**) has a small contiguous enhancing focus that extends into the hypotympanum.

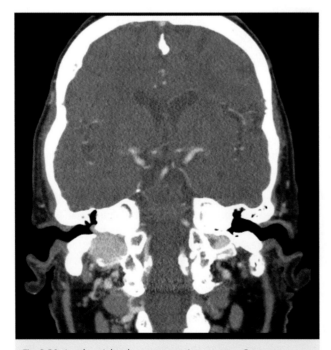

**Fig. 3.20** Another right glomus tympanicum tumor. Contrast-enhanced coronal CT shows a large mass within the jugular fossa with a small superolateral extension into the middle ear.

Indium-111 octreotide scanning is a useful adjuvant test to help detect multicentric, metastatic, or recurrent tumor and has greater sensitivity than iodine-123-metaiodobenzylguanidine.

Important imaging findings to communicate to the clinician includes the presence of multiple lesions, the intracranial and extracranial extent of the lesion (▸ Fig. 3.22), the presence of jugular bulb or sigmoid sinus involvement (▸ Fig. 3.23), erosion into the petrous bone (▸ Fig. 3.24) and involvement of the otic capsule and fallopian canal, and whether the carotid artery is intimately involved by the tumor (▸ Fig. 3.25). The rate of tumor growth over serial scans is also important.

For those patients who undergo radiation therapy, a glomus will not resolve completely. On CT, bone demineralization and erosions will persist. On MR, the following findings indicate local control:

- Stabilization or reduction in size.
- Decreased enhancement.
- Diminished flow voids.
- Reduced T2 signal intensity signifying the presence of fibrosis.[5,9]

## Prognosis and Treatment

Experienced skull base surgeons usually follow a wait-and-scan approach for glomus tumors that involve the skull base where

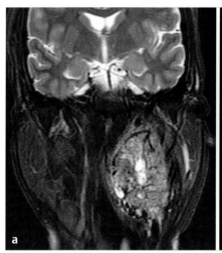
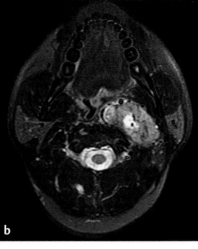

**Fig. 3.21** Coronal (**a**) and axial (**b**) T2-weighted images of a large left glomus vagale demonstrating multiple black flow voids ("pepper") and bright internal foci of thrombus ("salt").

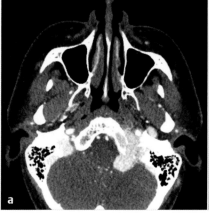
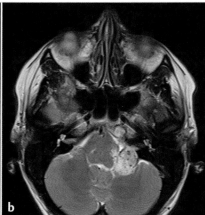

**Fig. 3.22** Contrast-enhanced axial CT (**a**) and a T2-weighted MRI (**b**) of a large left glomus jugulare tumor that has significant intracranial extension into the posterior fossa with mass effect upon the cerebellum and brain stem.

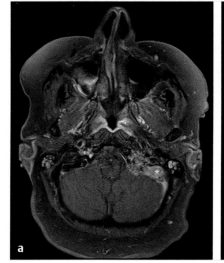
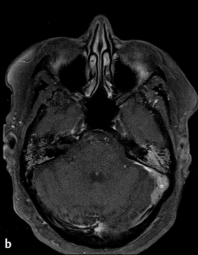

**Fig. 3.23** (**a,b**) Gadolinium-enhanced axial T1-weighted images of a left glomus jugulare. The heterogeneous tumor is abutting the adjacent cerebellum. There is also extension of tumor into the left sigmoid dural sinus (*asterisks*).

lower CN function is still intact. For isolated glomus tympanicum, surgery is usually done depending on the age of patients and often in an attempt to control the pulsatile tinnitus they experience. Imaging to determine the full extent of a glomus tympanicum tumor is very important in the surgical decision-making process.

Intervention is also considered for a rapidly growing tumor or if the tumor has already caused lower CN palsies. In the latter instance, there would be little further morbidity to swallowing or speaking from tumor resection. There, however, could be morbidity from facial nerve weakness/paralysis if the nerve was irreparably injured. The surgical risk could also include

The main reasons to avoid surgical resection are the presence of significant patient comorbidities or a patient's refusal to accept the potential comorbidities caused by surgery as mentioned earlier. Partial resection can be performed but may not necessarily have long-term benefits.

Since surgery for jugular foramen tumors can be associated with significant lower CN palsies, fractionated radiation therapy should be considered an option in all patients. Those tumors with large posterior fossa component and mass effect will require debulking and decompression. However, those tumors that are purely temporal lesions will frequently do well without progression for many years and radiation therapy represents a definite treatment option for these patients.

Long-term results with fractionated stereotactic radiation are excellent and with total dose of 45 to 54 Gy given (1.8–2.0 Gy/day), long-term local tumor control rates above 80% are observed without the risks associated with surgery.

## 3.2.5 Cerebellopontine Angle Meningioma

Meningiomas are tumors that arise from meningothelial arachnoid cap cells of the arachnoid granulations (villi) and not from the dura. These villi are most numerous in the large dural sinuses but also occur in smaller veins and along the root sleeves of exiting cranial and spinal nerves. Meningiomas are slow-growing neoplasms, usually with a wide attachment to the adjacent dura mater. WHO categorizes meningiomas into three types: typical (I) 90%, atypical (II) 7%, and anaplastic (III) 3%. There are also many histologic subtypes such as meningiothelial, fibrous, transitional, psammomatous, angiomatous, and miscellaneous types (microcystic, chordoid, clear cell, secretory, lymphoplasmocyte-rich, and metaplastic).

Meningiomas account for 20% of all primary intracranial tumors and are the most common primary nonglial tumor. Forty percent of meningiomas occur in the skull base. They are the second most common mass arising in the CPA after VS.[2,3,5,8] They are also the most common intracranial tumor to extend below the skull base.

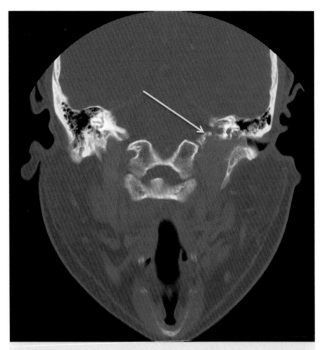

**Fig. 3.24** Coronal bone window image of a left glomus jugulotympanicum tumor. The expansile mass is filling the jugular fossa and extends into the left middle ear. Note also the erosion of the inferior aspect of the overlying petrous bone (*arrow*).

loss of the cochleovestibular activity if the inner ear is breached. This is why radiation therapy is an important clinical consideration.

Preoperative embolization can be considered if there is anticipation of high blood volume loss (1.5 L) during surgery. For tumors that are determined to be hormonally active, pre- and intraoperative administration of alpha- and beta-adrenergic blockers are required, as manipulation during surgery may result in release of neuropeptides and result in significant blood pressure changes.[5,8]

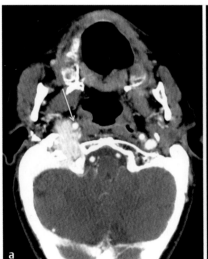
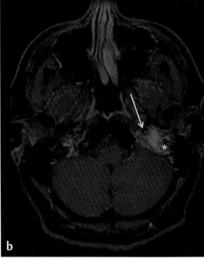

**Fig. 3.25** Two patients with glomus jugulare tumors. Contrast CT (**a**) shows an enhancing tumor that is partially encircling the right internal carotid artery (ICA; *arrow*). Gadolinium-enhanced T1-weighted MRI (**b**) in another patient with a left glomus tumor that is partially encasing the ICA flow void (*arrow*) and is also extending into the mastoid portion of the temporal bone (*asterisk*).

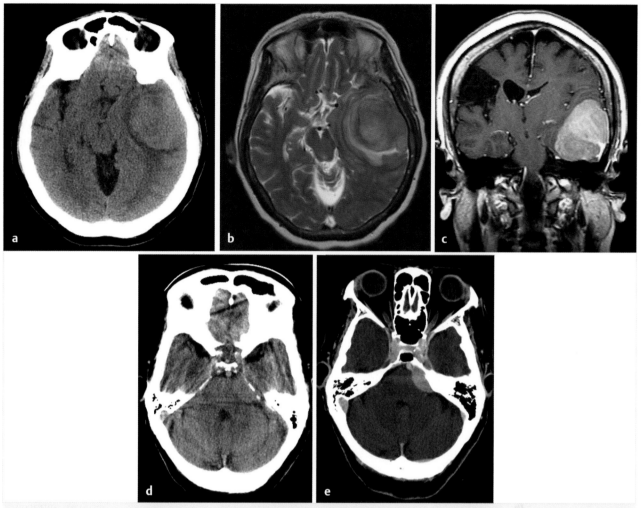

**Fig. 3.26** Series of intracranial meningiomas demonstrating the typical imaging features. Axial unenhanced CT (**a**) shows a left temporal meningioma which is mildly hyperdense to brain parenchyma. The same lesion on T2-weighted MRI (**b**) is seen to be intermediate in signal, while a coronal contrast T1-weighted image (**c**) shows marked enhancement of the mass. Axial CT images pre- (**d**) and postcontrast (**e**) of a left cerebellopontine angle meningioma show an isodense lesion that exhibits avid contrast enhancement.

Meningiomas have a distinct female predilection (with 2:1–4:1 ratios) and present primarily in middle age (peak at 45–55 years). NF2 gene mutation (long-arm deletion of chromosome 22) is a common association and is found in 60% of sporadic cases. Angiogenic factors such as fibroblast growth factor-2, vascular endothelial growth factor, and integrins are expressed by these tumors. Progesterone, prolactin, and growth hormone receptors may also be expressed. Multiple meningiomas occur in NF2. However, sporadic meningiomas can be multiple in 10% of cases.

Meningiomas arising in the CPA are generally much larger than VS at presentation. They are usually found incidentally but can cause cerebellar symptoms (disequilibrium, vertigo), obstructive hydrocephalus, or insidious CN 5, 7, and 8 palsies.[2,3,5,8]

## Imaging

Meningiomas in the CPA appear as extra-axial mass lesions applied along the cisternal face of the petrous portion of the temporal bone. On unenhanced CT, 70% of the tumors are hyperdense reflecting a high nuclear:cytoplasm ratio, while 30% of the tumors are isodense to gray matter (▶ Fig. 3.26). Calcifications are present in 25% of the tumors and can appear either very fine or very dense and coarse. Adjacent hyperostosis can arise along the petrous ridge. Hyperostosis is infrequent (15–20% of cases) but when present is very characteristic.[28] Meningiomas will typically show avid contrast enhancement on CT (▶ Fig. 3.26, ▶ Fig. 3.27).

On MRI, T1-weighted images show meningiomas to be isointense or slightly hypointense to brain (▶ Fig. 3.28). On T2-weighted images, meningiomas may appear extremely variable due to the histopathological variation of the many subtypes. Those that appear iso- or hypointense to brain on T2-weighted imaging tend to be composed of primarily fibrous or transitional elements. Hyperintensity on T2-weighted images reflects the presence of syncytial or angioblastic elements. Angioblastic meningiomas may demonstrate perilesional edema indicating a more aggressive/invasive behavior.

On T2* gradient-weighted images, marked dark internal signal blooming may be seen reflecting the presence of calcifications (▶ Fig. 3.27).

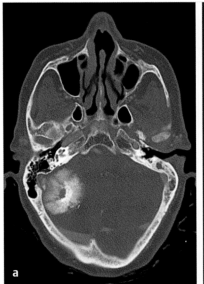
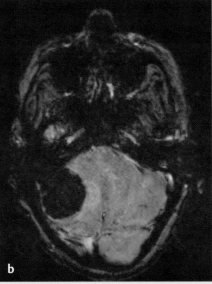
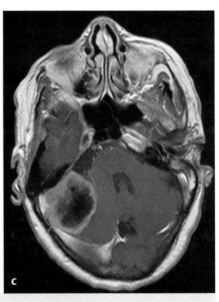

**Fig. 3.27** Axial images of a right cerebellopontine angle and lateral cerebellomedullary cistern meningioma. The lesion is densely calcified on the bone window CT (**a**) which manifests as a region of very low signal on the gradient MRI image (**b**). Postgadolinium-enhanced axial T1-weighted image shows compression and intimate contact with the right distal transverse and sigmoid sinus (**c**).

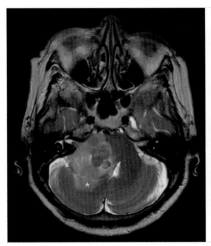
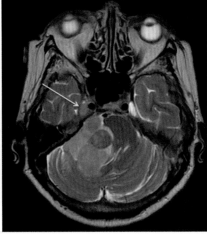

**Fig. 3.28** Axial T2-weighted images of a large lobulated cerebellopontine angle meningioma. The mass shows intermediate signal intensity. There is considerable mass effect on the adjacent brain parenchyma with associated vasogenic edema (*asterisk*). This lesion has extended into the internal auditory canal and is also infiltrating the right Meckel's cave as evidenced by the loss of normal fluid signal intensity (*arrow*).

As on CT, gadolinium-enhanced T1-weighted images will typically show avid enhancement. Meningiomas will also show mild diffusion restriction which reflects their high cellularity (▶ Fig. 3.29).

CPA meningiomas attach to the dura medial to the sigmoid sinus (▶ Fig. 3.27) below the superior petrosal sinus and above the jugular bulb. Unlike VS, meningiomas are centered eccentric to the porus (▶ Fig. 3.29, ▶ Fig. 3.30). Occasionally, extension into the IAC can occur, thus mimicking the appearance of VS (▶ Fig. 3.31). While VS will often enlarge and widen the IAC, this feature is rare with meningiomas. Other imaging features that help distinguish a CPA meningioma from VS are the obtuse angle that the former will make with the petrous ridge versus the acute angle that VS will develop. CPA meningiomas may also have an enhancing dural tail which is not seen with VS (▶ Fig. 3.30, ▶ Fig. 3.32).

On imaging, it is very important to delineate the full extent of the meningiomas. These lesions can occasionally herniate into the middle cranial fossa as well as extend into the cavernous sinus, sella, and even infiltrate the adjacent bone (▶ Fig. 3.33, ▶ Fig. 3.34).

As meningiomas can arise along the dural venous sinuses, MR or CT venography may be performed to formally assess for dural venous patency or invasion.

A catheter angiogram is rarely necessary for diagnostic purposes but, if performed, will show a dural vascular supply to the central aspect of the mass and pial vessels supplying the outer portion. A sunburst pattern of enlarged dural feeders is common. Prolonged vascular staining persisting into the venous phase is a characteristic feature of meningiomas.

Important imaging findings to communicate to the clinicians include the size of the tumor, location, and full extent of the tumor as these would influence the surgical planning. The presence of perilesional vasogenic edema is important, as this may reflect possible parenchymal invasion (▶ Fig. 3.35).

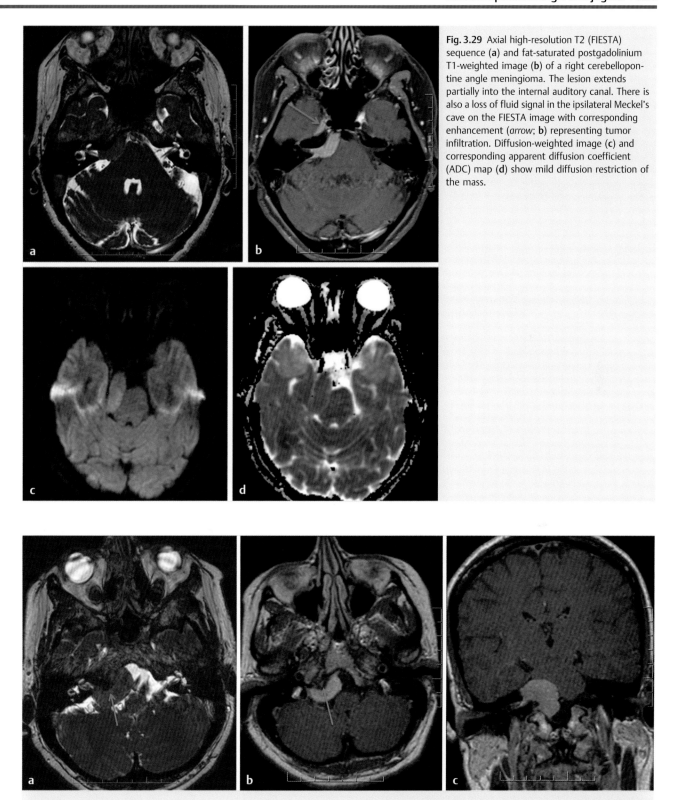

**Fig. 3.29** Axial high-resolution T2 (FIESTA) sequence (**a**) and fat-saturated postgadolinium T1-weighted image (**b**) of a right cerebellopontine angle meningioma. The lesion extends partially into the internal auditory canal. There is also a loss of fluid signal in the ipsilateral Meckel's cave on the FIESTA image with corresponding enhancement (*arrow*; **b**) representing tumor infiltration. Diffusion-weighted image (**c**) and corresponding apparent diffusion coefficient (ADC) map (**d**) show mild diffusion restriction of the mass.

**Fig. 3.30** Axial high-resolution T2 FIESTA (**a**) and axial (**b**) and coronal (**c**) T1-weighted postgadolinium sequences of a right cerebellopontine angle (CPA) meningioma. The mass is centered just anterior to the internal auditory canal. There is a small portion of tumor extending through the porus acusticus. A focal irregular ridge of hyperostosis is appreciated on the axial sequences (*arrows*; **a,b**) and there is also a small dural tail extending along the back of the clivus (**c**).

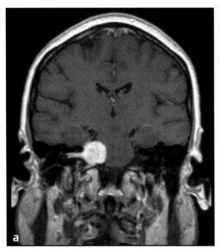
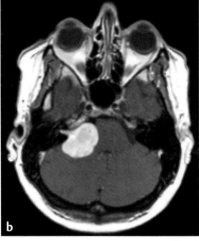

**Fig. 3.31** Gadolinium-enhanced coronal (**a**) and axial (**b**) T1-weighted images of a right cerebellopontine angle meningioma. This tumor shows avid enhancement and extension into the internal auditory canal without any significant widening.

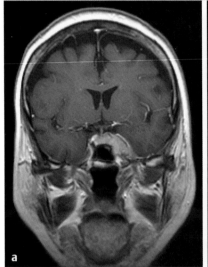
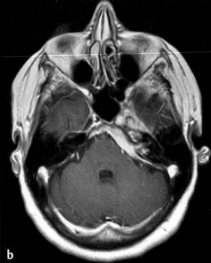
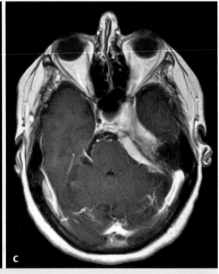

**Fig. 3.32** Coronal (**a**) and axial (**b**) contrast T1-weighted images of a left cerebellopontine angle meningioma. The lesion is rather elongated and has a long dural tail extending posteriorly. A small portion of the tumor is extending into the internal auditory canal. There is also extension into the left cavernous sinus which is abnormally enlarged. Note the absence of the normal left internal carotid artery flow void signifying very slow flow of thrombosis of this vessel. (**c**) Abnormal enhancement of the left petrous apex compatible with tumor infiltration into the bone.

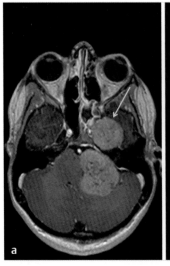
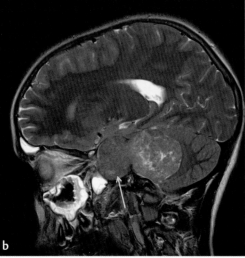

**Fig. 3.33** (**a**) Axial T1-weighted postgadolinium and (**b**) sagittal T2-weighted sequences. There is a bilobed spherical extra-axial mass in the left cerebellopontine angle with herniation into the left middle cranial fossa (*yellow arrow*). The tumor is predominantly solid and homogenous with central areas of cystic change. On pathology, this was a clear cell WHO Grade II meningioma.

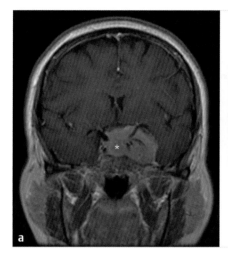
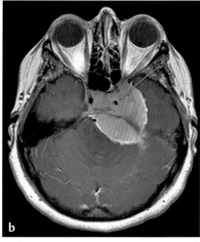

**Fig. 3.34** Gadolinium-enhanced coronal (**a**) and axial (**b**) T1-weighted images of an extensive cerebellopontine angle (CPA) and central skull base meningioma. The CPA component of the tumor is causing marked mass effect on the left aspect of the pons. This mass has contiguous extension into the left cavernous sinus and sella (*asterisk*; **a**). The mass is bulging laterally into the medial aspect of the left middle cranial fossa. Note the flow voids of the basilar artery which is in intimate contact with the mass. The left cavernous internal carotid artery is completely encased (*arrow*; **b**).

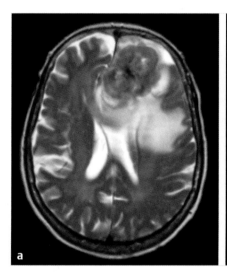
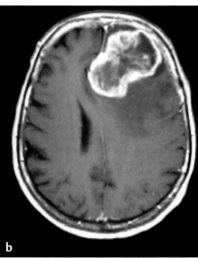

**Fig. 3.35** Axial T2 (**a**) and postcontrast T1-weighted (**b**) images of a large left frontal meningioma. Note the very heterogeneous appearance of the mass and the considerable adjacent brain edema. This was a pathologically proven WHO III meningioma with brain parenchymal invasion.

Involvement of the dural sinuses, JF (▶ Fig. 3.36), and the carotid and vertebrobasilar arteries is important, as these would also significantly complicate attempts at surgical resection. Giving the surgeon an estimate as to the degree of tumor vascularity as evidenced by the degree of contrast avidly and enhancement may predict a higher likelihood of excessive bleeding at surgery. Cross-sectional imaging may also reveal the presence of large intralesional vessels and flow voids that would indicate the presence of marked vascularity (▶ Fig. 3.37). In such instances, consideration can be made for presurgical embolization. Other features to note are the presence of brainstem compression and secondary obstructive hydrocephalus. The rate of growth over serial scans is also important to note.

## Prognosis and Treatment

Management of an incidental meningioma is a challenge. Meningiomas are usually slow growing. Intervention is considered in a rapidly growing tumor and/or the presence of progressive CN dysfunction or significant brainstem compression with obstructive hydrocephalus.

During surgery it is important to excise the tumor, dural tail, and any involved bone to decrease the risk of a recurrence.

The retrosigmoid paracerebellar approach is most commonly used for CPA meningiomas.

When there is tumor involving major arteries or draining venous sinuses, complete surgical resection is considered high risk, as there will likely be resultant stroke or central venous hypertension. In these cases, partial resection or radiation treatment can be considered.

The use of radiotherapy for CPA meningioma is largely dictated by the size and complexity of the lesion including the proximity to the optic apparatus. For well-defined lesions less than 3 cm, single fraction SRS (12–15 Gy) has well-defined long-term local control rates of approximately 80% at 10 years and a rate of serious adverse events of approximately 5%. For lesions closer than 2 mm from the chiasm and or optic nerves, large tumors of 3 cm or greater, complex lesions with irregular shapes, or postoperative cases such that the target cannot be clearly defined, the standard of care is fractionated SRT delivering 45 to 50 Gy over 5 to 6 weeks (1.8–2.0 Gy/day). This approach allows for maximal dosing of the tumor edge along critical structures that would otherwise be underdosed to

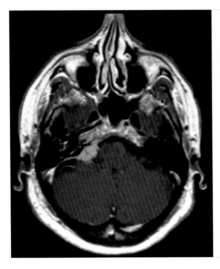
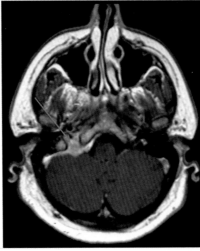

**Fig. 3.36** Axial gadolinium-enhanced T1-weighted images of a right cerebellopontine angle meningioma. The lesion is not overly large, but careful examination reveals that there is extension into the right jugular foramen (*arrow*).

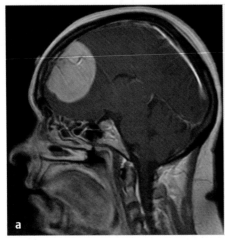
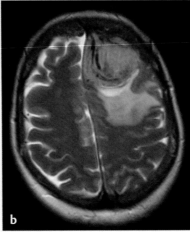

**Fig. 3.37** (a) Sagittal postcontrast T1 image and (b) axial T2-weighted images of a left frontal meningioma. The mass shows avid enhancement and both images also demonstrate the presence of large intralesional vessels indicating a very well-vascularized tumor.

respect tissue tolerance with single fraction SRS. For large tumors, fractionation is the safe option, as single fraction SRS could cause unacceptably high rates of radiation necrosis. For those lesions that could be treated with either SRS or fractionated SRT, local control rates are the same; however, toxicity rates are typically slightly more favorable for fractionated treatments. More recently, five fraction approaches are increasingly practiced (25–30 Gy) as a means to allow for the benefits of fractionation in a shorter time course to improve patient convenience. This approach is termed *hypofractionated SRS*. For grade II and grade III tumors, the standard is fractionated SRT delivering at least 60 Gy to the visible tumor, postoperative surgical tumor bed. A margin extending into the parenchymal tissue is needed to reduce the chance of recurrence. SRS to the tumor alone for grade II and III meningiomas yields higher marginal and distant failures and should be reserved for isolated failures following fractionated SRT.

### 3.2.6 Jugular Fossa Meningioma

Meningiomas of the JF arise from the arachnoid cap cells along the CNs within the jugular foramen. These tumors could also arise secondary to an inferior extension of a CPA meningioma.

Five percent of posterior fossa meningiomas are located in the JF. JF meningioma is the third most common JF mass after the paraganglioma and schwannoma. Sporadic and inherited cases can arise.

Risk factors for JF meningioma include prior skull base radiation, NF2, and female gender. They are more predominant in females (male-to-female ratio is 1:2) and usually present in the fifth to seventh decades of life.

These lesions are usually symptomatic causing CN 9 to 11 neuropathies and may also involve CN 7 and 8 if sufficiently large. Pulsatile tinnitus and a retrotympanic mass may be present.[2,5]

### Imaging

On unenhanced CT, JF meningiomas are typically greater than 3 cm at presentation, and will cause a permeative cortical erosion and sclerosis along the margins of the jugular foramen. Despite this, the bony foraminal margins are still better defined than with paraganglioma. The soft-tissue component is hyperdense on CT and internal calcification is uncommon (▶ Fig. 3.38). On enhanced CT, these lesions will show intense and uniform enhancement but will be less vascular than a JF region paraganglioma.

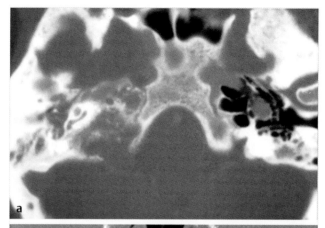

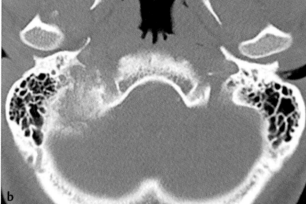

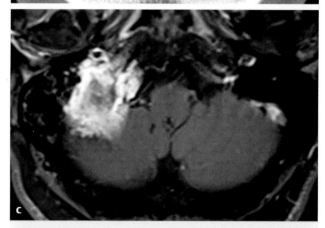

**Fig. 3.38** (a,b) Axial bone window CT and (c) T1-weighted fat-saturated postgadolinium images of a right jugular fossa meningioma. On CT, there is a mixed permeative and sclerotic expansion of the right jugular foramen. MRI shows a heterogeneously enhancing ill-defined mass.

JF meningiomas will demonstrate a radial pattern of spread in all directions from the foramen:
- Dural-based spread into the basal cisterns (most common).
- Pedunculation up into the CPA cistern (less common).
- Inferior extension into the nasopharyngeal carotid space with a dumbbell morphology.
- Superolateral extension into the middle ear mastoid. These lesions can grow into the hypotympanum, through the jugular vein and also into the posterior fossa.

- Lateral spread to involve the mastoid CN7.
- Anterior spread into the horizontal petrous ICA.
- Anteromedial extension into the petrous apex.

On MRI, T1- and T2-weighted images will show an iso- to slight hypointense mass compared to brain that is centered on the JF (▶ Fig. 3.39). On FLAIR-weighted images, perilesional edema can be present reflecting pial vessel recruitment. Following contrast injection, these lesions will show intense enhancement. A dural enhancing tail may be present. The typical salt-and-pepper appearance seen with glomus jugulare tumors will not be present. The smooth elongated enhancement and possible cystic change characteristic of a schwannoma is also not typically seen with a JF meningioma.

Larger lesions can potentially track along the jugular vein and MR venography can be performed to assess the patency of adjacent dural venous sinuses.

JF meningiomas will differ from meningiomas situated in other intracranial sites on digital subtraction angiography. These meningiomas will show minimal vascularity and will lack the typical prolonged cloudlike blush of enhancement.

Single photon emission computed tomography/positron emission tomography (SPECT/PET) [68]Gallium-labeled somatostatin analogs can be a useful adjunctive test as meningiomas may show increased uptake. The somatostatin analogs include [68Ga-DOTA0-Tyr3] octreotide (68Ga-DOTATOC, 68Ga-edotreotide), [68Ga-DOTA0–1NaI3] octreotide (68Ga-DOTANOC), and [68Ga-DOTA0-Tyr3] octreotate (68Ga-DOTATATE).[29]

Critical imaging findings to communicate to the clinician include the intracranial and extracranial extension of the lesion and its relationship to the ICA. It is also important to assess the ipsilateral sigmoid sinus and jugular bulb for patency and to see if they are the dominant draining venous sinus. One should also assess for possible extension to involve the mastoid segment of the facial nerve. The presence of significant brainstem compression should be communicated urgently, as it may necessitate emergent surgery. High-resolution T2-weighted imaging may also be a very useful test to assess the region for possible involvement of the lower CNs.

## Prognosis and Treatment

JF meningiomas are slow-growing lesions, but their locally invasive nature and location make them difficult to resect. However, complete resection is the goal in those cases that require removal.[2,5] If the lower CNs are not involved by the tumor and there are no compressive symptoms, a watch-and-wait approach is usually undertaken. Attempts to resect the tumor would likely cause lower CN palsies, particularly the facial nerve if an infratemporal fossa approach is contemplated.

Also, resection of these lesions can result in vascular injury to the ICA resulting in a stroke. Injury to a dominant sigmoid sinus/jugular bulb during surgery might result in thrombosis and cerebral venous hypertension. The patient has to be well informed about the potential complications of the surgery which could be worse than nonresection.

Other treatment options include radiation or surgical debulking with a planned subtotal tumor removal for any compressive symptoms.

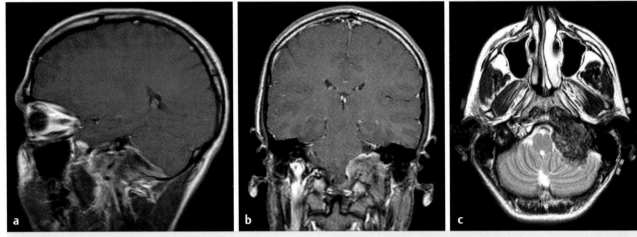

**Fig. 3.39** Sagittal (**a**) and coronal (**b**) gadolinium-enhanced T1-weighted images show a large heterogeneously enhancing mass centered on the left jugular fossa. Axial T2-weighted image (**c**) demonstrates a very low signal lesion. This jugular fossa meningioma mass extends inferiorly along the post-styloid parapharyngeal space and protrudes intracranially into the posterior fossa causing mass effect on the cerebellum. The T2-weighted image also shows signal change in the left aspect of the clivus. This can reflect a combination of reactive hyperostosis and/or tumor infiltration. The sagittal image shows the tumor tracking along the dura in the posterior fossa.

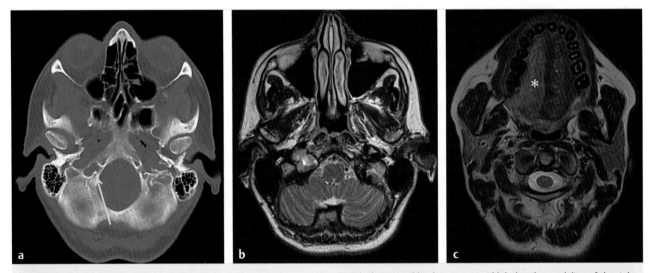

**Fig. 3.40** Axial images of a right hypoglossal schwannoma. On bone window CT (**a**), there is mild enlargement and lobulated remodeling of the right hypoglossal bony canal (*arrow*). T2-weighted MRI (**b,c**) shows a corresponding lobulated mass extending through the enlarged hypoglossal canal and ipsilateral tongue atrophy (*asterisk*; **c**).

Radiation is associated with long-term local tumor control without the associated morbidities of surgery. Stereotactic SRS typically range from 12 to 15 Gy, while fractionated SRT doses will consist of 45 to 54 Gy over 5 to 6 weeks for grade I meningioma. Atypical and malignant meningiomas require higher doses and are treated with stereotactic fractionated radiotherapy (60–70 Gy over 6–7 weeks).

### 3.2.7 Hypoglossal Schwannoma

Schwannomas arising from the hypoglossal nerve do not show any gender predilection and patients usually present in middle age. Patients presenting in the chronic stage of denervation will demonstrate ipsilateral tongue atrophy with deviation toward the site of the lesion upon tongue protrusion. In those presenting in the subacute stage of denervation, the presence of tongue fasciculation may be a dominant symptom. Hypoglossal schwannomas can also be seen as a manifestation of NF2.

Large lesions may compress upon adjacent CN 7 to 11 resulting in further deficits.[2]

### Imaging

CT imaging will demonstrate smooth remodeling and enlargement of the hypoglossal canal. Contrast MRI will show an elongated enhancing lesion extending along the course of the hypoglossal nerve. Associated fatty atrophy of the ipsilateral tongue may be visible reflecting the presence of denervation (▶ Fig. 3.40).

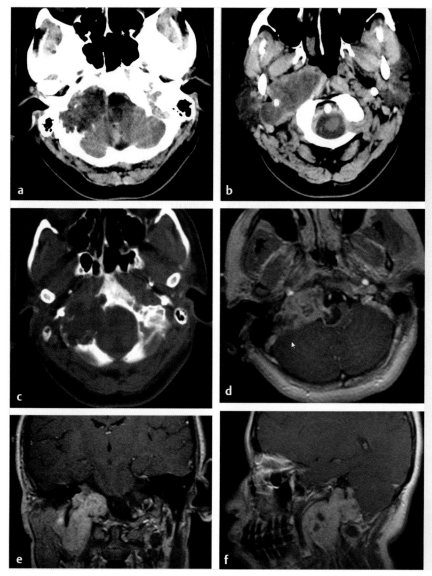

**Fig. 3.41** CT and MRI images of a large right hypoglossal schwannoma with significant intra- and extracranial components. Axial enhanced CT in soft tissue (**a,b**) and bone window (**c**) shows a large low attenuation mass centered on the right skull base. There is an expansile remodeling of the right lateral clivus and the adjacent occipital bone. There is a sizeable extracranial component extending into the upper neck. Axial (**d**), coronal (**e**), and sagittal (**f**) enhanced T1-weighted images show a heterogeneously enhancing mass. The lobulated intracranial component is causing mass effect on the medulla. The large extracranial component extends down the right poststyloid parapharyngeal space with displacement of the internal carotid artery anteriorly.

Large hypoglossal schwannomas can have sizable intracranial and extracranial components. The intracranial component can cause mass effect upon the posterior fossa contents while the extracranial component can extend along the poststyloid PPS (▶ Fig. 3.41).

Care should be taken when assessing for putative hypoglossal schwannoma, as asymmetric enhancement in the hypoglossal canal can be seen due to the presence of normal robust venous drainage or rarely a persistent hypoglossal artery. The differential diagnosis includes metastasis, paraganglioma, or meningioma.[2,5]

The most important imaging findings a skull base surgeon needs to know include the full intracranial and extracranial extent of the lesion and the relationship to the great vessels in the neck. The rate of growth on serial scans is also important to note in those patients who are being followed up without intervention.

### Prognosis and Treatment

If the tumor is small and not causing further morbidity, growth can be monitored with serial MRI. A rapidly growing tumor requires intervention. If there is extensive skull base involvement with an intimate tumor relationship to other CNs, the ICA, jugular bulb, and or the sigmoid sinus, surgical resection is often avoided as the procedure can cause further decline in hypoglossal nerve function, leading to additional lower CN palsies or vascular injury. When the tumor is unresectable, radiation can be considered. Typically, this is delivered as stereotactic fractionated radiotherapy (50–54 Gy in 5–6 weeks of 1.8–2.0 Gy/day). Fractionated stereotactic radiation gives rise to a low risk of cranial neuropathy (~5% or less) and achieves long-term tumor control of approximately 80–90% at 10 years.

## 3.2.8 Endolymphatic Sac Tumor

Endolymphatic sac tumors (ELSTs) are slow-growing, locally aggressive, low-grade malignances arising from the endolymphatic duct or sac.

Most ELSTs are sporadic, unilateral, and have no gender predilection. Patients with von Hippel-Lindau (VHL) disease have a higher incidence of ELST and VHL gene mutations have been shown to be present in both sporadic and VHL-associated ELST. A diagnosis of VHL should be considered in any patient with bilateral ELST. The average age at presentation for patients with ELST is 22 to 36 years.

These tumors tend to be quite large at presentation (> 3–5 cm) and can extend to involve the inner and middle ear cavities, the CPA cistern, and jugular foramen. One hundred percent of cases present with SNHL, which is acute in onset in 43% of cases. Other symptoms include facial nerve palsy (8%), pulsatile tinnitus (50–92%), and vertigo (20–62%).[2,5,29,30] Rarely, they can clinically mimic Meniere's syndrome as patients may presents with episodes of vertigo, tinnitus, aural fullness, and intermittent hearing loss.[31]

## Imaging

Unenhanced CT will show a local permeative process in the temporal bone centered in the fovea of the endolymphatic sac, presigmoid and retrolabyrinthine petrous portion of the temporal bone. Intratumoral calcific spicules and posterior rim calcification are reported to be present in 100% of the cases.[31] Permeative bony infiltration may extend to involve the posterolateral wall of the jugular foramen, the posterior wall of IAC, and the inner and middle ear cavity as well as extend into the mastoid portion of the temporal bone to invade the facial nerve.

ELST may show a characteristic intrinsic high T1 signal within the tumor (80–88%) related to the presence of protein, cholesterol, subacute blood products, or slow vascular flow.[2,32]

T2-weighted images will show a heterogeneous tumor with foci of low signal intensity that correspond to small bone fragments or hemorrhagic blood products. Foci of high signal intensity may also be present related to proteinaceous debris and or subacute blood product. Flow voids can be present when ELST are greater than 2 cm.

Gradient-weighted or susceptibility-weighted imaging will show areas of internal low signal corresponding to the presence of residual bone fragments and or blood products.

Contrast-enhanced MR or CT demonstrates an enhancing mass along the cisternal face of the temporal bone, usually centered at the vestibular aqueduct. Tumoral soft tissue may transgress the dura and invade into the brain parenchyma (▶ Fig. 3.42).

ELST receives blood supply via several external carotid artery branches (ascending pharyngeal, stylomastoid, and petrosal branch of middle meningeal artery). Larger lesions may also show additional supply from the ICA or posterior circulation vessels.[2,5,32,33]

MR or CT venography may be useful to assess the status of the adjacent dural venous sinuses.

Important imaging features to note are the exact extent of the tumor including the presence of involvement of the jugular foramen, IAC, the posterior fossa dural plate, and the rate of growth over serial scans. One should also assess for the presence of other lesions involved in the context of von Hippel-Lindau syndrome (such as cerebellar, spinal, or retinal hemangioblastomas and choroid plexus papillomas).

## Prognosis and Treatment

If the tumor is slow growing, then watchful waiting can be adopted. If the tumor is rapidly growing, then intervention should be considered to prevent further hearing loss. Prognosis is excellent if complete resection is achieved usually with wide

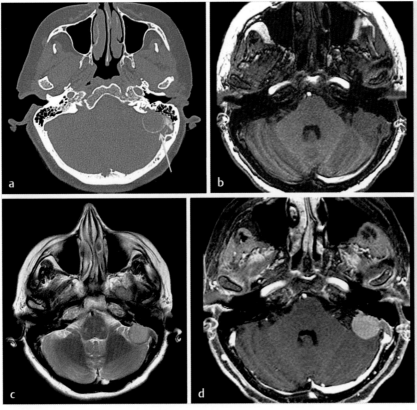

Fig. 3.42 Axial cross-sectional imaging of a left endolymphatic sac tumor. Axial enhanced CT in bone window (a) image shows a mass lesion causing erosion along the posterior margin of the petrous bone. The expansile mass has a peripheral shell of calcification (arrow). Axial T1- (b), T2- (c), and postcontrast T1-weighted (d) images show a corresponding enhancing lesion causing mass effect on the adjacent cerebellum and also extending into the vicinity of the left dural sigmoid sinus.

margins. Late recurrence may be possible.[2] Gamma-knife radiosurgery is performed for residual tumor.[33] If there is evidence of malignant transformation evident by the biological activity or suggested by pathology, radiation therapy and/or chemotherapy may be required.

## 3.2.9 Metastatic Disease Involving Bone, Jugular Foramen, and Leptomeningeal Tumor Seeding

Common primary cancers that can metastasize to the region include breast (40%), lung (14%), and prostate (12%). Myeloma, lymphoma, and leukemia are also common. The location of the metastatic disease can be bony, dural based, leptomeningeal, or a combination of any of these locations. In addition, primary central nervous system tumors such as glioblastoma multiforme and medulloblastoma can also result in CSF seeding to the leptomeninges.

Skull base bony metastases from extracranial primaries occur in 4% of cancer patients. Direct extension of malignancies from adjacent spaces is also possible (e.g., from the ear, parotid space, nasopharynx, or petrous apex). The differential diagnosis includes primary local tumors such as squamous cell carcinoma, chondrosarcomas, or ELST. In children and young adults, histiocytosis and embryonal rhabdomyosarcoma also need to be considered. Of note, malignant otitis externa and primary skull base osteomyelitis can have an aggressive appearance and mimic a malignancy.

Leptomeningeal carcinomatosis is the malignant infiltration of the pia, arachnoid, or both. The leptomeninges (arachnoid) extend along the cisternal and canalicular segments of the facial and vestibulocochlear nerves and metastases can seed into these locations.

Intracranial metastases are becoming increasingly common as the survival rate of cancer patients is improving. There is no gender predilection. Symptomatic cranial neuropathy is the most common presentation (e.g., rapidly progressive unilateral or bilateral CN 7 or 8 palsies) in those patients with leptomeningeal metastases.[2,5,9]

## Imaging

Imaging of metastatic disease can be quite variable resulting in solitary, multifocal, or diffuse disease.

### Bony metastases

On unenhanced CT, lesions can be lytic, permeative, or sclerotic depending on the primary tumor (▶ Fig. 3.43).

On MRI, T1-weighted images will show hypointense lesions in the marrow replacing the normal fatty/high signal in adults. On T2-weighted images, the lesions are typically hyperintense. If the metastasis gives rise to a sclerotic bony reaction, the lesions will show very low T1 and T2 signal.

On diffusion-weighted images (DWIs), osseous metastases may show diffusion restriction. Fat-saturated contrast-enhanced T1-weighted images will show an enhancing bone marrow mass with or without extraosseous soft tissue component.

### Dural-based metastases

Unenhanced CT may detect dural lesions if they are of significantly large size. These lesions will be better seen on contrast-enhanced studies.

On MRI, dural metastases are usually hypointense on T1-weighted imaging and hyperintensity on T2-weighted scans. On DWIs, there may be diffusion restriction if the primary tumor is cellular. Dural metastases will show enhancement following gadolinium injection (▶ Fig. 3.44).

### Leptomeningeal metastases

Unenhanced CT will not detect leptomeningeal disease unless they are sufficiently thick. Overall, contrast-enhanced CT has very low sensitivity for detecting leptomeningeal disease.

On MRI, T1-weighted images will reveal isointense meningeal thickening. On FLAIR-weighted images, lesions may give rise to abnormal high signal intensity within the sulci. Contrast-enhanced T1-weighted images will show multifocal, linear, nodular, or discrete leptomeningeal enhancement in the

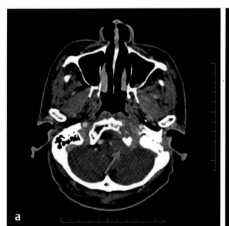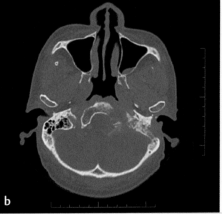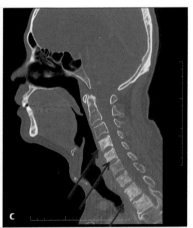

Fig. 3.43 Axial enhanced soft tissue (a), bone window (b), and sagittal bone window (c) CT images in a patient with advanced lung carcinoma. There are metastatic lesions situated in the left jugular fossa and laterally in the left petrous bone (*long arrow*; a). There are extensive permeative erosive changes in the left petroclival junction with erosion of the left jugular tubercle and extension into the left hypoglossal canal (*short arrow*; b). Multilevel sclerotic metastases to the cervical and upper thoracic vertebral bodies are also present (*red arrows*; c).

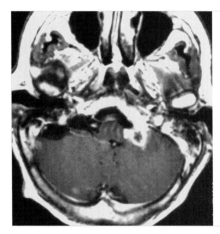
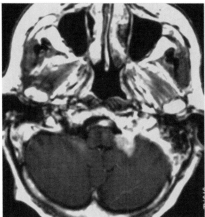

**Fig. 3.44** Axial gadolinium-enhanced T1-weighted images show a dural-based lung carcinoma metastasis in the left cerebellomedullary region with extension into the left jugular foramen. This patient initially presented with a left vocal cord paralysis of unknown cause. (Images courtesy of Dr. C. Douglas Phillips.)

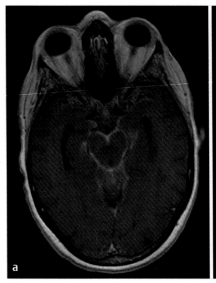
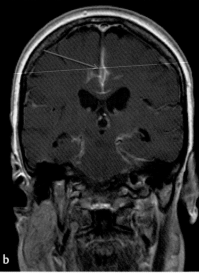

**Fig. 3.45** T1-weighted gadolinium-enhanced axial (**a**) and coronal (**b**) images show diffuse leptomeningeal carcinomatosis secondary to metastatic breast carcinoma. There is abnormal enhancement within the interhemispheric fissure (*arrow*; **b**) and circumferentially along the midbrain and basal cisterns.

cerebral and cerebellar sulci, within the CPA-IAC and in other basal cisterns (▶ Fig. 3.45, ▶ Fig. 3.46, ▶ Fig. 3.47).

### Prognosis and Treatment

Skull base, dural, or leptomeningeal metastases are often late events in the disease course and indicate a poor prognosis. Overall survival is variable depending on the tumor type. No curative treatment is available. Instead, therapy is aimed at preserving neurological function and improving or maintaining quality of life. Radiotherapy or chemotherapy can be undertaken depending on the tissue type. Surgery is rarely considered only for either excisional biopsy or decompression of a tumor mass effect.[2,9] Great vessel involvement is thought to be a contraindication to surgery.

Radiation is the dominant therapy for leptomeningeal disease. In the brain, typical treatment consists of whole brain radiation, while in the spine, regions demonstrating gross disease are radiated as there is morbidity associated with bone marrow function that could preclude patients from systemic therapy. Typical doses range from 20 Gy in 5 fractions to 30 Gy in 10 fractions as a short course palliative approach.

## 3.3 Benign Tumors and Mimics

### 3.3.1 Cholesterol Granuloma

Cholesterol granulomas are the result of a chronic foreign body reaction to cholesterol aggregates that are produced by the degradation of erythrocytes. Pathologically, cholesterol granulomas are pseudocysts containing cholesterol crystals, inflammatory cells including macrophages, and multinucleated giant cells encased by a fibrous capsule. Cholesterol granulomas of the petrous apex are relatively aggressive lesions and are the most common primary lesion of the petrous apex accounting for approximately 60% of lesions in this location.[34,35] The most common entity is the tympanomastoid cholesterol granuloma which is more indolent and occurs as a result of chronic otitis media.[36] We will focus discussion on the petrous apex cholesterol granuloma, as these lesions can enlarge and extend into the CPA.

Cholesterol granulomas occur most commonly in young to middle-aged adults without apparent sexual predilection. Two hypotheses have been put forward regarding the pathophysiology of cholesterol granulomas. The classical obstruction-vacuum

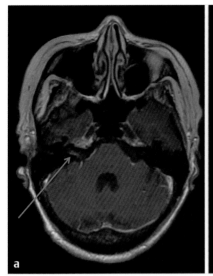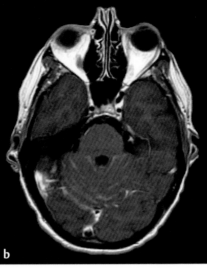

**Fig. 3.46** Axial T1-weighted enhanced images in a patient with metastatic breast (**a**) and lung (**b**) carcinoma. The *arrow* shows leptomeningeal cancer seeding into the right internal auditory canal. (**b**) Abnormal leptomeningeal seeding along the cerebellar folia manifesting as diffuse enhancement.

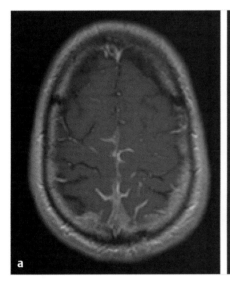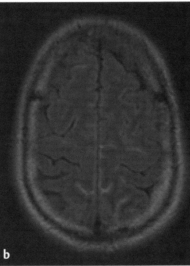

**Fig. 3.47** Axial gadolinium-enhanced T1-weighted (**a**) and FLAIR (**b**) images showing leptomeningeal leukemic infiltrates. There is abnormal enhancement within multiple cerebral sulci over the convexities (▶ Fig. 3.45a) with corresponding abnormal high signal on the FLAIR image.

hypothesis postulates that cholesterol granulomas arise from a process of air trapping in the small air cells of the petrous apex with subsequent gas resorption, vacuum formation, and bleeding into unventilated air cells.[37,38] Blood products are slowly converted to cholesterol by anaerobic metabolism which leads to a foreign body granulomatous reaction. Recently, a new line of thinking suggests an exposed marrow hypothesis.[36] During development, mucosa-lined tracts replace hematopoietic marrow elements in the petrous apex leading to exposed vascular marrow which has a propensity to bleed. The hemorrhage occludes outflow resulting in trapped blood products, anaerobic metabolism into cholesterol and granulomatous reaction. As the pseudocyst expands, bone erosion continues leading to new hemorrhage and continuation of the cycle.

The clinical presentation of cholesterol granulomas is variable depending on the size and local extent of the lesion. In one cohort of 90 patients with petrous apex cholesterol granulomas, the most common symptom was headache (56.7%) followed by dizziness (35.6%) and facial pain or paresthesia (12.2%).[39] A smaller percentage of patients presented with asymmetric SNHL or facial nerve palsy secondary to inner ear extension or nerve compression.

## Imaging

The imaging modality of choice for diagnosing cholesterol granulomas is MRI. Petrous apex cholesterol granulomas are well-circumscribed, nonenhancing, expansile lesions which show erosion of underlying bony trabeculae which is best shown on CT. The key imaging feature on MRI is signal hyperintensity on noncontrast T1-weighted fat-saturated images which is the result of blood degradation products (methemoglobin) within the lesion. Fat suppression allows distinction of the intrinsic T1 hyperintense fatty marrow within the petrous apex, from the T1 hyperintense blood degradation products of the cholesterol granuloma. On T2-weighted images (including FLAIR), these lesions are typically hyperintense centrally but may show a low T2 signal rim secondary to hemosiderin lining the periphery (▶ Fig. 3.48). On DWI, these lesions are hypointense and do not show water diffusion restriction as is the case

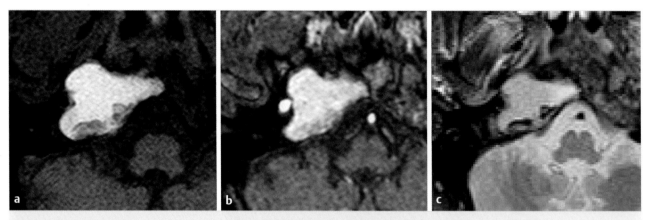

**Fig. 3.48** Axial MR of petrous apex cholesterol granuloma. **(a)** Precontrast T1-weighted fat-saturated image shows lobulated intrinsically T1-hyperintense lesion in right petrous apex. **(b)** After gadolinium administration, there is no appreciable contrast enhancement. **(c)** T2-weighted image shows lesion to be predominantly T2 hyperintense with some T2 hypointense material (presumably blood products) within the dependent portion of the lesion.

for cholesteatomas. There may be minimal enhancement of the fibrous capsule, but there should not be any significant internal enhancement. There are several lesions of the petrous apex that should be included in the differential diagnosis and can be distinguished from cholesterol granulomas based on imaging features (▶ Table 3.1).

High-resolution T2-weighted sequences such as CISS (constructive interference into steady state) or FIESTA (fast imaging employing steady-state acquisition) and high-resolution CT are useful to evaluate for the extension of disease into or compression of critical structures such as the otic capsule, facial nerve canal, carotid canal, and vestibulocochlear nerve. Furthermore,

for surgical management (see later), high-resolution temporal bone CT is required for planning and to screen for anatomical variants such as an aberrant course of the ICA, persistent stapedial artery, or high-riding jugular bulb which may pose problems during surgical approach.

## Prognosis and Treatment

Historically, asymptomatic patients were managed with primary observation and symptomatic patients were treated surgically. Given the indolent nature of many cholesterol granulomas, there is now growing support for observation in many cases,

**Table 3.1** Petrous apex lesions

| | T1 | T2 | Enhancement | Key features |
|---|---|---|---|---|
| *Cholesterol granuloma* | Hyperintense | Hyperintense centrally with hypointense rim | Mild peripheral occasionally | T1 hyperintensity on fat-saturated images |
| *Cholesteatoma* | Hypointense (rarely hyperintense) | Hyperintense | Mild peripheral occasionally | Diffusion restriction |
| *Apical petrositis* | Hypointense | Hyperintense | More solid enhancement (phlegmon) and peripheral enhancement (abscess) | Clinical presentation Abscess may show restricted diffusion |
| *Simple effusion* | Hypointense | Hyperintense | None | Trabeculae intact on CT |
| *Mucocele* | Hypointense or hyperintense | Generally hyperintense | None | Expansile on CT, T1 hyperintense mucoceles may be difficult to distinguish from cholesterol granulomas but do not have T2 hypointense rim |
| *Aneurysm* | Thrombosed components may be hyperintense, central flow void on spin echo sequences | Complex, central flow void on spin echo sequences | Avid enhancement of nonthrombosed component | Avid arterial enhancement, continuity with ICA on angiography, pulsation artifact on MR |
| *Encephalocele/meningocele* | Meningocele is hypointense, encephalocele follows brain signal | Meningocele is hyperintense, encephalocele follows brain signal or may be hyperintense if gliotic | Encephalocele may show enhancement | Show bony defect with CT and connection with subarachnoid space or brain with high-resolution MRI |

Abbreviations: CT, computed tomography; ICA, internal carotid artery; MRI, magnetic resonance imaging.

reserving surgical intervention for patients with lesions causing or with the potential to cause neurological symptoms either via mass effect or invasion of critical structures.[39]

Surgical approach will depend on the presence of residual hearing. In the past, a modified transcochlear approach with removal of the cochlea, cyst exposure, and fenestration was performed for patients with no serviceable hearing.[40] In patients with residual hearing, cyst drainage via infracochlear or infralabyrinthine approaches with insertion of drainage tube is preferred. For the infralabyrinthine approach, a simple mastoidectomy is performed with opening of the retrofacial space.[41] In the infracochlear approach, an approach through the space between the carotid artery, jugular bulb, and round window proximal to the entrance of the Eustachian tube is taken.[42] The choice of approach is dependent on surgeon's preference and the thickness of the wall separating the cyst from air cell tracts. If a transpetrous approach is not manageable, transsphenoidal or middle cranial fossa approaches are possible. The former can be taken for cysts that are adjacent to or extend into the sphenoid sinus and can be performed endoscopically.[43] For large cholesterol granulomas extending into the middle cranial fossa, complete excision of the lesion through the middle cranial fossa is recommended.[40] During surgical resection, great care is taken to not breach the dural space to avoid the possibility of chemical meningitis.

## 3.3.2 Petrous Apex Cholesteatoma/ Epidermoid

Cholesteatomas are also known as epidermoid cysts and can be generally classified as acquired or congenital. Acquired cholesteatomas commonly arise within the middle ear cavity as a result of previous otitis media, tympanic membrane perforation, or surgery and are typically small and generally do not extend to the petrous apex or CPA. Congenital cholesteatomas can arise intradurally and, in 20% of cases, extradurally.[44] The most common intradural location is the CPA or middle cranial fossa which is described separately in the next section on CPA epidermoid. The most common extradural location for congenital cholesteatomas is the temporal bone and these lesions can be found in a number of locations including the middle ear cavity, the petrous apex, the mastoid and squamous portions of the temporal bone, and the tympanic membrane or EAC. Congenital cholesteatomas arise from epithelial rests, also known as epidermoid formations, which are found in the fetal or postnatal temporal bone and normally regress at approximately 33 weeks of age.[45] These epithelial rests form squamous epithelial-lined cysts which grow slowly through desquamation

of the epithelial lining and contain concentric layers of keratin and stratified squamous epithelial cells.

Petrous apex cholesteatomas comprise approximately 4 to 9% of all petrous apex lesions[35] and are more commonly found in children and young adults. The clinical presentation of congenital cholesteatomas of the temporal bone depends on the size and extent of the lesion. With middle ear invasion and ossicular involvement, petrous apex cholesteatomas can result in conductive hearing loss. This is typically not a significant problem as conductive hearing loss can be surgically corrected. Petrous apex cholesteatomas can erode into the bony labyrinth, invade the auditory canal, and enter the CPA resulting in an array of symptoms including facial nerve palsy, SNHL, and vertigo. Otic capsule involvement typically results in profound SNHL and once this is identified, surgical resection can be more aggressive with resection via a transcochlear or transotic approach in addition to the traditional translabyrinthine, infra-/supralabyrinthine approaches. These lesions may also invade into vital structures including the carotid canal and sigmoid sinus.

### Imaging

On temporal bone CT, cholesteatomas of the petrous apex are well-marginated, expansile, low attenuating lesions that do not show any evidence of an internal matrix (▶ Fig. 3.49). CT is useful for evaluating local disease extension and bone erosion. The key to diagnosis of a cholesteatoma is diffusion restriction or high signal on diffusion-weighted MRI. Other MRI features are less specific and include intermediate signal on T2 FLAIR images, hyperintensity on T2-weighted images, and hypointensity on T1-weighted images. These lesions may show minimal peripheral enhancement but should not show any significant central enhancement. There is a shared primary differential of petrous apex cholesteatomas and cholesterol granulomas which is outlined in ▶ Table 3.1.

### Prognosis and Treatment

The mainstay of treatment of petrous apex cholesteatomas is total resection, as lesion residual will result in disease recurrence. Unfortunately, complete resection is difficult as removal of tumor from CNs, dura, venous sinuses, and the ICA is challenging. In cases where structures such as petrous carotid or venous sinuses are involved, subtotal resection with exteriorization of any remnant is performed which can be observed over time. Treatment and surgical approach will depend on residual hearing on the affected and contralateral side, facial nerve function, and extent of lesion and the possibility of CSF leaks after resection. Petrous apex cholesteatoma affecting the only

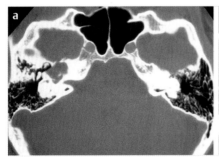
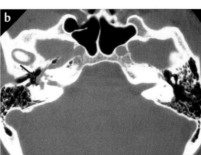

**Fig. 3.49 (a,b)** Axial CT of right petrous apex cholesteatoma. This patient presented with right facial weakness. Imaging revealed an expansile soft-tissue lesion (**a**) in the right petrous apex. This was a primary petrous apex cholesteatoma that had extended to track along the tympanic segment of the facial nerve (*arrow*; **b**).

hearing ear can be treated conservatively with observation and follow-up imaging. For patients with no residual hearing, a lateral transtemporal approach with removal of the otic capsule allows good surgical exposure for radical lesion excision. Facial nerve function is crucial to the patient, and for patients with normal preoperative facial nerve function, prognosis for facial nerve function is good.[46] Careful dissection of disease and nerve decompression is recommended for these patients. However, if preoperative facial nerve dysfunction exists, postoperative nerve function is unlikely to recover and, in this case, more aggressive management can be considered with the possibility for facial-to-facial end-to-end anastomosis, facial to hypoglossal end-to-side anastomosis, or other nerve repair techniques. Middle fossa approaches can be used for large petrous apex lesions. There is growing interest in the use of an endoscopic transsphenoidal approach for resection of petrous apex cholesteatomas with the potential for a faster recovery and a shorter postoperative hospitalization.

### 3.3.3 CPA Epidermoid

Intracranial epidermoid cysts are pathologically the same as cholesteatomas and are squamous epithelium-lined cysts that contain desquamated epithelium and keratin. The CPA is the most common location accounting for approximately 40 to 50% of intracranial epidermoid cysts.[47] With regard to CPA lesions, epidermoids are the third most common lesion after CPA schwannomas and meningiomas and account for approximately 5 to 10% of lesions in this location.[48] CPA epidermoids are congenital lesions that arise from ectodermal inclusions which arise from cells of the first branchial cleft.[47] On gross pathology, the classic appearance is that of a soft, lobulated, shiny "mother of pearl" tumor which insinuates around vessels and CNs. There is no sex predilection and these lesions typically present between the third and fifth decades of life.[49] The clinical presentation is variable with the most common presenting symptom being headache. Hearing impairment and trigeminal neuralgia are common presenting symptoms and facial nerve symptoms are less common. Rarely, these lesions can present with pyramidal or cerebellar symptoms.

### Imaging

The CT appearance of CPA epidermoids is that of a low attenuating (near CSF density) lesion that more often insinuates around structures in the cistern rather than displacing them and can occasionally invaginate into the brainstem. Occasionally, the lesion may contain calcifications. Very rarely, epidermoid cysts can appear hyperdense on CT owing to internal hemorrhage or high protein content or fatty attenuation due to triglyceride content. The primary differential consideration on CT is a CPA arachnoid cyst. As with petrous apex cholesteatomas, MRI is diagnostic with characteristic diffusion restriction (▶ Fig. 3.50). On T2 FLAIR, CPA epidermoids show signal intensity slightly greater than CSF. On T2-weighted images, these lesions are typically iso-hyperintense to CSF but can occasionally be hypointense due to protein content or hemorrhage. Most commonly, these lesions are T1 hypointense but rarely can be hyperintense (the so-called white epidermoids) due to high internal triglyceride and fatty acid content, protein content, or hemorrhage.[50] Unlike typical epidermoids, these white epidermoids may not demonstrate diffusion restriction.[51] On postgadolinium imaging, there is generally no enhancement, although there may be minimal enhancement of the margins of the lesion. There should be no internal solid enhancement which should raise suspicion for an alternative diagnosis or malignant degeneration of an epidermoid into squamous cell carcinoma which can rarely occur.[52]

### Prognosis and Treatment

As with petrous apex cholesteatomas, the mainstay of treatment of CPA epidermoids is complete or subtotal surgical resection. The retrosigmoid approach is commonly employed and allows good exposure of the lesion and important structures in the

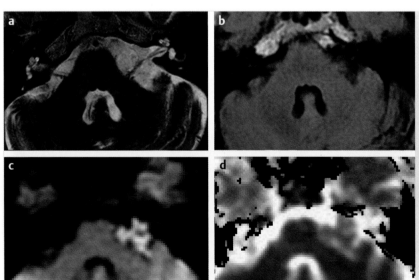

**Fig. 3.50** Axial MR of cerebellopontine angle (CPA) epidermoid. **(a)** T2-weighted image shows expansion of left CPA by a T2 hyperintense lesion causing mass effect on the left pons, brachium pontis, and cerebellum. **(b)** T2 FLAIR shows subtle hyperintensity within the lesion, suggesting that this is not simply a cerebrospinal fluid–containing structure such as an arachnoid cyst. **(c)** Diffusion-weighted imaging and **(d)** corresponding apparent diffusion coefficient (ADC) map demonstrate the lesion to restrict water diffusion confirming the diagnosis of a CPA epidermoid.

CPA.[49] Subtemporal and suboccipital approaches can be used for tumors with supratentorial extension into the middle cranial fossa. Hearing can sometimes be improved after resection of CPA epidermoids and so a translabyrinthine approach is typically reserved for patients with otic capsule involvement and significant SNHL on the affected side. As with petrous apex cholesteatomas, ossicular involvement can be dealt with using reconstruction techniques and subtotal resection with exteriorization of any remnant is performed when disease involves vital vascular structures such as the carotid canal or the dural venous sinuses.

The tendency of epidermoids to adhere to structures in the CPA makes complete surgical resection difficult and adds to the morbidity that can be seen after surgical resection. Worsening of preoperative CN deficits is common after surgery and new CN deficits can also occur.[49] Lower CN deficits will lead to significant morbidities for patients. Facial nerve paresis/paralysis can be cosmetically and functionally quite devastating as well. Good disease control can be achieved after surgical resection; however, these lesions have a tendency to recur and postoperative surveillance with MRI is required to evaluate for disease recurrence.

### 3.3.4 Apical Petrositis

Apical petrositis is an infection of the petrous apex which typically results from spread of infection from otitis media into the pneumatized petrous apex.[35] Subsequent obstruction of drainage can result in abscess formation. Infection can spread beyond air cells and into the bone of the petrous apex resulting in an osteomyelitis. Spread beyond bone into adjacent structures such as the carotid canal, venous sinuses, meninges, and brain can result in arteritis, pseudoaneurysm, thrombophlebitis, venous thrombosis, meningitis, cerebritis, and brain abscess.

Causative organisms include *Streptococcus pneumonia, Haemophilus influenza,* and *Staphylococcus aureus.* Clinical presentation is the key to diagnosis. Patients are typically unwell and present with fever, otalgia, and otorrhea. Depending on disease extension, there may be other clinical symptoms such as CN palsies. Sometimes patients may present with the Gradenigo triad of otomastoiditis, facial pain secondary to trigeminal involvement, and diplopia secondary to lateral rectus palsy from abducens involvement as infection spreads from petrous apex to Meckel's cave and Dorello's canal, respectively. Apical petrositis occurs in children as an acute complication of otitis media. In adults, it occurs as a chronic complication of otomastoiditis or as a postoperative complication.

### Imaging

CT typically shows evidence of otomastoiditis with opacification of petrous apex air cells and cortical or trabecular bony erosion which are seen later in the disease process. MRI provides better evaluation of soft tissues and complications. Fluid signal is observed in petrous apex air cells characterized by high T2 and low T1 signals. After administration of (gadolinium—could be other contrast as well. Better just to say contrast) contrast, heterogeneous enhancement of the petrous apex can be observed compatible with phlegmon. As infections become organized into an abscess, peripheral enhancement and diffusion restriction can be seen (▶ Fig. 3.51). As disease extends outside of bone, dural enhancement can be observed. MR can show other complications such as carotid arteritis/thrombosis, cavernous or venous sinus thrombosis, leptomeningeal enhancement with meningitis, cerebritis, and a brain abscess. Gallium-67 SPECT can be useful in detecting skull base infection and has been used to monitor response to treatment.[53]

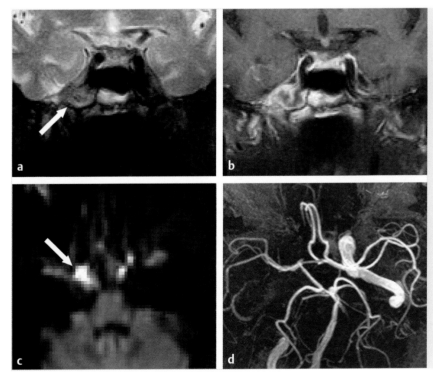

**Fig. 3.51** MR of apical petrositis. **(a)** Coronal T2-weighted image shows a heterogeneously hyperintense lesion in right petrous apex (*white arrow*). **(b)** Postgadolinium T1-weighted image shows avid peripheral enhancement of the right petrous apex lesion. **(c)** Axial diffusion-weighted imaging shows high signal representing abscess (*white arrow*). **(d)** Time-of-flight MRA shows occlusion of the right internal carotid artery—a complication of infection.

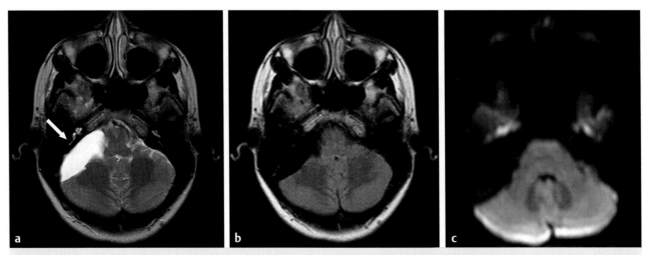

**Fig. 3.52** Axial MR of right cerebellopontine angle (CPA) arachnoid cyst. (**a**) Axial T2-weighted image shows a hyperintense lesion in right CPA (*white arrow*). (**b**) T2 FLAIR shows nulling of signal within the lesion consistent with cerebrospinal fluid (CSF) composition. (**c**) Diffusion-weighted imaging shows no restricted diffusion confirming CSF composition and excluding epidermoid cyst.

## Prognosis and Treatment

While some cases of apical petrositis have been managed conservatively with antibiotic treatment alone,[54] many cases require antibiotics plus surgery for drainage, debridement, and permanent drainage of apical air cells. Typically, if standard intravenous antibiotic therapy fails and there is continued disease progression present on both clinical and radiological imaging, adjuvant surgical intervention can be added. This has traditionally been accomplished with a mastoidectomy with sacrifice of the inner ear. More recently, other hearing-sparing surgical approaches have been explored with promising results.[55]

## 3.3.5 Arachnoid Cyst

Arachnoid cysts are benign CSF-containing cysts lined by a layer of arachnoid cells. Most arachnoid cysts result from anomalies of meningeal development when the embryonic endomeninges fail to merge resulting in a duplicated arachnoid layer.[47] The cyst fills with CSF formed by the layer of arachnoid cells comprising the cyst wall. Most arachnoid cysts are found in the supratentorium and the majority of these are within the middle cranial fossa. About 10 to 15% of arachnoid cysts occur in the posterior fossa and the majority of these arise in the CPA. Arachnoid cysts are the second most common cystic lesion of the CPA after epidermoid cysts. A recent epidemiological study revealed a slight female predominance of CPA arachnoid cysts.[56] While CPA arachnoid cysts can be asymptomatic, they can present with a number of symptoms, including CN deficits, headache, and vertigo. Sensorineural hearing loss can occur and facial nerve weakness has also been described.

## Imaging

CT shows a CSF attenuation cystic lesion which displaces rather than engulfs adjacent structures such as CNs and vessels. Occasionally, arachnoid cysts may become complicated with hemorrhage which can be seen on CT. CT cisternography performed by the intrathecal administration of iodinated contrast can show communication of the subarachnoid space with the cyst interior. The major differential consideration for CPA arachnoid cyst is an epidermoid cyst. MRI is diagnostic and shows arachnoid cysts to be low signal (CSF intensity) on T2 FLAIR and nonrestricting on DWI (▶ Fig. 3.52). CSF pulsation artifact can sometimes result in areas of high signal within arachnoid cysts on T2 FLAIR. After intravenous gadolinium administration, arachnoid cysts should not enhance. High-resolution T2-weighted sequences such as FIESTA or CISS may be useful to delineate the cyst wall and mass effect on small structures such as CNs. Phase contrast MRI can be used to demonstrate CSF flow between the cyst and subarachnoid space which can be useful when treatment by cyst fenestration is being considered.[57]

## Prognosis and Treatment

Treatment is usually reserved for symptomatic lesions. Surgical intervention for arachnoid cysts includes craniotomy for cyst removal, fenestration, or cystoperitoneal shunting; however, less invasive procedures such as endoscopic cyst fenestration and endoscopic cystocisternostomy or ventriculocystomies provide a safe and effective alternative treatment. In patients with symptoms such as SNHL and facial nerve palsy, symptoms can be relieved after surgery.[58] There is growing support for more widespread conservative management for symptomatic CPA arachnoid cysts based on studies showing radiographic and clinical stability of these lesions.[59]

## 3.3.6 Facial Nerve Hemangioma

Hemangiomas of the facial nerve are rare lesions accounting for 0.7% of all intratemporal tumors.[60] In the past, there has been debate as to whether these lesions represent true neoplasms of the facial nerve or vascular malformations. Today, the general consensus is that these lesions more closely resemble vascular malformations.[61] Classically, four histological subtypes have been described: capillary, cavernous, mixed capillary-cavernous, and venous based on the appearance of

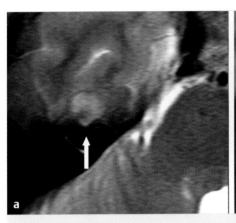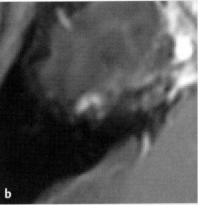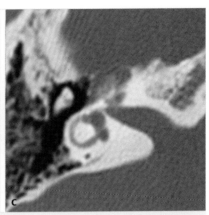

**Fig. 3.53** Axial MR and CT of facial nerve hemangioma. **(a)** Axial T2-weighted image shows a hyperintense lesion centered in right geniculate ganglion (*white arrow*). **(b)** Postgadolinium enhanced images show avid enhancement. **(c)** CT shows an expansile lesion with calcified matrix (honeycomb appearance) which is a classic appearance of a facial nerve hemangioma.

the vascular spaces.[62] Facial nerve hemangiomas can arise from any segment of the facial nerve, but the most common location is the geniculate ganglion followed by the IAC and mastoid segment of the facial nerve.[60] These lesions can present with progressive or sudden facial nerve symptoms (paresis, paralysis, or hemifacial spasm) or SNHL with symptoms that are disproportionate to the size of the lesion. One explanation for this discordance is that these lesions result in vascular steal resulting in neural ischemia affecting the facial and cochlear nerves. Direct compression of the facial and vestibulocochlear nerve within the IAC is also a likely mechanism resulting in CN dysfunction.

## Imaging

Gadolinium-enhanced MR of the IAC, middle ear, and parotid is recommended to detect facial nerve hemangiomas and other possible pathologies involving the facial nerve. On T2-weighted imaging, these lesions are typically hyperintense and iso- to slightly hypointense to brain on T1-weighted images. After gadolinium contrast, these lesions avidly enhance. The primary differential consideration is a facial nerve schwannoma which may be difficult to differentiate from facial nerve hemangioma on MRI. Discordance between lesion size and patient symptoms should raise suspicion for a facial nerve hemangioma. Additionally, facial nerve hemangiomas of the geniculate ganglion do not typically demonstrate significant extension along the facial nerve, and extension to the IAC or beyond the cochleariform process is rare. CT may be useful in distinguishing these two entities and for detecting very small lesions that cannot be detected on MRI. Unlike schwannomas which show well-circumscribed margins, geniculate ganglion hemangiomas typically demonstrate irregular or ill-defined margins on high-resolution CT of the temporal bone. Facial nerve hemangiomas can also show internal mineralization giving these lesions a "honeycomb" appearance on CT which is a classic appearance (ossifying hemangiomas; ▶ Fig. 3.53). Hemangiomas of the IAC typically produce remodeling of the IAC which is similar in appearance to schwannomas. CT is also useful for the evaluation of local disease extension including cochlear fistula formation.

## Prognosis and Treatment

The mainstay of treatment for symptomatic facial nerve hemangiomas is complete surgical excision.[63] In cases where the lesion is tightly adhered to the facial nerve or geniculate ganglion, complete excision with nerve repair should be considered over partial lesion excision, given the rare possibility of disease recurrence with a subtotal resection. The timing of surgery is debatable but generally, early detection and resection are recommended as there is a suggestion that this leads to better functional outcomes.

## 3.3.7 Aneurysm

Petrous ICA aneurysms are a rare but important differential consideration for lesions involving the petrous apex. These are typically fusiform-type aneurysms and may be quite large at the time of diagnosis. These may arise by a number of mechanisms and may be congenital, posttraumatic, or postinfectious.[64] The majority of these lesions are asymptomatic, but patients may present with a range of symptoms including Horner's syndrome, pulsatile tinnitus, diplopia, or headache.

## Imaging

On CT, these are well-circumscribed lesions of the petrous apex centered on the carotid canal which may be dehiscent. With contrast, these lesions demonstrate arterial enhancement and contiguity with the carotid artery which is the key to diagnosis. CTA is the imaging modality of choice to demonstrate these features and evaluate the arterial anatomy which is necessary for treatment planning. MRI appearance is quite variable depending on the amount of thrombosis and nature of flow within the lesion. On T1- and T2-weighted spin echo sequences, the aneurysm may appear as a complex mixed signal mass with a central hypointense flow void. Mural thrombus can be hyperintense on T1-weighted images and can mimic cholesterol granuloma (▶ Table 3.1). Occasionally, pulsation artifact propagating in the phase encode direction is a clue that the lesion has arterial flow which is characteristic. After gadolinium contrast, these lesions will show arterial contrast enhancement and will show

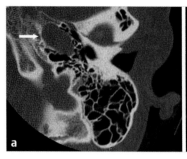
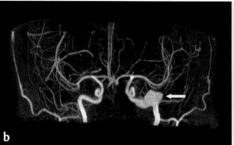

**Fig. 3.54** Petrous apex aneurysm. (**a**) Axial temporal bone CT shows a well-circumscribed ovoid lytic lesion in left petrous apex (*white arrow*) which was contiguous with the carotid canal. (**b**) MRA confirms the lesion to be an aneurysm of the left petrous internal carotid artery (*white arrow*). (Images courtesy of Dr. Aditya Bharatha.)

contiguity with the carotid artery. Contrast-enhanced MRA is preferred over time of flight MRA, as the latter can suffer from turbulence-related artifact which can underestimate the size of the residual aneurysmal sac (▶ Fig. 3.54).

## Prognosis and Treatment

Small asymptomatic aneurysms of the petrous ICA can be followed without treatment. Larger and asymptomatic aneurysms are treated either with endovascular or surgical approaches.[64]

# 3.4 Conclusion

This chapter has reviewed the most important neoplastic and nonneoplastic entities that can arise in the CPA and JF region. Many of these can give rise to similar symptoms such as tinnitus and hearing loss. Cross-sectional imaging has an important role in helping establish a correct diagnosis as well as the evaluation of key features that determine tumor resectability.

# 3.5 High Yield Summary

- The four most common tumors of the CPA are the VS, meningiomas, epidermoid cysts, and non-VS.
- MRI with contrast is the best imaging test to detect VS.
- Closely evaluate the course of the facial nerve for enhancement and enlargement—especially the labyrinthine segment and geniculate ganglion in putative cases of VS to rule out the possibility of a facial nerve schwannoma.
- The circumneural venous plexus around the facial nerve can lead to normal enhancement on imaging; the portions of the facial nerve that should not enhance are the cisternal, canalicular, and segment distal to the stylomastoid foramen.
- In some patients, one can normally see quite robust normal enhancement through the hypoglossal canal.
- Paragangliomas and schwannomas are two lesions that arise in the CS and both can be elongated in configuration.
- Key distinguishing features between these two include the presence of smooth borders and smooth bony remodeling and internal cystic change that can arise with schwannomas; paragangliomas are avidly enhancing, may show the presence of vascular flow voids, and will cause permeative bony erosion as it travels through the JF.
- Key imaging features to note for all CPA and JF region lesions include extent of intracranial disease and mass effect on the brain parenchyma, secondary hydrocephalous, degree of involvement/encasement of the carotid, jugular vessels and

dural venous sinuses, and proximity to/involvement of the cochleovestibular apparatus.
- Always assess and report any aberrant anatomy: aberrant ICA, aberrant course of the facial nerve, high-riding, and dehiscent jugular bulb, as these may influence the ease of surgery and surgical approach.
- Clinical features such as the presence and severity of any lower CN palsies play an important role in the decision-making process in patient with CPA and JF lesions; patients with serviceable hearing who also require surgery will significantly influence surgical approach in the case of VS.

# References

[1] Yasargil MG. Microneurosurgery: Volume 1: Microsurgical Anatomy of the Basal Cisterns of the Brain, Diagnostic Studies, General Operative Techniques and Pathological Consideration of the Intracranial Aneurysms. Stuttgart, Germany: Thieme; 1984:5–53

[2] Harnsberger HR, Wiggins RH III, Hudgins PA, Davidson HC, eds Diagnostic Imaging: Head and Neck. 1st ed. Salt Lake City, UT: Amirsys; 2008:126–366, 816–832

[3] Smirniotopoulos JG, Yue NC, Rushing EJ. Cerebellopontine angle masses: radiologic-pathologic correlation. Radiographics. 1993; 13(5):1131–1147

[4] Harnsberger HR, Swartz JD. Temporal bone vascular anatomy, anomalies, and diseases, emphasizing the clinical-radiological problem of pulsatile tinnitus. In: Swartz JD, Harnsberger HR. Imaging of the Temporal Bone. 3rd ed. New York, NY: Thieme; 1998:170–239

[5] Som PM, Curtin HD, eds. Head and Neck Imaging. 5th ed. St Louis: Mosby; 2011:1264–1402

[6] Clemis JD, Ballad WJ, Baggot PJ, Lyon ST. Relative frequency of inferior vestibular schwannoma. Arch Otolaryngol Head Neck Surg. 1986; 112(2):190–194

[7] Komatsuzaki A, Tsunoda A. Nerve origin of the acoustic neuroma. J Laryngol Otol. 2001; 115(5):376–379

[8] Bernstein M, Berger M. Neuro-Oncology: The Essentials. 3rd ed. New York, NY: Thieme; 2014:194–197, 391–384, 430–437

[9] https://my.statdx.com. Accessed January 31, 2015

[10] Kasantikul V, Netsky MG, Glasscock ME, III, Hays JW. Acoustic neurilemmoma. Clinicoanatomical study of 103 patients. J Neurosurg. 1980; 52(1):28–35

[11] Valvassori GE. The abnormal internal auditory canal: the diagnosis of acoustic neuroma. Radiology. 1969; 92(3):449–459

[12] Wu EH, Tang YS, Zhang YT, Bai RJ. CT in diagnosis of acoustic neuromas. AJNR Am J Neuroradiol. 1986; 7(4):645–650

[13] Schmalbrock P, Chakeres DW, Monroe JW, Saraswat A, Miles BA, Welling DB. Assessment of internal auditory canal tumors: a comparison of contrast-enhanced T1-weighted and steady-state T2-weighted gradient-echo MR imaging. AJNR Am J Neuroradiol. 1999; 20(7):1207–1213

[14] Krassanakis K, Sourtsis E, Karvounis P. Unusual appearance of an acoustic neuroma on computed tomography. Neuroradiology. 1981; 21(1):51–53

[15] Held P, Fellner C, Seitz J, Graf S, Fellner F, Strutz J. The value of T2(*)-weighted MR images for the diagnosis of acoustic neuromas. Eur J Radiol. 1999; 30(3): 237–244

[16] Sughrue ME, Kaur R, Kane AJ, et al. Intratumoral hemorrhage and fibrosis in vestibular schwannoma: a possible mechanism for hearing loss. J Neurosurg. 2011; 114(2):386–393

[17] Nakamura H, Jokura H, Takahashi K, Boku N, Akabane A, Yoshimoto T. Serial follow-up MR imaging after gamma knife radiosurgery for vestibular schwannoma. AJNR Am J Neuroradiol. 2000; 21(8):1540–1546

[18] Norén G, Arndt J, Hindmarsh T. Stereotactic radiosurgery in cases of acoustic neurinoma: further experiences. Neurosurgery. 1983; 13(1):12–22

[19] Hajioff D, Raut VV, Walsh RM, et al. Conservative management of vestibular schwannomas: third review of a 10-year prospective study. Clin Otolaryngol. 2008; 33(3):255–259

[20] Brändle P, Satoretti-Schefer S, Böhmer A, Wichmann W, Fisch U. Correlation of MRI, clinical, and electroneuronographic findings in acute facial nerve palsy. Am J Otol. 1996; 17(1):154–161

[21] Chiofalo MG, Longo F, Marone U, Franco R, Petrillo A, Pezzullo L. Cervical vagal schwannoma. A case report. Acta Otorhinolaryngol Ital. 2009; 29(1):33–35

[22] Glenner G, Grimley P. Tumors of the extraadrenal paraganglion system (including chemoreceptors). In: Firminger H, ed. Atlas of Tumor Pathology. Vol. 9. Washington, DC: Armed Forces Institute of Pathology; 1974:13–75

[23] Nelson MD, Kendall BE. Intracranial catecholamine secreting paragangliomas. Neuroradiology. 1987; 29(3):277–282

[24] Rao AB, Koeller KK, Adair CF, Armed Forces Institute of Pathology. From the archives of the AFIP. Paragangliomas of the head and neck: radiologic-pathologic correlation. Radiographics. 1999; 19(6):1605–1632

[25] Handley TP, Miah MS, Majumdar S, Hussain SS. Collet-Sicard syndrome from thrombosis of the sigmoid-jugular complex: a case report and review of the literature. Int J Otolaryngol. 2010; 2010:203487

[26] Hunt WE, Meagher JN, Lefever HE, Zeman W. Painful opthalmoplegia. Its relation to indolent inflammation of the cavernous sinus. Neurology. 1961; 11:56–62

[27] Keane JR. Cavernous sinus syndrome. Analysis of 151 cases. Arch Neurol. 1996; 53(10):967–971

[28] Stein SC, Hurst RW, Sonnad SS. Meta-analysis of cranial CT scans in children. A mathematical model to predict radiation-induced tumors. Pediatr Neurosurg. 2008; 44(6):448–457

[29] Choyke PL, Glenn GM, Walther MM, Patronas NJ, Linehan WM, Zbar B. von Hippel-Lindau disease: genetic, clinical, and imaging features. Radiology. 1995; 194(3):629–642

[30] Lonser RR, Kim HJ, Butman JA, Vortmeyer AO, Choo DI, Oldfield EH. Tumors of the endolymphatic sac in von Hippel-Lindau disease. N Engl J Med. 2004; 350 (24):2481–2486

[31] Raghunandhan S, Vijaya Krishnan P, Murali S, Anand Kumar RS, Kameswaran M. Endolymphatic sac tumor: a neoplastic cause for Meniere's syndrome. Indian J Otolaryngol Head Neck Surg. 2014; 66 Suppl 1:352–355

[32] Patel NP, Wiggins RH, III, Shelton C. The radiologic diagnosis of endolymphatic sac tumors. Laryngoscope. 2006; 116(1):40–46

[33] Yang X, Liu XS, Fang Y, Zhang XH, Zhang YK. Endolymphatic sac tumor with von Hippel-Lindau disease: report of a case with atypical pathology of endolymphatic sac tumor. Int J Clin Exp Pathol. 2014; 7(5):2609–2614

[34] Tringali S, Linthicum FH, Jr. Cholesterol granuloma of the petrous apex. Otol Neurotol. 2010; 31(9):1518–1519

[35] Razek AA, Huang BY. Lesions of the petrous apex: classification and findings at CT and MR imaging. Radiographics. 2012; 32(1):151–173

[36] Jackler RK, Cho M. A new theory to explain the genesis of petrous apex cholesterol granuloma. Otol Neurotol. 2003; 24(1):96–106, discussion 106

[37] Friedmann I. Epidermoid cholesteatoma and cholesterol granuloma; experimental and human. Ann Otol Rhinol Laryngol. 1959; 68(1):57–79

[38] Beaumont GD. The effects of exclusion of air from pneumatized bones. J Laryngol Otol. 1966; 80(3):236–249

[39] Sweeney AD, Osetinsky LM, Carlson ML, et al. The natural history and management of petrous apex cholesterol granulomas. Otol Neurotol. 2015; 36(10):1714–1719

[40] Mosnier I, Cyna-Gorse F, Grayeli AB, et al. Management of cholesterol granulomas of the petrous apex based on clinical and radiologic evaluation. Otol Neurotol. 2002; 23(4):522–528

[41] Gherini SG, Brackmann DE, Lo WW, Solti-Bohman LG. Cholesterol granuloma of the petrous apex. Laryngoscope. 1985; 95(6):659–664

[42] Ghorayeb BY, Jahrsdoerfer RA. Subcochlear approach for cholesterol granulomas of the inferior petrous apex. Otolaryngol Head Neck Surg. 1990; 103(1):60–65

[43] Montgomery WW. Cystic lesions of the petrous apex: transsphenoid approach. Ann Otol Rhinol Laryngol. 1977; 86(4, Pt 1):429–435

[44] Robert Y, Carcasset S, Rocourt N, Hennequin C, Dubrulle F, Lemaitre L. Congenital cholesteatoma of the temporal bone: MR findings and comparison with CT. AJNR Am J Neuroradiol. 1995; 16(4):755–761

[45] Pisaneschi MJ, Langer B. Congenital cholesteatoma and cholesterol granuloma of the temporal bone: role of magnetic resonance imaging. Top Magn Reson Imaging. 2000; 11(2):87–97

[46] Aubry K, Kovac L, Sauvaget E, Tran Ba Huy P, Herman P. Our experience in the management of petrous bone cholesteatoma. Skull Base. 2010; 20(3):163–167

[47] Osborn AG, Preece MT. Intracranial cysts: radiologic-pathologic correlation and imaging approach. Radiology. 2006; 239(3):650–664

[48] deSouza CE, deSouza R, da Costa S, et al. Cerebellopontine angle epidermoid cysts: a report on 30 cases. J Neurol Neurosurg Psychiatry. 1989; 52(8):986–990

[49] Safavi-Abbasi S, Di Rocco F, Bambakidis N, et al. Has management of epidermoid tumors of the cerebellopontine angle improved? A surgical synopsis of the past and present. Skull Base. 2008; 18(2):85–98

[50] Chen CY, Wong JS, Hsieh SC, Chu JS, Chan WP. Intracranial epidermoid cyst with hemorrhage: MR imaging findings. AJNR Am J Neuroradiol. 2006; 27(2):427–429

[51] Law EK, Lee RK, Ng AW, Siu DY, Ng HK. Atypical intracranial epidermoid cysts: rare anomalies with unique radiological features. Case Rep Radiol. 2015; 2015:528632

[52] Solanki SP, Maccormac O, Dow GR, Smith S. Malignant transformation of residual posterior fossa epidermoid cyst to squamous cell carcinoma. Br J Neurosurg. 2016 Jan;13:1-2.

[53] Lee YH, Lee NJ, Kim JH, Song JJ. CT, MRI and gallium SPECT in the diagnosis and treatment of petrous apicitis presenting as multiple cranial neuropathies. Br J Radiol. 2005; 78(934):948–951

[54] Burston BJ, Pretorius PM, Ramsden JD. Gradenigo's syndrome: successful conservative treatment in adult and paediatric patients. J Laryngol Otol. 2005; 119(4):325–329

[55] Kantas I, Papadopoulou A, Balatsouras DG, Aspris A, Marangos N. Therapeutic approach to Gradenigo's syndrome: a case report. J Med Case Reports. 2010; 4:151

[56] Helland CA, Lund-Johansen M, Wester K. Location, sidedness, and sex distribution of intracranial arachnoid cysts in a population-based sample. J Neurosurg. 2010; 113(5):934–939

[57] Algin O, Hakyemez B, Gokalp G, Korfali E, Parlak M. Phase-contrast cine MRI versus MR cisternography on the evaluation of the communication between intraventricular arachnoid cysts and neighbouring cerebrospinal fluid spaces. Neuroradiology. 2009; 51(5):305–312

[58] Olaya JE, Ghostine M, Rowe M, Zouros A. Endoscopic fenestration of a cerebellopontine angle arachnoid cyst resulting in complete recovery from sensorineural hearing loss and facial nerve palsy. J Neurosurg Pediatr. 2011; 7(2):157–160

[59] Alaani A, Hogg R, Siddiq MA, Chavda SV, Irving RM. Cerebellopontine angle arachnoid cysts in adult patients: what is the appropriate management? J Laryngol Otol. 2005; 119(5):337–341

[60] Mangham CA, Carberry JN, Brackmann DE. Management of intratemporal vascular tumors. Laryngoscope. 1981; 91(6):867–876

[61] Benoit MM, North PE, McKenna MJ, Mihm MC, Johnson MM, Cunningham MJ. Facial nerve hemangiomas: vascular tumors or malformations? Otolaryngol Head Neck Surg. 2010; 142(1):108–114

[62] Arts HA. Tumors of the Ear and Temporal Bone. Philadelphia, PA: Lippincott Williams & Wilkins; 2000

[63] Dai C, Li J, Zhao L, et al. Surgical experience of nine cases with intratemporal facial hemangiomas and a brief literature review. Acta Otolaryngol. 2013; 133(10):1117–1120

[64] Liu JK, Gottfried ON, Amini A, Couldwell WT. Aneurysms of the petrous internal carotid artery: anatomy, origins, and treatment. Neurosurg Focus. 2004; 17(5):E13

# 4 Petroclival and Lateral Skull Base

*Rickin Shah, Gregory J. Basura, and Ashok Srinivasan*

## 4.1 Surgical Anatomy of the Petroclival Region and Lateral Skull Base

The petroclival region can be defined as the region that includes the upper clivus and the anterior third of the petrous pyramid anterior to the internal acoustic meatus. It can be considered more as a surgical entity rather than an anatomical one, primarily due to the predilection of specific diseases such as petroclival tumors. The petroclival region or parasagittal skull base incorporates the greater sphenoid wing, cavernous sinus, branches of the trigeminal nerve, and the petroclival synchondrosis. The lateral skull base includes the far lateral aspect of the greater sphenoid wing, the lateral temporal bone, and the temporomandibular joint. When tumors affect the clival dura mater, they may also spread to the cavernous sinus, Gasserian ganglion, sphenoidal sinus, the sella, tentorial incisura, the porus, and the ventral edge of the foramen magnum. A lateral transpetrosal approach to the petroclival region is favored when exposure is needed beyond the lateral cavernous carotid and, even more so, the petrous apex and the Gasserian area. This lateral approach creates considerably broader exposure than other approaches and is also associated with reduced cerebral retraction. Since this region contains critical neurovascular structures, it is important to evaluate the anatomy accurately with noninvasive imaging prior to any surgical intervention.[1,2,3,4,5,6,7,8]

## 4.2 Imaging Modalities for Evaluation of Petroclival and Lateral Skull Base Lesions

Given the complex and intricate anatomy of the skull base, high-resolution cross-sectional imaging is the mainstay for evaluating tumors in the petroclival region and lateral skull base. It is important to realize that computed tomography (CT) and magnetic resonance imaging (MRI) are complementary. Both of these modalities can help narrow the differential diagnosis based on evaluation of the site of origin, growth pattern, and the imaging features.[9] Cross-sectional imaging also provides an assessment of the extent and accurate delineation of tumor margins, and the precise relationship between the tumor and important surrounding structures.[9]

MR imaging is the gold standard to assess the soft-tissue components, as it can routinely and accurately depict the intracranial extent of tumor. Specifically, it is helpful in evaluating for dural or leptomeningeal involvement, brain parenchymal invasion, and whether there is perineural tumor spread.[9,10,11] Both CT and MRI are useful in evaluating osseous involvement, but CT is the gold standard to define the complex anatomy of the skull base and illustrate destructive change to the thin cortical margins of the skull base neural foramina, depict calcification, and assess bony growth rate and aggressiveness.[9,10,12] The

more permeative and erosive bone changes frequently indicate aggressive neoplastic lesions, while bone expansion, remodeling, and cortical thinning usually indicate a more benign indolent neoplastic lesion.[9,12] It is important to remember that infectious processes can mimic both bone patterns.

The typical MR protocol to image the skull base will require the three orthogonal imaging planes utilizing T1- and T2-weighted images, and gadolinium-enhanced T1-weighted images with and without fat suppression. Gradient echo (T2*) imaging is useful to detect the presence of absence of paramagnetic substances, including calcification, blood degradation products, and melanin.[11,13,14] A high-resolution heavily T2-weighted sequence performed in the steady-state equilibrium will illustrate the relationships between the tumor and cisternal segments of the adjacent cranial nerves.[10,12] The conventional spin echo T1-weighted sequence can provide information on bone marrow invasion with loss of the normal fat.[11] If not contraindicated, administration of gadolinium contrast agents is essential to delineate the tumor extent and invasion as the tumor usually will demonstrate maximal enhancement signal and the other surrounding structures will enhance to a lesser degree.[10,11,14] Additional useful information is provided with utilization of fat suppression to increase the conspicuity of the enhancement on postcontrast T1-weighted sequences. However, depending on the technique, it is important to be mindful of the pitfalls with fat suppression. For example, using frequency selective fat suppression techniques, there can be failure or inadequate fat suppression along the multiple interfaces in the skull base yielding false-positive results.[9,12,15] This pitfall has increased the use of inversion recovery sequences (STIR) or Dixon-based fat suppression. Increased susceptibility effects can be seen at the skull base due to multiple air–soft tissue interfaces which has the potential for obscuring neural foramina; this can be mitigated to some extent by employing parallel imaging. Diffusion-weighted imaging provides high sensitivity to detect impeded water proton movement, which can be helpful to identify areas of increased tumor cellularity. As tumors can involve the intracranial compartment, additional whole brain evaluation with axial FLAIR and axial postcontrast sequences are also commonly employed. Utilization of parallel imaging and high field strength (3 tesla and beyond) can help in improved visualization of the finer details of the cranial nerves and cavernous sinus anatomy.

The typical CT protocol on a multidetector CT involves acquisition of the images at 0.625 mm that allows reconstructions in all three orthogonal planes with isotropic resolution. It is important to reconstruct the images using both a soft tissue and a bone algorithm to be able to depict the complex bony anatomy and detect small areas of cortical thinning or destruction. As lesions in the petroclival region and lateral skull base are better depicted using MRI, contrast-enhanced CT is typically employed for preoperative planning and not for purely diagnostic reasons.

[18]F-fluorodeoxyglucose positron emission tomography is very helpful in the posttreatment follow-up imaging protocol but plays no role in the initial diagnosis or evaluation of skull

base tumors. Catheter angiography is primarily used to assess the patency of the circle of Willis when carotid artery sacrifice is being considered. While CT angiography may be sufficient for the initial workup of vascular anatomy, catheter angiography provides a dynamic way of assessing collateral flow and performs test occlusions. When appropriate, preoperative embolization of certain highly vascular tumors has the potential for reducing surgical mortality and morbidity.[9,10,16]

## 4.3 Neoplastic Pathology of the Petroclival and Lateral Skull Base Regions and Their Imaging Features

Meningiomas occur throughout central nervous system with about 2% occurring in the petroclival region. They are most commonly found in women around the age of 50 years.[17] Although centered in the petroclival region, they can exert mass effect or compromise the surrounding structures due to the various sizes and configurations. These structures include the internal auditory canal (IAC), Meckel's cave, cavernous sinus, jugular foramen, parasellar region, foramen magnum, and brainstem. They are almost always well-defined and circumscribed masses abutting the dura.

As with most meningiomas, they are typically hyperattenuating on CT with about 25% containing calcifications.[17] The calcifications may be diffuse, focal, globular, or "sunburst" in appearance. It is not uncommon to see hyperostosis on CT which accounts for 20 to 40% of cases.[17] A majority of these lesions display intense homogenous enhancement on CT. When they grow large enough, they could demonstrate necrosis or cystic change, but hemorrhage is rare within the lesions. On MR, wherever possible, it is important to detect the cerebrospinal fluid (CSF) or vascular cleft between the tumor and brain parenchyma to ensure it is extra-axial in location. Up to 80% of meningiomas may demonstrate an enhancing "dural tail."[17] It is important to realize that the "dural tail" is not specific as it may be seen with other lesions such as a metastasis or schwannoma. They are isointense on T1-weighted images, hyperintense on T2-weighted

images, and display avid homogenous enhancement unless there is necrotic or cystic change. Heavily calcified meningiomas may exhibit T1 and T2 hypointensity with variable enhancement, sometimes termed as a *burned-out* meningioma. The FLAIR sequence is useful to detect the perilesional reactive edema/gliosis in the surrounding parenchyma, while the gradient recalled echo or T2*sequence can illustrate the calcification. When clinically indicated, a MR venography can evaluate the dural venous sinus for invasion, thrombus, and/or occlusion. Catheter angiography is reserved for preoperative embolization which can reduce blood loss.[17] The angiography will demonstrate a "sunburst" or radial appearance of arterial opacification within the tumor with the classic prolonged capillary "stain."

Schwannomas and neurofibromas can affect any cranial nerve. In the petroclival region, the trigeminal nerve is the most common affected nerve. Schwannomas are well-defined soft-tissue lesions which are hypointense on T1-weighted images and intermediate to hyperintense on T2-weighted images.[18,19] They may have homogenous or heterogeneous enhancement after gadolinium administration (▶ Fig. 4.1).[18,19] The larger tumors can show peripheral cysts and necrotic areas.[18,19] These usually present as a single lesion but when encountering multiple schwannomas, it is important to consider neurofibromatosis type 2 or schwannomatosis.[13] Neurofibromas are also well-defined soft-tissue lesions which are hypointense on T1-weighted images and intermediate to hyperintense on T2-weighted images.[18,19] After gadolinium administration, they demonstrate avid homogenous enhancement.[18,19] As schwannomas and neurofibromas grow along the nerve, they produce smooth enlargement of the nerve and exhibit spread both antegrade and retrograde along the trigeminal nerve.[18,19,20] There can be focal or segmental enlargement with skip areas.[20] These are usually benign; however, malignant schwannomas and neurofibromas exist and are most commonly seen in patients with neurofibromatosis type 1.[13,19] The more malignant tumors are more aggressive and infiltrative lesions.[16,19] While distinction between schwannomas and neurofibromas may not always be possible, the former are more frequently associated with hemorrhage, cyst formation, and fatty degeneration and are more eccentric and rounded, as opposed to the latter which are commonly fusiform and concentric.

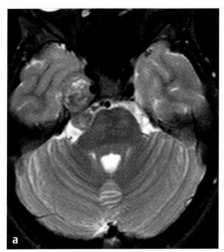 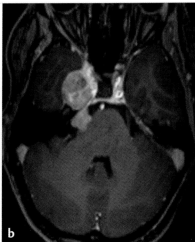

**Fig. 4.1** Axial T2-weighted (**a**) and postcontrast T1-weighted (**b**) images in a 45-year-old female patient demonstrate an enhancing lesion with heterogeneous signal on the T2-weighted image that involves the cisternal segment of the right trigeminal nerve and extends anteriorly over the petrous apex into the right middle cranial fossa. This was pathologically proven to be a trigeminal schwannoma.

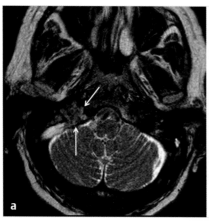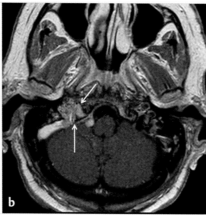

**Fig. 4.2** Axial T2-weighted (**a**) and postcontrast T1-weighted (**b**) images in a 66-year-old female patient demonstrate a lesion (*arrows*) that is of mixed signal and partly hypointense on T2-weighted images and has intense contrast enhancement in the right jugular foramen, which was proven to represent a glomus jugulare (paraganglioma).

Paragangliomas, also known as glomus tumors, can include the jugular foramen and vagus nerve. The paragangliomas that develop along the jugular foramen wall are called *glomus jugulare*, while the ones that develop along the vagus nerve are called *glomus vagale*. When they occur at the cochlear promontory, they are called *glomus tympanicum* and arise from the paraganglia along the Jacobson nerve. Their MR features include hyperintense signal on T2-weighted images mixed with T2 hypointense foci ("salt and pepper" appearance) with avid enhancement (▶ Fig. 4.2).[21] On CT, there can be permeative-destructive bony changes, particularly at the jugular foramen which distinguishes these tumors from meningiomas.[21] Glomus jugulare tumors characteristically cause dehiscence of the hypotympanum of the middle ear. Most occur as a solitary lesion and are considered benign, despite their well-known predilection for invasion of adjacent structures. The lesions are considered malignant if metastases are identified associated with the lesion. On imaging, there are no reliable imaging features to distinguish the malignant from the benign forms other than identification of a metastatic lesion.[21] MR and digital subtraction angiography is used preoperatively to assess the collateral cerebral blood flow and contralateral sigmoid sinus and internal jugular vein if the ipsilateral vessels will need to be sacrificed.[21]

Chondroid tumors including chondromyxoid fibroma and chondrosarcomas occur from the cartilaginous remnants at the petroclival synchondrosis.[13,22] These chondroid tumors contain a typical chondroid matrix of arc and ringlike calcifications which are best seen by CT.[22,23] On MR imaging, they demonstrate very high hyperintense signal on T2-weighted images which is a distinctive feature and are of low to intermediate signal on T1-weighted images (▶ Fig. 4.3).[22,23] The MR signal of the calcifications is variable depending on the size and calcium crystal composition.[22,23] MR imaging of the skull base routinely includes fat-saturated sequences to define the tumor margins. Chondromyxoid fibroma is rare but presents as an expansile, noninfiltrating mass.[24] These can demonstrate ground-glass density on CT.[24] Chordomas and plasmacytomas occur at the skull base but are typically more midline in location. Chondroblastoma or chondromatous giant cell tumor is very rare but occasionally can originate in the lateral skull base.[25]

Among all the neoplastic skull base lesions, metastasis is the most common tumor in the adult population.[12] They are usually within the marrow space due to the increased vascularity. Common primary malignancies include lung, breast, prostate, and kidney.[10,16] The CT and MR appearances can be quite variable; hence, diffuse bony metastatic disease can be confused with Paget's disease or other fibro-osseous disease. The more hypervascular metastases can be confused with hypervascular primary lesions, including paragangliomas, hemangiopericytomas, and meningiomas. Metastasis can also present as perineural spread from squamous cell, adenoid cystic, and mucoepidermoid carcinomas.[18]

A plasmacytoma-related multiple myeloma is an expansile and destructive lytic lesion that occurs in the skull base but more commonly midline in location.[13,16] They are hyperattenuating on CT and demonstrate intermediate signal on T1- and T2-weighted images.[13,16] This is typical for hypercellular tumors with small round cells and a high nuclear–cytoplasmic ratio.[13,16]

Cutaneous malignancies such as squamous cell carcinoma (▶ Fig. 4.4) and basal cell carcinoma can also invade the underlying temporal bone and necessitate large surgical resection with or without radiation therapy. Endolymphatic sac tumors are rare tumors that have high association with Von Hippel–Lindau disease, especially when they are bilateral. Their location along the posterior aspect of the petrous temporal bone along with a moth-eaten appearance on CT is an important clue toward the diagnosis (▶ Fig. 4.5).

While tumors are not uncommon entities in this region of the skull base, they have to be distinguished from nontumor entities such as infection, fibroosseous abnormalities, and Paget's disease. Appropriate history of a short clinical course with imaging clues of bone destruction and significant periosseous enhancement are clues toward making a diagnosis of skull base osteomyelitis (▶ Fig. 4.6) or necrotizing otitis externa; however, tissue diagnosis may need to be obtained when the clinical and imaging pictures are indeterminate. Fibrous dysplasia has a characteristic ground-glass appearance on CT (▶ Fig. 4.7), while Paget's disease typically presents with a mixed lytic-sclerotic appearance with or without coarsened trabeculae, thickened cortices, and bone hypertrophy in late stages (▶ Fig. 4.8). The

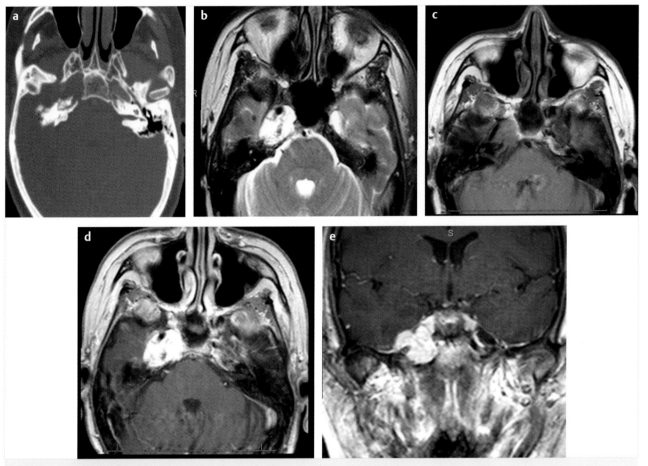

**Fig. 4.3** Axial CT image displayed using bone window settings (**a**) in a 59-year-old male patient with pathologically-proven chondrosarcoma demonstrates an expansile lytic lesion in the right petroclival region with an internal chondroid matrix. T2-weighted (**b**) as well as precontrast (**c**) and postcontrast (**d,e**) T1-weighted MRI images in the same patient demonstrate a lesion with intermediate signal on T1- and high signal on T2-weighted images that enhance after administration of contrast in the same location, with effacement of the right Meckel's cave.

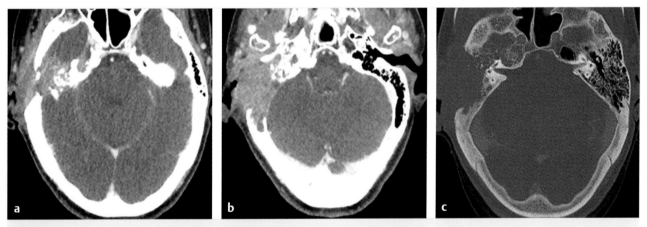

**Fig. 4.4** Axial contrast-enhanced CT images displayed using soft tissue (**a,b**) and bone window settings (**c**) demonstrate abnormal soft tissue in the right external auditory canal in an 81-year-old male with significant destruction of the lateral temporal bone, including the sigmoid sinus plate and intracranial invasion. There was also apical cochlear involvement by this squamous cell carcinoma that was presumed to be of skin origin.

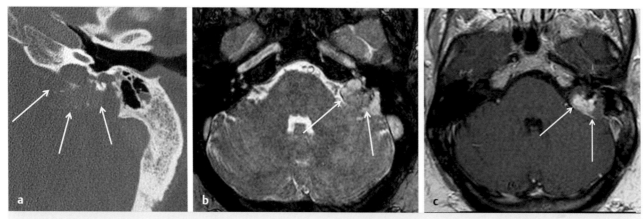

**Fig. 4.5** Axial CT image displayed using bone window settings (**a**) as well as axial T2-weighted (**b**) and postcontrast T1-weighted (**c**) MRI images in a patient with Von Hippel–Lindau syndrome demonstrate a destructive lesion (*arrows*) with heterogeneous signal on T2-weighted images and intense enhancement along the posterior aspect of the temporal bone in the expected location of the endolymphatic sac. This was an endolymphatic sac tumor on pathology.

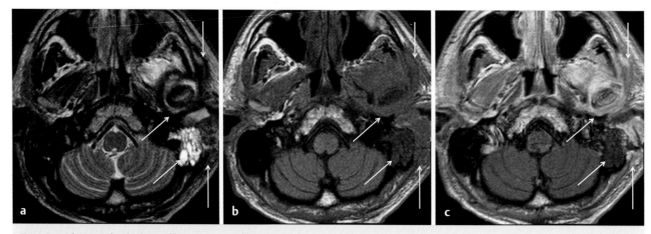

**Fig. 4.6** Axial T2-weighted (**a**) as well as precontrast (**b**) and postcontrast T1-weighted (**c**) MRI images in a 65-year-old diabetic patient demonstrate abnormal signal in the left mastoid air cells with overlying bone erosion, abnormal fat effacement in the left masticator space and subcutaneous fat, and patchy postcontrast enhancement, all of which are suspicious for osteomyelitis with extraosseous inflammation (*arrows*). The extraosseous tissue was sampled and grew *Staphylococcus aureus*, and the patient was managed nonsurgically with antibiotic therapy.

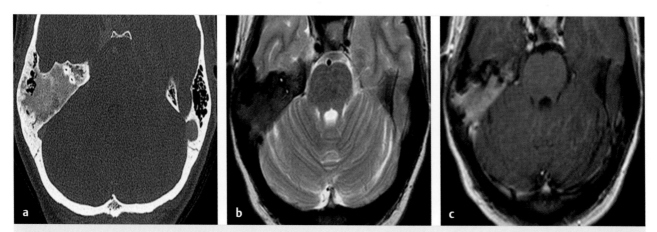

**Fig. 4.7** Axial CT displayed using bone window settings (**a**), axial T2-weighted (**b**) and postcontrast T1-weighted (**c**) MRI images in a 24-year-old male demonstrate ground-glass appearance involving nearly the entire right temporal bone with low T2 signal and intense postcontrast enhancement. These imaging features are characteristic of fibrous dysplasia.

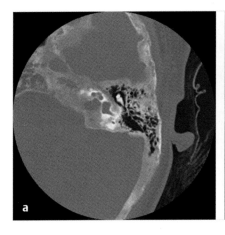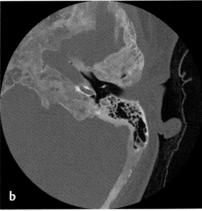

**Fig. 4.8** (a,b) Axial CT images of the left temporal bone displayed using bone window settings in a 72-year-old male demonstrate patchy rarefaction involving nearly the entire temporal bone (with sparing of most of the otic capsule) and middle cranial fossa with osseous expansion. These features are classic for Paget's disease.

imaging characteristics of common neoplastic pathologies seen in these locations are summarized in ▶ Table 4.1.

Irrespective of the disease entity that affects the petroclival region and the lateral skull base, it is important for the radiologist to comment on the status of critical structures in their dictations. These include the presence or absence of abnormalities along the course of the facial nerve, inner ear labyrinth, sigmoid sinus, and jugular bulb. Involvement of the intratemporal nerve by malignancy implies that total surgical resection may not be possible. If the inner ear labyrinth is involved by tumor, there is significant risk for hearing loss after radiation therapy. Involvement of sigmoid sinus and jugular bulb may imply intracranial invasion in some patients and preclude surgical resection; these features also place the patient at a higher risk of venous sinus thrombosis and resulting brain parenchymal complication of venous hypertension and hemorrhage.

Treatment of lesions in the petroclival region and lateral skull base often includes medical intervention (chemotherapy), radiation therapy, surgery, or a combination thereof. When lesions are surgically unresectable or when only subtotal resection can be performed, radiation therapy or stereotactic radiosurgery can be used for primary treatment or as adjuvant therapy after subtotal surgical resection. Chemotherapy can also be used as a

primary or adjunctive treatment of many skull base tumors based on the specific pathology of the tumor.

# 4.4 Surgical Approaches for Petroclival Lesions and Postsurgery Follow-Up[26]

Surgical approaches to the petroclival region are challenging due to the medial location of the skull floor and the proximity of important neural and vascular structures including the brain, cavernous sinus, and internal carotid artery. The medial portion of the petrous ridge is the petrous apex. Anatomically, this area is bounded laterally by the otic capsule and medially by the clivus with which it articulates at the petroclival synchondrosis. Many indications for surgery of the petrous apex involve access to lesions, tumors, and cystic structures (i.e., cholesterol granulomas, petrous apicitis) and therefore the approach demands the creation of a conduit between the lesion and the middle ear or mastoid, bypassing the inner ear structures. These procedures are classified as a petrous apicotomy versus a petrous apicectomy. The latter of the two actually involves the resection of the

**Table 4.1** Imaging features of petroclival and lateral skull base tumors

| Diagnosis | CT | T1 | T2 | Postcontrast | Additional features |
|---|---|---|---|---|---|
| Meningiomas | Hyperdense, homogeneous enhancement | Isointense | Variable | Avid homogeneous enhancement | Causes hyperostosis, can calcify, dural tail often present |
| Schwannomas | Isodense, heterogeneous enhancement | Iso/Hypointense | Hyperintense | Heterogeneous or peripheral enhancement | "Dumbbell" shaped |
| Neurofibromas | Isodense | Isointense | Hyperintense | Avid, sometimes heterogeneous enhancement | Infiltrative with NF-1, solitary without NF-1 |
| Paragangliomas | Isodense, homogeneous enhancement | Mixed | Mixed hyperintense | Intense enhancement | "Salt and pepper," permeative bone destruction |
| Chondrosarcomas | Slightly hyperdense, heterogeneous enhancement | Iso/Hypointense | Hyperintense | Heterogeneous enhancement | Characteristic chondroid matrix |
| Metastasis | Isodense, homogeneous enhancement | Hypointense | Hyperintense | Homogeneous enhancement | Infiltrative, perineural, or dural based |
| Plasmacytoma | Hyperdense, mild enhancement | Iso/Hypointense | Isointense | Moderate homogeneous enhancement | |

petrous apex, typically indicating for tumors of the petrous apex (i.e., chondrosarcomas, clival chordomas) or for approaches to cholesterol granulomas or basilar tip aneurysms that are not amenable to other surgical approaches. Chondrosarcomas are the most common malignancy arising from the cartilaginous component of the petroclival synchondrosis that may extend to erode into the inner ear and clivus. Other common tumors in this region include lateral extensions of clival chordomas or erosive lesions including metastatic squamous cell carcinoma.

The typical surgical approach to the petrous apex for surgical extirpation of tumor initially begins with a subtemporal craniotomy. Subsequent extradural elevation of the ipsilateral temporal lobe allows for visualization of the medial and anterior aspects of the petrous ridge. Using the landmarks including the IAC and Meckel's cave for identification of the trigeminal nerve ganglion, the tumor can be approached and resected. To adequately approach the tumor in this area, the greater superficial petrosal nerve is often sacrificed resulting in ipsilateral chronic dry eye. Further dissection medial to Meckel's cave must also take into consideration the course of the abducens nerve that travels through Dorello's canal. The limits of dissection along the floor of the petrous apical resection include the horizontal segment of the internal carotid artery.

Deeper approaches to the medial clivus typically require a combined middle and posterior fossa craniotomy.[26] Surgically, this typically consists of a retrolabyrinthine approach combined with a middle cranial fossa (MCF) craniotomy joined by the division of the tentorium. This combined approach provides optimal access to medial depths of the petrous apex for tumors located anterior and lateral to the brainstem. By pursuing this approach, tumor resection is completed between the jugular foramen (cranial nerves IX–XI) and between cranial nerves VII and VIII, near the root entry zone of the trigeminal nerve. As a result, intraoperative nerve monitoring of the trigeminal, facial, and lower cranial nerves is commonly performed to avoid any untoward events that could leave the patient with considerable head and neck dysfunction. Postoperatively, these patients are admitted to the neurosurgical intensive care unit for 24 to 48 hours of hourly neurological evaluations, pain control, and hemodynamic monitoring. Once patients have cleared the first 24 to 48 hours of care, they are typically transferred to the floor units where physical therapy begins and normalization of activities of daily living (i.e., bowel, bladder, and ambulation) ensues. Postoperative imaging following tumor resection or cyst drainage varies depending on clinical pathology as well as the potential need for postresection radiation.

# 4.5 Surgical Approaches for Lateral Skull Base Lesions and Postsurgery Follow-Up

Three surgical approaches (MCF, retrosigmoid (RS)/suboccipital, or translabyrinthine [TL]) to the lateral cranial base/temporal bone are typically employed for tumor extirpation (▶ Table 4.2). Each approach is individually selected based on the nature of the pathology and tumors that includes tumor size, location, preoperative hearing status, patient preference, and individual medical comorbidities. The MCF approach is typically reserved for small tumors confined to the medial aspects of the IAC with optimal characteristics for hearing preservation.[27] The RS approach is used for large cerebellopontine angle (CPA) tumors with or without considerable brainstem compression or for all tumors except those isolated to the lateral IAC. The TL approach is hearing ablative as it provides a direct route through the inner ear to the IAC and CPA without brain retraction. This approach provides ideal access and visualization of the lateral IAC for complete tumor extirpation and early facial nerve (FN) identification.[28]

## 4.5.1 Middle Cranial Fossa Approach

With availability of thinner sections and increased spatial resolution in MR imaging, identification of small (< 1.5 cm) tumors in patients with normal or near-normal hearing has increased in the last few years. In younger, healthy patients with serviceable hearing and a medially positioned tumor within the IAC, a MCF approach is indicated (▶ Fig. 4.9, ▶ Fig. 4.10). DeMonte and Gidley[29] outlined the ideal patients for a MCF approach and VS resection with hearing preservation to include those with tumors with 1 cm or less extension into the CPA located in the medial end of the IAC with a hearing loss no greater than 40 dB on pure tone average testing and a word recognition score of at least 80% (AAO-HNS Class A and upper Class B hearing). They also identified those younger than 65 years as dural elevation becomes more difficult in older patients.

The surgical approach begins following a supra-auricular incision that leads to a downward displacement of the temporalis muscle and a squamous temporal bone craniotomy. The temporal lobe is elevated off the floor of the petrous temporal bone in the extradural plane and retracted. During the elevation, care must be exercised to avoid facial nerve

**Table 4.2** Comparison of the different surgical techniques for resection of lateral skull base lesions

| Approach | Advantages | Disadvantages | Structures at risk |
|---|---|---|---|
| MCF | 1. Hearing preservation approach<br>2. Balance function can be potentially spared | 1. Brain retraction<br>2. Facial nerve superior in internal auditory canal; injury prone | 1. Temporal lobe retraction<br>2. Cochlea and labyrinth<br>3. Facial nerve |
| TL | 1. No brain retraction<br>2. Facial nerve location optimal for identification to minimize injury | 1. Destroys residual hearing and balance<br>2. Requires large abdominal fat graft | 1. Facial nerve in temporal bone<br>2. Sigmoid, superior petrosal sinus, and jugular bulb |
| RS | 1. Hearing preservation approach<br>2. Less bony drilling required | 1. Brain retraction<br>2. Intradural drilling if IAC component; more headache | 1. Cerebellar retraction<br>2. Facial nerve in cerebellopontine angle cistern |

Abbreviations: IAC, internal auditory canal; MCF, middle cranial fossa; RS, retrosigmoid; TL, translabyrinthine.

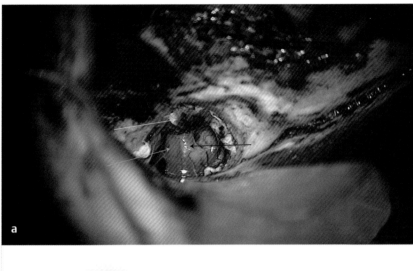

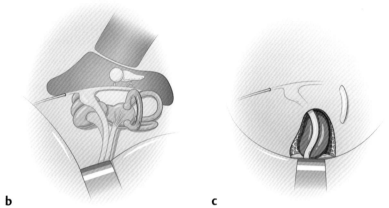

**Fig. 4.9** Middle cranial fossa approach to internal auditory canal vestibular schwannoma as a hearing preservation approach. (**a**) Photograph shows surgical removal of the roof of the internal auditory canal with the temporal lobe of the brain elevated off the floor of the skull (bottom of picture with retractor in place). Notice the facial nerve (*green arrow*) positioned in the anterior superior quadrant of the internal auditor canal making it vulnerable to injury upon opening of the canal dura and during tumor resection. The superior vestibular nerve (SVN; *long black arrow*) is oriented in the posterior superior quadrant of the canal with the inferior vestibular nerve (posterior and inferior to the SVN), which is free of the vestibular schwannoma (*yellow arrow*), which is lateral in the internal auditory canal and likely arising from the SVN. Note the relationship of the greater superficial petrosal nerve within the anterior petrous ridge (*short black arrow*). This approach is also illustrated on the schematic diagrams (**b,c**). (Part **a** is courtesy of Karl Storz, Endoscopy, Tuttlingen, Germany.)

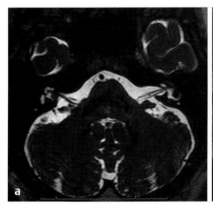

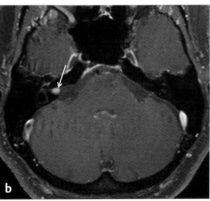

**Fig. 4.10** Axial high-resolution heavily T2-weighted (**a**) and postcontrast T1-weighted (**b**) images in a 60-year-old male patient demonstrate an enhancing lesion (*arrow*) confined to the right internal auditory canal without extracanalicular extension. A middle cranial fossa surgical approach would be ideal in this situation, especially for hearing preservation.

injury to a potentially dehiscent geniculate ganglion or greater superficial petrosal nerve (GSPN). Anterior exposure must also respect the trigeminal ganglion in Meckel's cave and the middle meningeal artery in foramen spinosum. Once the temporal lobe has been elevated to the medial edge of the petrous bone adjacent to the superior petrosal vein, bone removal begins. The dome of the superior semicircular canal (SSCC) must be identified first to establish the posterolateral boundary of the dissection where the medial "safe triangles" can then be drilled adjacent to the porus acusticus of the IAC between the SSCC and the petrous apex. Knowing the course

of the IAC being delineated by a line bisecting an angle made between the SSCC dome and the GSPN, the medial triangles can then be planned. Once the dura of the IAC has been identified at the porus acusticus, the dissection then proceeds from medial to lateral along the IAC, identifying the labyrinthine segment of the facial nerve and the cochlea. Once the IAC has been skeletonized at least 270 degrees around, the dura can be opened and tumor removal may begin. The durotomy following tumor resection is typically sealed with abdominal fat to prevent CSF leaks and the craniotomy bone flap secured with plates and screws.

Any intracranial surgery that involves brain retraction has potential surgical risks that include epidural hematoma, brain edema, pneumocephalus, CSF leak, meningitis, seizure, and wound complications/infections. Specific to MCF surgery are temporal lobe injury (if dominant lobe could lead to transient aphasia/dysphasia), CSF leak, hearing loss, and FN injury. With more improved surgical technique leading to shorter operative and brain retraction time, many complications secondary to MCF surgery are largely limited to CSF leak, FN injury, and hearing loss. One main disadvantage of the MCF approach is the proximity of the FN within the superior fallopian canal and manipulation of the nerve during tumor extirpation. Tumor size is therefore deemed to be the most important prognostic factor of postoperative FN outcome. At 1 year following MCF resection of tumors 1.5 cm or smaller, Arriaga et al[30] reported that 96% of patients retained normal or near-normal FN function (House-Brackmann grades I or II) with a more recent report of 94.5% retaining HB I–II following MCF resection of tumors smaller than 1 cm.[31] Other groups have reported similar findings with smaller IAC tumors.[32]

## 4.5.2 Retrosigmoid Approach

Of the noted surgical approaches to the CPA/IAC, the RS or suboccipital approach is the most commonly utilized and provides wide visualization of the CPA.[33] As such, it can be employed for small to medium sized tumors that have minimal extension within the IAC (▶ Fig. 4.11, ▶ Fig. 4.12) with the goal of hearing preservation (same AAO selection criteria as outlined for MCF approach earlier) and for large tumors, to alleviate brainstem and neurovascular compression. It is ideally utilized as a hearing sparing technique and provides ideal exposure of the brainstem and cranial nerves IV through XII.

Surgically, this approach involves making a RS craniotomy through a linear scalp incision behind the mastoid and sigmoid sinus near the temporal line. Following bone removal, the cerebellar cistern is entered and typically the evacuation of cisternal CSF allows for significant cerebellar brain relaxation that is amenable to retraction. Following placement of the retractor, tumor is often encountered and debulked up to the porus acusticus. If tumor does extend into the porus and the IAC, bone removal over the medial IAC is often performed. Following the creation of dural cuts and reflections near the posterior porus, the bone is removed along the posterior aspect of the IAC up to the limits of the dissection, the endolymphatic duct, and the posterior semicircular canal. This bone removal will provide for adequate access to remove any components of tumor that may course through the IAC.

Like the MCF approach, the RS also involves brain retraction and may therefore be fraught with similar surgical complications, including brain (brainstem and cerebellar) edema, hematoma, dural venous sinus congestion, vascular and/or lower

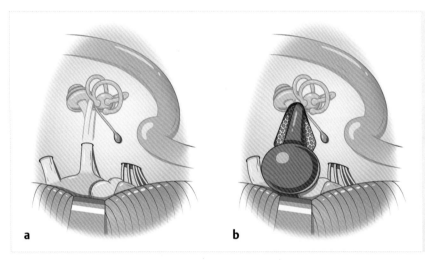

**Fig. 4.11 (a,b)** Schematic diagrams illustrating the retrosigmoid (RS) surgical approach.

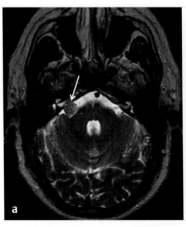
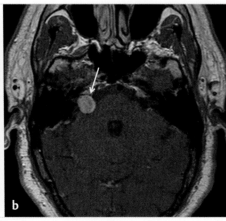

**Fig. 4.12** Axial T2-weighted (**a**) and postcontrast T1-weighted (**b**) MRI images in a 70-year-old female patient demonstrate an enhancing lesion (*arrow*) mostly confined to the right cerebellopontine angle with mild mass effect on the pons. A RS approach in this situation can be optimal, as it provides wide visualization of this anatomical region with hearing preservation.

cranial nerve injury, chronic headache from intradural drilling, CSF leak, FN injury, and hearing loss. Given the posterior approach for larger tumors, the FN is often found on the anterior surface of the tumor and is therefore not at immediate risk of injury as it is in the MCF approach. However, the cisternal segment of the FN lacks a true epineurium and is therefore prone to splaying with mass effect from larger tumors, which may place the nerve at greater risk for stretch or transection injury often leading to subtotal tumor resection.

### 4.5.3 Translabyrinthine Approach

The TL approach is often utilized for larger CPA/IAC tumors when preoperative hearing is poor or in cases where the chance of sparing hearing during surgery would be unlikely (▶ Fig. 4.13, ▶ Fig. 4.14). As with the MCF and RS approaches, there are advantages and disadvantages. One main advantage of the TL approach is that it provides the most direct route to the CPA and exposes the IAC in its entirety. This is accomplished without brain retraction and the FN can be easily located and unmolested due to the vast exposure of the IAC and translocation if required. The TL approach therefore provides ideal tumor exposure and a safe and reliable tissue plane between the tumor and the FN. In addition to VS, the TL approach may be used for other lesions of the CPA including meningiomas, epidermoid cysts, glomus tumors, lipomas, metastatic lesions, and choroid plexus papillomas.[28] The main disadvantages of the TL approach lie in the obliteration of residual hearing and balance function for the ipsilateral ear and the need for a fat graft repair to prevent CSF leaks postoperatively.

Surgically, the TL approach begins with a widely exposed intact canal wall mastoidectomy identifying and exposing the mastoid antrum, horizontal semicircular canal, temporal lobe dura, the sigmoid sinus, and the posterior fossa dura. Once the mastoid segment of the facial nerve has been identified, a labyrinthectomy is performed and all bone lining the pre- and postsigmoid sinus dura and temporal lobe of the brain is removed. The IAC is then identified extending at the level of the inner ear vestibule and superior and inferior bony troughs are drilled above the IAC to the level of the skull base and inferiorly down to the jugular bulb. Once the IAC dura is identified, bone is removed above and below down to the dura which then is extended posteriorly to the presigmoid, endolymphatic sac. Following bone removal, the dura is opened along the presigmoid region with dissection extending into the IAC to outline the CPA tumor for extirpation. Following tumor removal, the CPA is filled with abdominal fat and a watertight primary closure of the periosteum to prevent CSF leak.

As with the MCF and RS techniques, surgical complications also exist for the TL approach. Since the TL approach obliterates

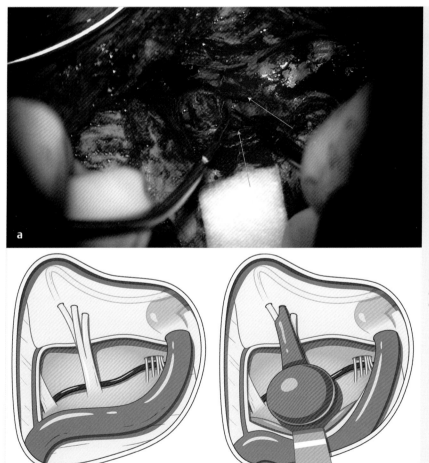

**Fig. 4.13** Vestibular schwannoma resection using a hearing-ablative translabyrinthine approach to the internal auditory canal and cerebellopontine angle. (a) Photograph shows the temporal bone following mastoidectomy, labyrinthectomy, and removal of the deeper bone over the posterior fossa dura and temporal lobe of the brain. The bone overlying the internal auditory canal (*black arrow*) has been removed revealing gross schwannoma filling the canal. The tumor extends into the cerebellopontine angle deep to the posterior fossa dura (*green arrow*) that will be opened to provide a panoramic view within the cerebellopontine angle and cistern for tumor removal. Note the proximity of the internal auditory canal (formerly deep to the bony labyrinth) to the second genu and descending portion of the facial nerve (*yellow arrow*) that must be accounted for to prevent injury when performing the labyrinthectomy. This approach is also illustrated by schematic diagrams (**b,c**). (Part **a** is courtesy of Karl Storz Endoscopy, Tuttlingen, Germany.)

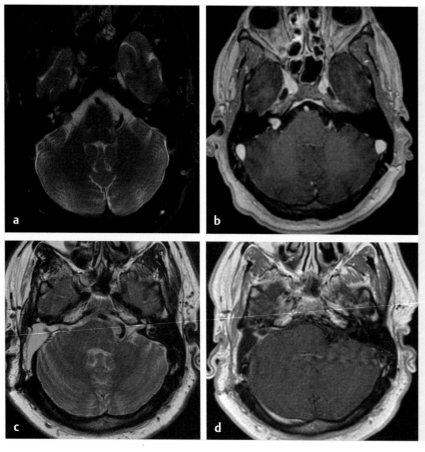

**Fig. 4.14** Axial T2-weighted (**a**) and postcontrast T1-weighted (**b**) images in a 56-year-old female patient demonstrate an enhancing lesion involving nearly the entire right internal auditory canal with medial extension into the cerebello-pontine angle cistern. A translabyrinthine approach in this situation provides ideal access and visualization of the lateral IAC for complete tumor extirpation and early facial nerve identification without brain retraction but is hearing ablative. Postoperative axial T2-weighted (**c**) and postcontrast T1-weighted (**d**) images in the same patient show a large surgical cavity involving the mastoid and petrous temporal bones and the absence of the major inner ear structures.

the inner ear, residual hearing and balance function are sacrificed entirely and are therefore expected outcomes rather than surgical complications. Owing to the lack of brain retraction required for this approach, complications are largely limited to FN injury, bleeding, CSF leak, meningitis, and wound complications/infections.

## 4.6 Summary

In conclusion, many different types of tumors can involve the lateral skull base and petroclival region. Radiologists should not only strive to provide an appropriate differential diagnosis based on the imaging features but also focus on describing the entire extent of the lesion, as this information is crucial for the surgeons to determine which surgical approach may be the most appropriate for an individual patient.

## References

[1] Cho CW, Al-Mefty O. Combined petrosal approach to petroclival meningiomas. Neurosurgery. 2002; 51(3):708–716, discussion 716–718

[2] Day JD, Fukushima T, Giannotta SL. Microanatomical study of the extradural middle fossa approach to the petroclival and posterior cavernous sinus region: description of the rhomboid construct. Neurosurgery. 1994; 34(6): 1009–1016, discussion 1016

[3] Day JD, Fukushima T, Giannotta SL. Cranial base approaches to posterior circulation aneurysms. J Neurosurg. 1997; 87(4):544–554

[4] Day JD, Giannotta SL, Fukushima T. Extradural temporopolar approach to lesions of the upper basilar artery and infrachiasmatic region. J Neurosurg. 1994; 81(2):230–235

[5] Dolenc VV. Microsurgical Anatomy and Surgery of the Central Skull Base. New York, NY: Springer, Wien; 2003

[6] Lasjaunias P, Merland JJ, Théron J, Moret J. Vascularisation meningee de la fosse cerebrale moyenne. [Dural vascularization of the middle fossa (author's transl)]. [Article in French]. J Neuroradiol. 1977; 4(4):361–384

[7] Matsushima T, Rhoton AL, Jr, de Oliveira E, Peace D. Microsurgical anatomy of the veins of the posterior fossa. J Neurosurg. 1983; 59(1):63–105

[8] Mercier P, Cronier P, Mayer B, Pillet J, Fischer G. Microanatomical study of the arterial blood supply of the facial nerve in the ponto-cerebellar angle. Anat Clin. 1982; 3(3):263–270

[9] Borges A. Skull base tumours part I: imaging technique, anatomy and anterior skull base tumours. Eur J Radiol. 2008; 66(3):338–347

[10] Casselman JW. The skull base: tumoral lesions. Eur Radiol. 2005; 15(3):534–542

[11] Fischbein NJ, Kaplan MJ. Magnetic resonance imaging of the central skull base. Top Magn Reson Imaging. 1999; 10(5):325–346

[12] Curtin HD, Chavali R. Imaging of the skull base. Radiol Clin North Am. 1998; 36(5):801–817, v-vi

[13] Lufkin RB, Borges A, Nguyen K, et al. MRI of the Head and Neck. 2nd ed. Philadelphia, PA: Lippincott Williams & Wilkins; 2001

[14] Lufkin RB, Borges A, Villablanca P. Teaching Atlas of Head and Neck Imaging. 1st ed. New York, NY: Thieme; 2000

[15] Borges AR, Lufkin RB, Huang AY, Farahani K, Arnold AC. Frequency-selective fat suppression MR imaging. Localized asymmetric failure of fat suppression mimicking orbital disease. J Neuroophthalmol. 1997; 17(1):12–17

[16] Borges A. Skull base tumours Part II. Central skull base tumours and intrinsic tumours of the bony skull base. Eur J Radiol. 2008; 66(3):348–362

[17] Hunter JB, Weaver KD, Thompson RC, Wanna GB. Petroclival meningiomas. Otolaryngol Clin North Am. 2015; 48(3):477–490

[18] Borges A, Casselman J. Imaging the cranial nerves: part II: primary and secondary neoplastic conditions and neurovascular conflicts. Eur Radiol. 2007; 17 (9):2332–2344

[19] Majoie CB, Hulsmans FJ, Castelijns JA, et al. Primary nerve-sheath tumours of the trigeminal nerve: clinical and MRI findings. Neuroradiology. 1999; 41(2): 100–108

[20] Williams LS. Advanced concepts in the imaging of perineural spread of tumor to the trigeminal nerve. Top Magn Reson Imaging. 1999; 10(6):376–383

[21] Gjuric M, Gleeson M. Consensus statement and guidelines on the management of paragangliomas of the head and neck. Skull Base. 2009; 19(1):109–116

[22] Rosenberg AE, Nielsen GP, Keel SB, et al. Chondrosarcoma of the base of the skull: a clinicopathologic study of 200 cases with emphasis on its distinction from chordoma. Am J Surg Pathol. 1999; 23(11):1370–1378

[23] Neff B, Sataloff RT, Storey L, Hawkshaw M, Spiegel JR. Chondrosarcoma of the skull base. Laryngoscope. 2002; 112(1):134–139

[24] Keel SB, Bhan AK, Liebsch NJ, Rosenberg AE. Chondromyxoid fibroma of the skull base: a tumor which may be confused with chordoma and chondrosarcoma. A report of three cases and review of the literature. Am J Surg Pathol. 1997; 21(5):577–582

[25] Bui P, Ivan D, Oliver D, Busaidy KF, Wilson J. Chondroblastoma of the temporomandibular joint: report of a case and literature review. J Oral Maxillofac Surg. 2009; 67(2):405–409

[26] Jackler RK, Brackmann DE. Neurotology. Portland, OR: Elsevier Health Sciences; 2004

[27] Quesnel AM, McKenna MJ. Current strategies in management of intracanalicular vestibular schwannoma. Curr Opin Otolaryngol Head Neck Surg. 2011; 19(5):335–340

[28] Arriaga MA, Lin J. Translabyrinthine approach: indications, techniques, and results. Otolaryngol Clin North Am. 2012; 45(2):399–415, ix

[29] DeMonte F, Gidley PW. Hearing preservation surgery for vestibular schwannoma: experience with the middle fossa approach. Neurosurg Focus. 2012; 33(3):E10

[30] Arriaga MA, Luxford WM, Berliner KI. Facial nerve function following middle fossa and translabyrinthine acoustic tumor surgery: a comparison. Am J Otol. 1994; 15(5):620–624

[31] Fayad JN, Brackmann DE. Treatment of small acoustic tumors (vestibular schwannomas). Neurosurg Q. 2005; 15(2):127–137

[32] Satar B, Jackler RK, Oghalai J, Pitts LH, Yates PD. Risk-benefit analysis of using the middle fossa approach for acoustic neuromas with > 10 mm cerebellopontine angle component. Laryngoscope. 2002; 112(8, Pt 1):1500–1506

[33] Elhammady MS, Telischi FF, Morcos JJ. Retrosigmoid approach: indications, techniques, and results. Otolaryngol Clin North Am. 2012; 45(2):375–397, ix

# 5 Open and Endoscopic Approaches to the Sinonasal Cavity and Skull Base

*Nidal Muhanna, Christopher J. Chin, Allan D. Vescan, and John R. de Almeida*

## 5.1 Introduction

Surgical access to the sinonasal cavity and skull base is intrinsically challenging given their proximity to critical anatomy and neurovascular structures. The ideal surgical approach to the sinonasal cavity and skull base should provide adequate exposure for complete surgical resection and subsequently for appropriate reconstruction. Cancers of the nasal cavity and paranasal sinuses make up a small subset of these head and neck tumors, but given their location and proximity to important structures, they may be some of the most difficult to manage. The underlying goal of treatment remains gross total tumor eradication, whether through surgery, radiation, chemotherapy, or a combination of modalities. As surgical, radiation and imaging techniques have improved, so have survival, functional outcomes, and quality of life.

More recently, endoscopic endonasal approaches have been adopted as a strategy in surgical management of these tumors. Endoscopic endonasal approaches offer improved visualization and the avoidance of external facial incisions and external bony osteotomies for tumor access. As experience with endoscopic techniques and technology have progressed, an increasing amount of skull base tumors have become accessible. However, the ultimate goals of surgical management, which include the extirpation of tumors, with negative surgical margins while maintaining patient quality of life, have not changed.

## 5.2 Skull Base Pathology

### 5.2.1 Frontal Sinus

Isolated frontal sinus pathology is rare. Most commonly these include inflammatory sinus disease. Other processes include complications of inflammatory sinus disease such as mucocele, benign pathology such as osteomas, traumatic cerebrospinal fluid (CSF) leaks associated with frontal sinus fractures, and rarely isolated sinus malignancy.

### 5.2.2 Anterior Cranial Base

Pathology of the anterior cranial base includes sinonasal malignancies and metastatic disease. Benign histopathology includes osteomas, cavernous hemangiomas, and inverted papillomas, among others. Anterior cranial base meningiomas of the olfactory groove, planum sphenoidale, or tuberculum sellae also arise in this location. Iatrogenic, congenital, or idiopathic injuries or deficiencies in the skull base resulting in CSF leak and/or meningoencephaloceles may arise here.

### 5.2.3 Sella/Suprasellar

Sellar pathology most commonly arises in the pituitary gland in the form of pituitary adenomas. Other pathology in these locations includes craniopharyngiomas, Rathke's cysts, and meningiomas.

### 5.2.4 Nasopharynx/Clivus

Nasopharyngeal carcinoma is the most common pathology of the nasopharynx, although other rare pathologies such as Tornwaldt cysts and minor salivary gland tumors may arise here. Clival tumors chordomas, chondrosarcomas, as well as other infectious processes such as skull base osteomyelitis can develop in this location.

### 5.2.5 Upper Cervical Spine

Pathology of the upper cervical spine may be accessed by endoscopic techniques in rare instances, but commonly requires open procedures. Pathologies of this location include chordomas and inflammatory processes such as rheumatoid panus associated with basilar invagination.

### 5.2.6 Petrous Apex

Petrous apex pathologies include inflammatory disease such as cholesterol granulomas and malignant processes such as chondrosarcoma and metastatic disease.

## 5.3 Endoscopic Surgical Anatomy

Endoscopic anatomy, from the surgical perspective, is conceptualized differently than traditional open surgical approaches and has been termed "inside out anatomy." For surgeons facile with open transfacial or transcranial approaches, this involves an understanding of nasal and paranasal sinus anatomy as the focal point of surgical access. With endoscopic approaches, skull base pathology is approached through corridors usually created by the surgeon.

Endoscopic surgical anatomy maybe conceptualized as approaches of the "sagittal plane" and those of the "coronal plane." "Because of the structures in the mediolateral plane, coronal plane approaches may be associated with more potential collateral damage associated with the surgical approach. As such, it has been suggested that surgeons undertaking these procedures adopt a graduated approach beginning with cases involving the sagittal plane early in their experience before undertaking cases involving the coronal plane.[1,2] The sagittal plane is divided into several surgical modules including transfrontal, transcribriform, transplanum, transsellar, transclival, and transodontoid approaches (▶ Fig. 5.1). The coronal plane may be subdivided into anterior, middle, and posterior coronal planes.[2] The anterior coronal plane is primarily composed of the transorbital approach. The middle coronal plane is composed of transpterygoid, infrapetrous, and suprapetrous approaches, as well as approaches to the cavernous sinus.

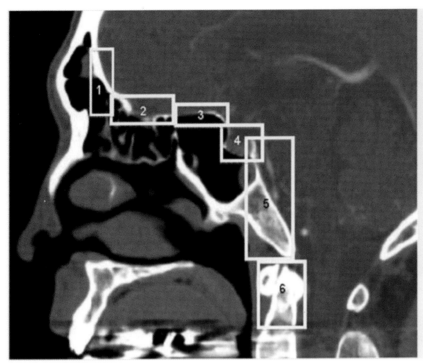

**Fig. 5.1** Endoscopic endonasal approaches in the sagittal plane. Approaches can be divided into (1) transfrontal, (2) transcribriform, (3) transplanum, (4) transsellar, (5) transclival, and (6) transodontoid approaches. (Used with permission from Snyderman CH, Pant H, Carrau RL, et al. What are the limits of endoscopic sinus surgery? The expanded endonasal approach to the skull base. Keio J Med. 2009;58(3):152–160.)

The posterior coronal plane includes approaches to the parapharyngeal space and jugular foramen.

Anatomically, endoscopic access to the frontal sinus may be limited anteriorly and pathologies at the anterior and superior aspects of the frontal sinus often require open approaches. The frontal sinus outflow tract or frontal recess is bordered medially by the middle turbinate, anteriorly by the frontal process of the maxilla and frontal bone (frontal beak), laterally by the lamina papyracea, and posteriorly by the bulla ethmoidalis. The agger nasi air cell is the most anterior ethmoidal air cell and lies anterolateral to the frontal recess. Enlargement of the frontal recess often requires skeletonizing this air cell.

The roof of the anterior skull base is formed by the cribriform plate medially and the fovea ethmoidalis laterally. The cribriform plate is often located inferior to the plane of the fovea ethmoidalis. These two structures are connected by an oblique bone known as the lateral lamella of the cribriform plate. Because of its relatively thin structure, the lateral lamella is often an area susceptible to iatrogenic injury and resultant CSF leaks. The risk for injury to this structure is thought to be related to its vertical height. The classification system of Keros describes the height of the lateral lamella, or the difference in height of the fovea ethmoidalis and the cribriform plate, as either type 1 (depth of 1–3 mm), type 2 (depth of 4–7 mm), or type 3 (8–16 mm).[3] The greater the depth, the higher the risk of iatrogenic injury. Also, an asymmetrical skull base (between the left and right sides) poses a higher risk for iatrogenic injury.

More posteriorly located is the sphenoid sinus which drains anteriorly into the nasal cavity through the sphenoethmoidal recess. The sphenoid ostium is located medial to the superior turbinate. The sphenoid sinus is the central point for many endoscopic skull base approaches. Also intimate with the sphenoid sinus are several critical structures such as the sella turcica, the internal carotid artery, and the optic nerve.

The sphenoid sinus pneumatization may vary from individual to individual. The pneumatization of the sphenoid may be classified as a sellar, presellar, or conchal pneumatization pattern.[4] The most pneumatized of these patterns is the sellar pattern, followed by presellar and conchal. Conchal pneumatization may pose challenges for surgical access in that anatomic landmarks are not readily visualized and the sella, carotid arteries, and optic nerves are often hidden in bone. When planning surgical approaches that require opening of the sphenoid sinus, surgeons must be aware of the presence of Onodi air cells. Onodi cells are posterior ethmoidal air cells that pneumatize superiorly and laterally above the sphenoid sinus. These cells, when present, can place certain anatomic structures, particularly the optic nerve, at risk.

There are several limits to endoscopic approaches (▶ Fig. 5.2, ▶ Fig. 5.3, ▶ Fig. 5.4). Anteriorly, the anterior table of the frontal sinus may be difficult to access. Although the posterior table is often accessible, this may provide challenges in terms of tumor resection and reconstruction. Superolaterally, the midline of the orbit is generally considered the farthest lateral access that can be achieved with an endoscopic approach. Inferolaterally, access to the pterygopalatine fossa, infratemporal fossa, and middle cranial fossa can be achieved through an endonasal approach. Further lateral access can be achieved with a Denker's modification or with a Caldwell-Luc modification (these modifications are described in section "Endoscopic Lateral Approaches"). Inferiorly, the palate serves as the inferior border of dissection. Lesions involving the palate often require open approaches for complete resection. The inferior limit of dissection posteriorly is limited by fixed bony structures with the nasal bones superiorly and the hard palate posteroinferiorly. The so-called nasopalatine line is an imaginary line connecting these two anatomic structures and serves as a theoretical boundary for inferior dissection (▶ Fig. 5.4).[5]

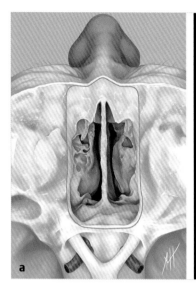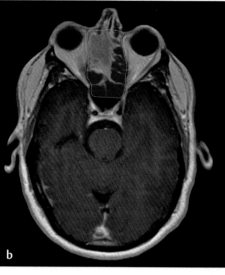

Fig. 5.2 Axial view of endoscopic limits of resection at the level of the cribriform plate and orbits in (a) graphic image and (b) axial imaging (magnetic resonance imaging [MRI]). The lateral extent of resection depicted here is the lamina papyracea bilaterally. Further lateral surgical access can be gained to the meridian of the orbit by removing the bony lamina papyracea.

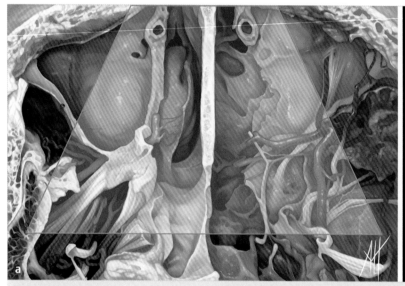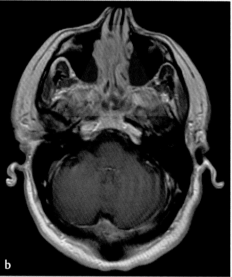

Fig. 5.3 Axial view of endoscopic limits of resection at the level of the maxillary sinus in (a) graphic image and (b) axial imaging (magnetic resonance imaging). Access to the lateral wall of the maxillary sinus as depicted in the above figure is limited but may be improved with a Caldwell-Luc approach or a Denker's approach. The endoscopic approach provides good access to the pterygopalatine fossa and infratemporal fossa and can be further enhanced with the previous two modifications.

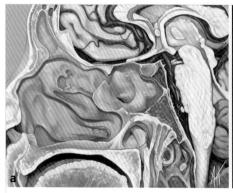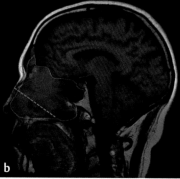

Fig. 5.4 Sagittal view of endoscopic limits of resection in (a) graphic image and (b) sagittal imaging (magnetic resonance imaging). The anterior extent of surgical access is the posterior table of the frontal sinus. Tumor extension into the anterior table of the frontal sinus is often difficult to access endoscopically. Anterior extension of tumors into the soft tissues of the nose and nasal bones often requires open approaches for access. The posterior extent depicted here are for malignant sinonasal tumors. Further posterior access to the planum, tuberculum, and clivus is possible. Similarly, superior extension depicted here is for malignant sinonasal tumors. Further superior dissection is possible. The *dotted line* depicts the nasopalatine line.

## 5.4 Open Surgical Anatomy

Understanding of the anatomy for open surgical approaches requires understanding of the function of the anatomic structures in the surgical field, as well as the course of critical neurovascular structures, and the potential spaces in which these structures may reach a confluence.

The nasal cavity warms and humidifies air, while functioning to also filter out larger particles. The nasal septum, made up of cartilage and bone, comprises the midline structure of the nose. Attached on the lateral walls are the paired inferior, middle, and superior turbinates. Occasionally, a supreme turbinate is also present. Olfactory mucosa helps in the detection of odors, and is located along the skull base and superior septum. The nasal cavity meets the nasopharynx at the choana posteriorly, where the adenoid tissue is located.

Classically, there are four paired air-filled sinuses: the maxillary, ethmoid, frontal, and sphenoid sinuses. The maxillary sinus ("antrum of Highmore") drains into the middle meatus, specifically the infundibulum. The entrance to the infundibulum is the crescent-shaped hiatus semilunaris, formed by the uncinate process and the bulla ethmoidalis. Ohngren's line represents an imaginary line that divides the maxillary sinus into anterior and posterior compartments. It is formed by drawing a line from the medial canthus to the angle of the mandible. Tumors inferior to this line are prognostically more favorable and generally referred to as infrastructural tumors, whereas tumors above this line are generally referred to as suprastructural tumors.

Beyond the posterior wall of the maxillary sinus is a fat-filled space known as the pterygopalatine fossa. This fossa contains several important structures including the internal maxillary artery, the pterygopalatine ganglion, the Vidian nerve, the infraorbital nerve and V2 nerve, the palatovaginal nerve, and the descending palatine nerve. There are seven foramina that communicate with this space, all of which provide potential routes of tumor spread. These foramina include foramen rotundum (V2), Vidian canal, the palatovaginal canal, inferior orbital fissure, sphenopalatine foramen, the pterygomaxillary fissure, and the greater palatine canal. Lateral to the pterygopalatine fossa is the infratemporal fossa. This is separated from the pterygopalatine fossa by the pterygomaxillary fissure. The borders of this space include the maxillary tuberosity anteriorly, the temporal bone posteriorly, the greater wing of the sphenoid bone superiorly, the medial pterygoid muscle inferiorly, the mandibular ramus laterally, and lateral pterygoid plate medially.

## 5.5 Skull Base and Sinonasal Imaging

Diagnostic imaging of the skull base is critical to adequately delineate tumor extent, as well as relationships between tumors and critical anatomy. Cross-sectional imaging can be obtained with either computed tomography (CT) and/or magnetic resonance imaging (MRI). CT provides detailed imaging of bony structures as well as information about bony erosion, remodeling, and/or invasion of bony structures surrounding the paranasal sinuses and nasal cavities. Structures such as the walls of the maxillary sinus, orbits, pterygoid plates, hard palate, or the clivus and skull base should be examined for bony erosion or invasion. CT may further aid in identifying dehiscence of the internal carotid artery or optic nerves and bony erosion or invasion of the skull base and all the cranial nerve foramina. Contrast-enhanced CT scans may add further detail to noncontrast studies and are useful in staging the neck for regional spread of tumors.

MRI adds superior soft-tissue delineation in comparison to CT. T1-weighted imaging may help identify bone invasion particularly in marrow-rich bone such as the clivus. MRI will also show muscle denervation secondary to cranial neuropathies. Fatty infiltration of the pterygoid or temporalis muscles, for example, may suggest a loss of function of the motor branch of the trigeminal nerve due to chronic denervation. T2-weighted imaging can also help differentiate between trapped mucous secretions and soft-tissue tumor. Secretions are typically hyperintense on T2-weighted imaging in comparison to solid tumor, which is mildly hyperintense to intermediate in signal. Contrast-enhanced MRI with gadolinium will also help delineate sinonasal tumors with enhancement of the lesion. Contrast may further aid in detecting perineural spread of nerves intracranially. The addition of special sequences such as the fast imaging employing steady-state acquisition (FIESTA) may aid in detecting cranial nerve tumor spread. Other sequences such as the fluid attenuated inversion recovery (FLAIR) sequence are used to identify brain edema secondary to parenchymal invasion. Orbital invasion can also be seen on MRI (▶ Fig. 5.5).

The short tau inversion recovery (STIR) sequence may be used to detect orbital fat invasion. Tumor adjacent to the periorbita, extraocular muscle involvement, and orbital fat obliteration may suggest orbital invasion.[6] Periorbita is typically hypointense on T2 and contrast-enhanced T1-weighted images relative to tumor. Loss of this plane on MRI may further suggest orbital invasion.

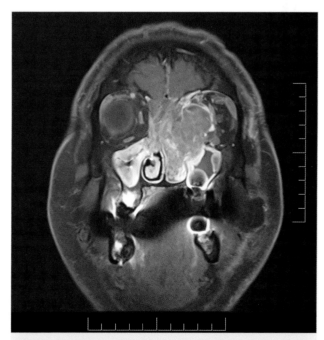

**Fig. 5.5** T1-weighted magnetic resonance imaging with gadolinium showing a sinonasal tumor extending into the left orbit.

Imaging of the chest to rule out pulmonary metastases at presentation should be performed. CT has a higher sensitivity in detecting pulmonary lesions in comparison to conventional radiography.

Positron emission tomography (PET)/CT scanning with 18F-fluorodeoxyglucose (FDG) can be used both in staging and re-staging tumors. PET scans are commonly used in the detection of recurrences in the surveillance setting, particularly in health care settings where it is readily available.

Special nuclear imaging such as technetium-99 m, gallium-67, indium-111 scans can also be helpful in certain situations to better help delineate infectious processes such as osteomyelitis of the skull base. Technetium-99 bone scans are typically positive focally shortly after an acute infection. These scans, however, may remain positive long after the clearance of the infectious process. Gallium-67 scans, on the other hand, may be helpful in monitoring responses to therapy and may be used to monitor the progress of infectious processes. Indium-111-labeled scans are helpful in identifying acute or chronic processes but may be more specific than the other two modalities in identifying infection.

# 5.6 Surgical Approaches
## 5.6.1 Endoscopic Surgical Approaches

Advantages of the endoscopic approach include superior tumor visualization with high definition magnification of the surgical field. In addition, entirely endonasal approaches avoid external facial incisions. Compared to the open approach, endoscopic approaches may be associated with fewer complications and shorter hospital stays.[7,8,9] The ideal candidates for an endoscopic resection are those patients with a tumor confined to the nasal cavity or ethmoid sinuses with limited anterior, lateral, and inferior extension. Tumor erosion through the posterior wall of the frontal sinus may be resectable, but extensive tumor extension into the frontal sinus abutting the anterior wall requires an open approach through either a frontal craniotomy or an osteoplastic flap. To access lateral tumors, a Denker's maxillotomy or a Caldwell-Luc approach can be combined with endoscopic approaches to reach the lateral wall of the maxillary sinus, pterygopalatine fossa, and infratemporal fossa.

### Endoscopic Anterior Craniofacial Resection

Endoscopic anterior craniofacial resection is typically used for midline tumors of the nasal cavity or ethmoid sinuses with skull base involvement.[10,11,12,13,14] Preliminary experience with this approach was developed around the management of esthesioneuroblastomas (olfactory neuroblastoma) because of their favorable location and biology. However, many sinonasal malignancies as well as anterior skull base meningiomas may now be accessed with this approach. The endoscopic anterior craniofacial resection combines an endoscopic approach (▶ Fig. 5.6) along with the access of the traditional transfacial/transcranial open craniofacial resection. This allows for resection of skull base pathology as well as intracranial resection when necessary. Limits of resection for this approach include the frontal sinus anteriorly, the planum sphenoidale posteriorly, and the midline of the orbits laterally. Clinical and/or imaging findings

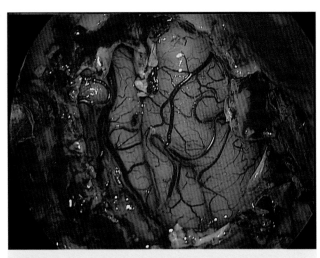

**Fig. 5.6** Intraoperative view of endoscopic anterior craniofacial resection.

that preclude the use of an endoscopic resection (thus requiring an open approach) include the following:
1. Involvement of the anterior table of the frontal sinus.
2. Tumor invasion of the nasal bones.
3. Extensive dural involvement laterally over the orbit.
4. Invasion of the palate.
5. Invasion of the facial skin.
6. Invasion of the orbit.

For anterior skull base meningiomas, relative contraindications include meningiomas with extensive encasement of critical vascular structures (i.e., carotid artery).

The principles of the endoscopic craniofacial resection for sinonasal malignancies generally involve debulking of tumor to the pedicle point followed by resecting a margin around the tumor pedicle and achieving negative surgical margins. Intraoperative frozen sections may help confirm the absence of microscopic residual disease at the margins of resection. Resection of the bony skull base is necessary for tumors pedicled on the skull base, and often resection of dura is also necessary for adequate clearance of the margins, although this is dependent on the structures involved by the tumor and the biology of the tumor. The anterior limit of the procedure is the posterior table of the frontal sinus and therefore a Draf III frontal sinusotomy (modified endoscopic Lothrop procedure) is performed. This entails wide opening of the frontal recess from the lamina papyracea of one orbit to the other side. The floor of the frontal sinuses, the intersinus septum, and the superior nasal septum are removed. The lamina papyracea is skeletonized bilaterally, and may be removed depending on tumor extent. The ethmoid sinuses are resected such that the skull base can be visualized superiorly. On the nasal aspect of the tumor, the lesion may be debulked up to the pedicle point on the skull base. Ligation and division of the anterior and posterior ethmoidal arteries is usually necessary to reduce the blood supply to tumor on the skull base and to facilitate resection of the bony skull base. Posteriorly, the planum sphenoidale is the limit of resection for sinonasal malignancies. The sphenoid sinus is opened bilaterally. The tumor is resected with the skull base. Osteotomies are performed with a drill, along the defined limits. Once the bony cuts have been made, the underlying dura and olfactory nerves are resected if it is suspected they are involved with tumor.

A meningioma that spans the anterior cranial fossa floor is approached slightly differently, with the basic tenet of internal debulking followed by a capsular dissection. Meningiomas are approached after resection of the bony skull base and dura. They are then typically debulked internally and then approached by a capsular dissection after allowing the tumor and surrounding dura to descend intranasally.

## Endoscopic Lateral Approaches

Tumors with lateral extension can now also be approached endoscopically.[2] Nasal tumors with extension into the maxillary sinus may be approached with an endoscopic medial maxillectomy. The archetypal tumor for this approach is the inverted papilloma. More posterior tumors or pathology with extension into the pterygopalatine fossa, infratemporal fossa, lateral recess of sphenoid, or Meckel's cave may also be accessed. Removal of the posterior wall of the maxillary sinus and drilling of the pterygoid plates may facilitate access to these areas. Examples of pathology in these locations include CSF leaks or encephaloceles of the lateral recess of the sphenoid, tumors with perineural extension along V2 or V3, or schwannomas of the trigeminal nerve. An important landmark in the expanded endonasal approach is the Vidian nerve.[15] The anterior genu of the petrous carotid artery is superior and medial to the Vidian canal. Therefore, by following the nerve, the internal carotid artery can be located and protected during dissection.

A Denker's maxillotomy may further facilitate endonasal access laterally. This approach is performed by making an incision in the nasal vestibular mucosa over the piriform aperture and drilling the bone of the piriform aperture to enlarge the working area and facilitate lateral access. More posteriorly, the inferior turbinate may be resected and the nasolacrimal duct transected. A Caldwell-Luc approach can be used to facilitate access to the lateral maxillary sinus. A gingivobuccal incision is made and the face of the maxillary sinus is exposed. A bony window is then made into the maxillary sinus, which can be used for the endoscope or for instrumentation. Patients should be warned about the potential for injury to the infraorbital nerve and potential cheek paresthesia.

## Transorbital Approach

Advances in endoscopic techniques now allow for surgical access to both intraconal and extraconal pathology of the orbit. This pathology is most accessible and safely dealt with if it is medial to the optic nerve. In this approach, a wide maxillary antrostomy is made, exposing the bone of the orbital floor. An anterior ethmoidectomy is then performed, skeletonizing the lamina papyracea. This bone is carefully removed, thus exposing the periorbita. The orbit can then be entered by incising the periorbita. As the orbital fat is dissected, the medial rectus and inferior oblique muscles are visualized. Careful, blunt dissection allows access to the orbital pathology. Identification of the medial rectus and inferior oblique muscles may be facilitated by dissection of these muscles through small periorbital incisions and careful mobilization.

The transorbital neuroendoscopic surgery approach (TONES) may also provide access to the anterior and middle cranial fossa.[16] These approaches rely on approaches to the orbit such as the precaruncular, preseptal lower eyelid, superior eyelid crease, and lateral retrocanthal approaches. This approach may be used for access to tumors, encephaloceles, and skull base trauma.

## 5.6.2 Open Surgical Approaches

Open surgical approaches may be used to access several areas of the cranial base and can be divided into transfacial or transcranial approaches. These approaches require careful incision placement and bony osteotomies either for extirpation of tumors or for surgical access. These approaches may be used when patients have contraindications for endoscopic approaches, or depending on surgeon comfort and experience.

### Bicoronal

A bicoronal incision extending from the root of the helix of one ear to the contralateral root of the helix (▶ Fig. 5.7) is used to access sinonasal tumor with skull base invasion, when a craniotomy may be required. Undermining of the tissue in the subgaleal or subperiosteal plane is then performed. The bicoronal approach can be used for frontal craniotomies or frontolateral craniotomies. A bicoronal incision may also be used to harvest a pericranial flap for skull base reconstruction.

### Lateral Rhinotomy Approach

The lateral rhinotomy approach involves making an incision from the medial canthus down to the nasal ala (▶ Fig. 5.8). It is used for access to the midface, and it can be extended to include a lip-splitting incision or a subciliary incision. It provides excellent access to the midfacial skeleton and allows the surgeon to perform a medial or infrastructure maxillectomy.

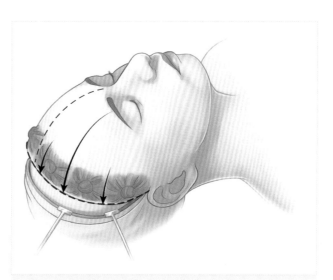

**Fig. 5.7** Schematic diagram shows the placement of the bicoronal incision.

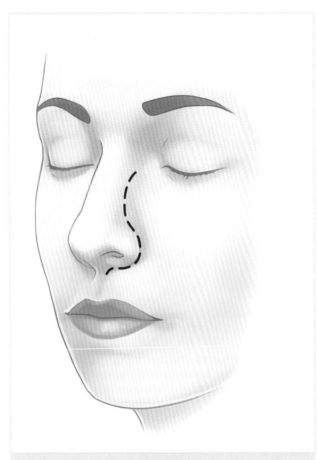

**Fig. 5.8** Schematic diagram shows the incision lines for a classic left lateral rhinotomy.

## Weber-Ferguson Approach

This approach involves a lateral rhinotomy incision that is extended superiorly with a subtarsal or subciliary incision (► Fig. 5.9). A subtarsal incision is typically more obvious than a subciliary incision, but it has a lower risk of ectropion (which is a potential disadvantage of this approach).[17] The Weber-Ferguson approach affords improved access to the maxilla when compared to the standard lateral rhinotomy (► Fig. 5.10).

## Midfacial Degloving

This approach involves bilateral sublabial or gingivobuccal incisions from the maxillary tuberosity on one side to the contralateral maxillary tuberosity (► Fig. 5.11). Intercartilaginous incisions are needed to deglove the tissue off of the nasal framework. The advantage of this approach is the avoidance of any external facial scars. It can be combined with LeFort 1 osteotomies and provides good access to the anterior nasal cavity, but poor access to the skull base superiorly.

## Infratemporal Fossa Approaches

Both the preauricular and postauricular approaches can be utilized for access to the infratemporal fossa (► Fig. 5.12, ► Fig. 5.13, ► Fig. 5.14, ► Fig. 5.15). For disease in the sinonasal cavity, often a preauricular approach is used; this can be extended inferiorly into a cervical incision and superiorly into a hemicoronal incision. The root of the zygoma, the zygomaticofrontal suture, and the zygomaticomaxillary suture are osteotomized and the bone flap is temporarily removed if access to the infratemporal fossa is needed. Often facial nerve dissection and preservation of the nerve, with removal of the parotid

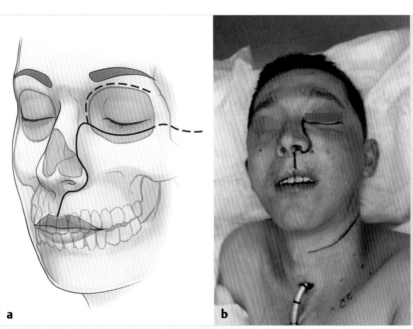

a   b

**Fig. 5.9 (a)** Schematic illustration and **(b)** intraoperative photograph of the Weber-Ferguson incision. (Part **b** is courtesy of Dr. de Almeida.)

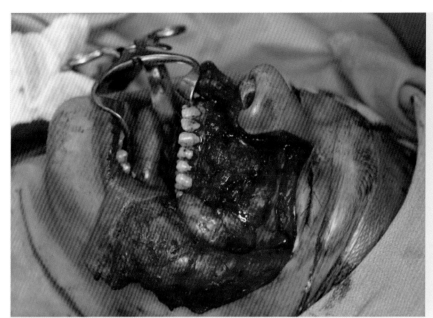

Fig. 5.10 Weber-Ferguson access.

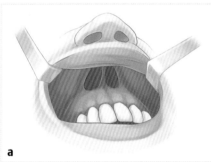

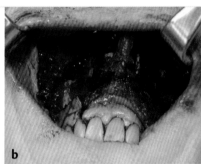

Fig. 5.11 (a) Schematic illustration and (b) intraoperative photograph of midfacial degloving incisions. (Part b is courtesy of Dr. de Almeida.)

**a**  **b**

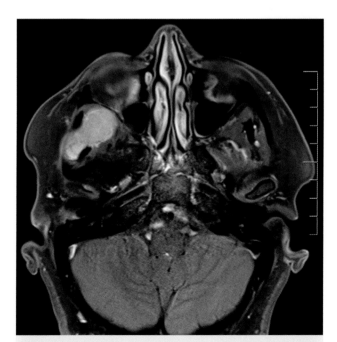

Fig. 5.12 Axial magnetic resonance imaging T1-weighted with gadolinium showing sarcoma in the infratemporal fossa abutting the posterior maxilla and lateral orbital wall.

gland, are required for access and visualization. Dislocation of the mandibular condyle, or occasionally a mandibulotomy, can improve visualization and access. Alternatively, an anterior facial translocation approach may be used to access the infratemporal fossa. In this approach, a Weber-Ferguson incision is extended laterally from the lateral canthus until the preauricular incision is reached.

## Medial Maxillectomy

A medial maxillectomy can be performed either endoscopically or via an open approach for sinonasal tumors that arise from the middle meatus. With this procedure, the lateral nasal wall is resected, as well as the ethmoid sinuses and the medial orbital floor (medial to the infraorbital nerve; ▶ Fig. 5.16). After the bone has been dissected from the soft tissue, four osteotomies are performed, which are followed by three anterior to posterior osteotomies. The anterior cuts are (1) through the infraorbital rim (with preservation of the infraorbital nerve), (2) through the anterior wall of the maxillary sinus, (3) from the floor of the sinus to the piriform aperture, and (4) through the frontal process of the maxilla. Following this, the anterior to posterior osteotomies are as follows: (1) along the medial orbital floor; (2) along the floor of the lateral nasal wall; and (3) along the superior aspect of the lateral nasal wall. Finally, a

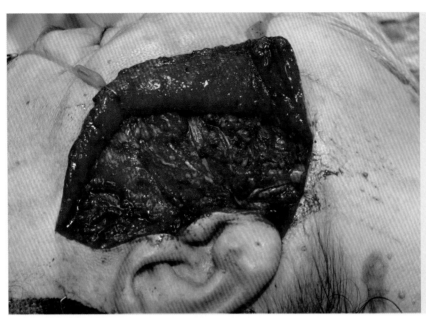

**Fig. 5.13** Initial skin incision and parotidectomy approach to identify facial nerve.

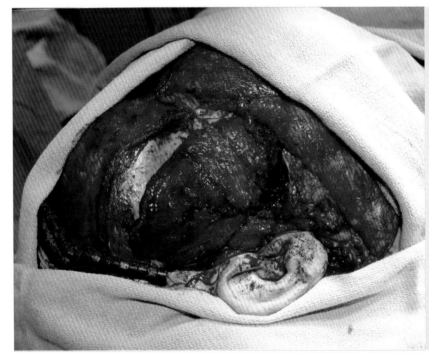

**Fig. 5.14** Extension of preauricular incision to bicoronal incision to access temporal and infratemporal fossa.

final posterior vertical osteotomy is performed to release the specimen.

## Infrastructural Maxillectomy

When a tumor arises from the hard palate, or from the maxillary sinus, and erodes inferiorly into the oral cavity, an infrastructure maxillectomy can be used to resect the tumor. It can be performed entirely transorally, or through a lateral rhinotomy or midface degloving approach. After exposing the bone, three osteotomies are made: a medial osteotomy through the hard palate, a lateral osteotomy through the zygomaticomaxillary buttress, and a LeFort I superior osteotomy (▶ Fig. 5.17).

Once these are done, a final fourth posterior osteotomy is performed, freeing the specimen from the pterygoid plates.

## Total Maxillectomy

A total maxillectomy is typically approached through either a lateral rhinotomy or Weber-Ferguson incision. For disease involving the orbit, orbital incisions are required to include orbital exenteration. Resection of the entire orbital floor is required for suprastructural disease, in contrast to the infrastructure maxillectomy. In this procedure, the periorbita is dissected free from the medial orbital wall and the orbital floor. At this point, the surgeon can examine the tissue for potential

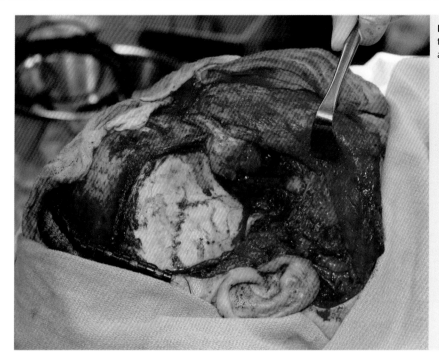

Fig. 5.15 Removal of tumor specimen including temporalis muscle, zygoma, lateral orbital wall, and posterior maxilla.

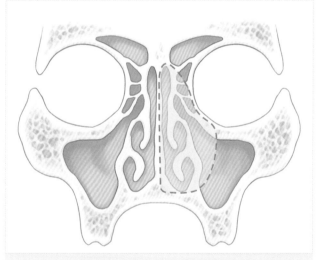

Fig. 5.16 Medial maxillectomy.

orbital or periorbital invasion and the nasolacrimal apparatus can be transected and marsupialized.

Multiple osteotomies are required for the total maxillectomy. Superior osteotomies are required through the frontal process of the maxilla (and/or medial orbital rim) and through the lateral orbital rim and zygomaticofrontal suture (▶ Fig. 5.18, ▶ Fig. 5.19). These osteotomies are then extended with anterior to posterior osteotomies through the medial and lateral orbital walls. Next, the floor of the orbit must be released with an osteotomy to release the superior aspect. Inferiorly, a palatal osteotomy and a lateral osteotomy through the zygomatico-maxillary buttress are made. The palatal osteotomy extends back to the hard and soft palate junction. Lastly, the specimen is released with a posterior vertical osteotomy behind the maxillary tuberosity with a curved osteotome. This anatomical region is very vascular containing the pterygoid venous plexus and the internal maxillary artery, and careful hemostasis must be achieved.

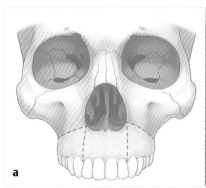
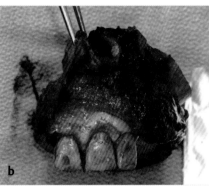

a          b

Fig. 5.17 (a) Schematic illustration and (b) intraoperative photograph of an infrastructure maxillectomy. (Part b is courtesy of Dr. de Almeida.)

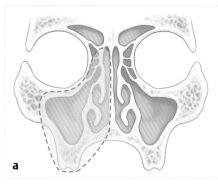
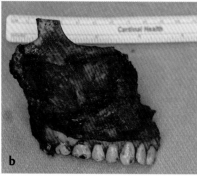

**Fig. 5.18 (a)** Schematic illustration and **(b)** intraoperative photograph of a total maxillectomy. (Part **b** is courtesy of Dr. de Almeida.)

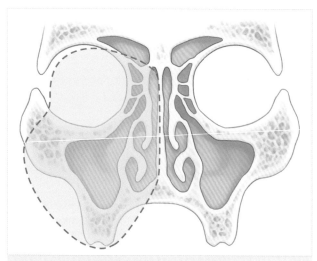

**Fig. 5.19** Total maxillectomy with orbital exenteration.

## Craniofacial Resection

Craniofacial resection involves the removal of the anterior skull base, typically via a combined frontal craniotomy and transfacial approach, or via an endoscopic approach. The open craniofacial resection was described by Smith et al[18] and popularized by Ketcham et al[19] in the 1960s. Typically a bicoronal incision is used. A pericranial flap can be harvested for reconstruction. Four osteotomies are used to free the specimen superiorly: a lateral osteotomy between the fovea ethmoidalis and the frontal bones on each side (two in total), a posterior osteotomy at the planum sphenoidale, and an anterior osteotomy behind the posterior table of the frontal sinus (▶ Fig. 5.20). A Weber-Ferguson or later rhinotomy approach is often used for transfacial access and a maxillectomy is performed to free the specimen from below. Alternatively, the inferior aspect can be performed endoscopically ("endoscopic assisted craniofacial resection") or the entire procedure (including superior osteotomies) can be performed endoscopically with no external cuts.

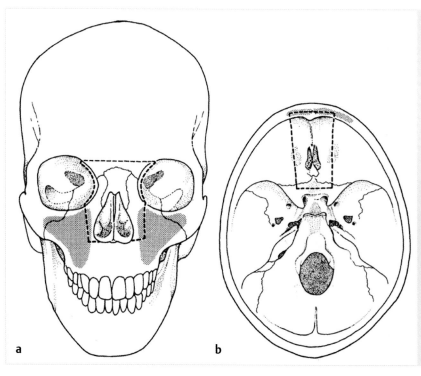

**Fig. 5.20 (a,b)** Craniofacial resection. (Used with permission from Som PM, Curtin HD, eds. Head and Neck Imaging. 4th ed. St. Louis, MO: Mosby-Elsevier Science; 2003.)

## Orbital Exenteration

Orbital exenteration involves removing all the orbital contents down to the bone and is performed when the periorbita has been breached by tumor. It should be differentiated from orbital evisceration or orbital enucleation. Evisceration entails removing the contents of the eye (typically with a curette) and is done for severe endophthalmitis. Enucleation involves removing the globe, but the extraocular muscles and the conjunctiva are preserved.

Exenteration is required for extrinsic malignant tumors with invasion of the orbit. Controversy exists as to the extent of orbital invasion requiring exenteration as some argue that invasion of the bony orbit without transgression of the soft tissues does not require an orbital exenteration, since the local control rates remain unchanged whether the eye is removed or not.[20] If the periorbita has limited involvement, but the underlying orbital fat appears normal, frozen sections can be taken to confirm the tumor has not extended into the orbit, and consideration of preserving the globe can be given.[21,22,23] If exenteration is to be performed, the eyelids can be preserved if there is no invasion of the skin. To do this, a circumferential skin incision is made around the superior and inferior lid lash line. Musculocutaneous flaps are raised superiorly and inferiorly to the orbital rims, and these flaps can be re-approximated after the exenteration. When the lid skin is involved, a circumorbital incision is made around the orbital rim. The periorbita is then dissected off of the bony orbit and the skin is removed en bloc with the orbital contents. The optic nerve is ligated and transected at the orbital apex. If there is concern about posterior extension, frozen section margins may be sent from the nerve at the orbital apex.

## 5.7 Reconstruction Approaches

Reconstruction following resection of skull base and midface tumors is important for a variety of reasons. The approach used, as well as the size and location of the defect, often helps dictate the reconstructive method chosen. Creating a water-tight seal between the nasal cavity and the intracranial cavity is essential to prevent CSF rhinorrhea and associated complications such as meningitis and intracranial abscess. Hard palate reconstruction can be performed with prosthodontics, or with autologous tissue (often free tissue transfer). Separation of the oral cavity from the nasal cavity is important for everyday functions, such as deglutition and speech. Obtaining appropriate projection of the maxilla is also very important for cosmesis.

### 5.7.1 Endoscopic Skull Base Reconstruction

Skull base reconstruction, like midface reconstruction, depends on the size and location of the defect. Traditionally, defects were closed with free mucosal grafts. These grafts can be harvested from septal mucosa, or from the resected middle turbinate. Oftentimes, the mucosa is used as an onlay graft. An inlay graft of fascia, or a synthetic dural substitute, can be placed under the graft if the defect is large enough.[24] Nowadays, more complex multilayered reconstructions are being performed (▶ Fig. 5.21). The nasoseptal flap ("NSF," "Hadad–Bassagasteguy flap," or "HB flap") supplied by the posterior septal branch of the sphenopalatine artery has been popularized for reconstruction following endoscopic endonasal surgery of the skull base.[25] This versatile flap can be used to reconstruct clival or sellar defects, as well as many cribriform defects.[26] The use of this vascularized flap has reduced the rate of CSF leak, when compared to other nonvascularized reconstructions. This flap can be harvested from the sphenoid face up to the nasal sill and the inferior cut can be taken down onto the nasal floor if the defect is expected to be large. The superior cut typically should be approximately 1 cm below the skull base to preserve olfactory function. This flap should not be harvested from the septum if it is involved with disease, limiting its use in cases when the

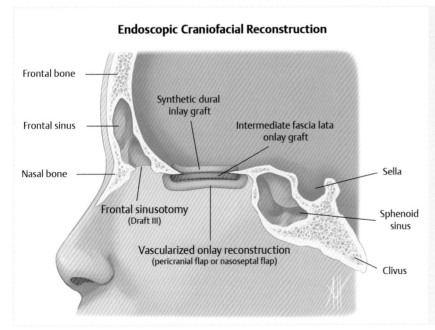

**Endoscopic Craniofacial Reconstruction**

Frontal bone

Synthetic dural inlay graft

Frontal sinus

Intermediate fascia lata onlay graft

Nasal bone

Sella

Frontal sinusotomy
(Draft III)

Sphenoid sinus

Vascularized onlay reconstruction
(pericranial flap or nasoseptal flap)

Clivus

**Fig. 5.21** Endoscopic skull base reconstruction. Graphic image showing the various layers used in the reconstruction of an anterior skull base defect.

tumor has bilateral extension. An alternative in these cases is the inferior turbinate flap and its variants.[27,28] This flap is limited by its arc of rotation and comparatively small surface area.

The pericranial flap is based on the supraorbital and supratrochlear arteries. It is a staple in reconstruction of most simple anterior skull base defects. It is often harvested using a bicoronal incision and can be used to achieve separation of the nasal cavity from the intracranial contents. Inset is through a frontal craniotomy or a nasal root osteotomy.

An advantage of this flap includes the fact that it is outside of the treatment field, and therefore if neoadjuvant radiotherapy was used, it should be spared. In addition, because it is extranasal, there is no fear about tumor seeding with it, which can be a concern with intranasal pedicled flaps. In addition to the pericranial flap, other pedicled options exists, such as the temporoparietal (TP) fascia flap and the buccinator flap.[29] The TP flap is based off of the superficial temporal artery and is ideal for defects in the nasopharynx; it is less suitable for reconstruction of cribriform defects because of the high degree of rotation needed to cover this area. The buccinator flap, based off of the facial artery, is another pedicled flap that can be used to close anterior defects if a pedicled flap is desired and the intranasal options are unavailable.

## 5.7.2 Open Approach for Reconstruction

The goals of maxillary reconstruction are to obtain oronasal separation, provide support for the orbit, allow dental restoration, and improve cosmesis. Maxillary reconstruction is complicated and there are many different classification systems and algorithms used to define the various defects.[20,21,22,23,24,25,26,27,28,29,30,31,32,33] Often, obturators can be used because of presence of the remaining supporting dentition. Alternatively, they may be reconstructed with a pedicled or free tissue flap with vascularized osseocutaneous or osseomyogenous flaps (such as a scapula free flap, fibular free flap, or iliac crest free flap) and subsequently be rehabilitated with a denture or implant-retained prosthesis. The decision to obturate or reconstruct with a free flap depends on surgeon preference, as well as patient factors.

## 5.8 Complications

Complications following surgery to the midface can be broadly divided into local, orbital, and cranial complications. Local complications such as bleeding may occur after maxillary surgery because of the highly vascular pterygoid plexus and due to injury of the sphenopalatine and/or internal maxillary arteries. Postoperative bleeding from maxillectomy cavities may be initially managed with packing or operative ligation of offending vessels. Other local complications would include secondary mucocele formation and sinusitis. Orbital complications include postoperative hematoma as well as injury to the nasolacrimal duct. If the anterior ethmoid arteries are injured during surgery, they can retract into the orbital fat and lead to bleeding. Injury to the nasolacrimal duct can lead to postoperative epiphora. It is usually treated with dacryocystorhinostomy. Other potential orbital complications include enophthalmos, diplopia, extraocular muscle injury, and orbital abscess.

Intracranial complications following surgery of the skull base can be devastating. Proper cranial base reconstruction is essential to avoid CSF leaks, pneumocephalus, meningitis, subdural empyema, and intracranial abscess.

# References

[1] de Lara D, Ditzel Filho LF, Prevedello DM, et al. Endonasal endoscopic approaches to the paramedian skull base. World Neurosurg. 2014; 82 (6 suppl):S121–S129

[2] Kassam AB, Gardner P, Snyderman C, Mintz A, Carrau R. Expanded endonasal approach: fully endoscopic, completely transnasal approach to the middle third of the clivus, petrous bone, middle cranial fossa, and infratemporal fossa. Neurosurg Focus. 2005; 19(1):E6

[3] Keros P. [On the practical value of differences in the level of the lamina cribrosa of the ethmoid]. Z Laryngol Rhinol Otol. 1962; 41:809–813

[4] Hammer G, Radberg C. The sphenoidal sinus. An anatomical and roentgenologic study with reference to transsphenoid hypophysectomy. Acta Radiol. 1961; 56:401–422

[5] de Almeida JR, Zanation AM, Snyderman CH, et al. Defining the nasopalatine line: the limit for endonasal surgery of the spine. Laryngoscope. 2009; 119 (2):239–244

[6] Eisen MD, Yousem DM, Loevner LA, Thaler ER, Bilker WB, Goldberg AN. Preoperative imaging to predict orbital invasion by tumor. Head Neck. 2000; 22 (5):456–462

[7] Suh JD, Ramakrishnan VR, Chi JJ, Palmer JN, Chiu AG. Outcomes and complications of endoscopic approaches for malignancies of the paranasal sinuses and anterior skull base. Ann Otol Rhinol Laryngol. 2013; 122(1):54–59

[8] Eloy JA, Vivero RJ, Hoang K, et al. Comparison of transnasal endoscopic and open craniofacial resection for malignant tumors of the anterior skull base. Laryngoscope. 2009; 119(5):834–840

[9] Wood JW, Eloy JA, Vivero RJ, et al. Efficacy of transnasal endoscopic resection for malignant anterior skull-base tumors. Int Forum Allergy Rhinol. 2012; 2 (6):487–495

[10] Manthuruthil C, Lewis J, McLean C, Batra PS, Barnett SL. Endoscopic endonasal management of olfactory neuroblastoma: a retrospective analysis of 10 patients with quality of life measures. World Neurosurg. 2016; 90:1–5

[11] Casiano RR, Numa WA, Falquez AM. Endoscopic resection of esthesioneuroblastoma. Am J Rhinol. 2001; 15(4):271–279

[12] Fu TS, Monteiro E, Muhanna N, Goldstein DP, de Almeida JR. Comparison of outcomes for open versus endoscopic approaches for olfactory neuroblastoma: a systematic review and individual participant data meta-analysis. Head Neck. 2016; 38 Suppl 1:E2306–E2316

[13] Higgins TS, Thorp B, Rawlings BA, Han JK. Outcome results of endoscopic vs craniofacial resection of sinonasal malignancies: a systematic review and pooled-data analysis. Int Forum Allergy Rhinol. 2011; 1(4):255–261

[14] Snyderman CH, Carrau RL, Kassam AB, et al. Endoscopic skull base surgery: principles of endonasal oncological surgery. J Surg Oncol. 2008; 97(8):658–664

[15] Vescan AD, Snyderman CH, Carrau RL, et al. Vidian canal: analysis and relationship to the internal carotid artery. Laryngoscope. 2007; 117(8):1338–1342

[16] Ramakrishna R, Kim LJ, Bly RA, Moe K, Ferreira M, Jr. Transorbital neuroendoscopic surgery for the treatment of skull base lesions. J Clin Neurosci. 2016; 24:99–104

[17] Ellis E III, Zide MF, eds. Transcutaneous approaches through the lower eyelid. In: Surgical Approaches to the Facial Skeleton. Philadelphia, PA: Lippincott Williams & Wilkins; 2006:9–40

[18] Smith RR, Klopp CT, Williams JM. Surgical treatment of cancer of the frontal sinus and adjacent areas. Cancer. 1954; 7(5):991–994

[19] Ketcham AS, Wilkins RH, Vanburen JM, Smith RR. A combined intracranial facial approach to the paranasal sinuses. Am J Surg. 1963; 106:698–703

[20] Carrau RL, Segas J, Nuss DW, et al. Squamous cell carcinoma of the sinonasal tract invading the orbit. Laryngoscope. 1999; 109(2, Pt 1):230–235

[21] Perry C, Levine PA, Williamson BR, Cantrell RW. Preservation of the eye in paranasal sinus cancer surgery. Arch Otolaryngol Head Neck Surg. 1988; 114 (6):632–634

[22] McCary WS, Levine PA, Cantrell RW. Preservation of the eye in the treatment of sinonasal malignant neoplasms with orbital involvement. A confirmation of the original treatise. Arch Otolaryngol Head Neck Surg. 1996; 122(6):657–659

[23] Essig GF, Newman SA, Levine PA. Sparing the eye in craniofacial surgery for superior nasal vault malignant neoplasms: analysis of benefit. Arch Facial Plast Surg. 2007; 9(6):406–411

[24] Ting JY, Metson R. Free graft techniques in skull base reconstruction. Adv Otorhinolaryngol. 2013; 74:33–41

[25] Hadad G, Bassagasteguy L, Carrau RL, et al. A novel reconstructive technique after endoscopic expanded endonasal approaches: vascular pedicle nasoseptal flap. Laryngoscope. 2006; 116(10):1882–1886

[26] Pinheiro-Neto CD, Ramos HF, Peris-Celda M, Fernandez-Miranda JC, Gardner PA, Snyderman CH, Sennes LU. Study of the nasoseptal flap for endoscopic anterior cranial base reconstruction. Laryngoscope. 2011; 121(12):2514–2520

[27] Choby GW, Pinheiro-Neto CD, de Almeida JR, et al. Extended inferior turbinate flap for endoscopic reconstruction of skull base defects. J Neurol Surg B Skull Base. 2014; 75(4):225–230

[28] Yip J, Macdonald KI, Lee J, et al. The inferior turbinate flap in skull base reconstruction. J Otolaryngol Head Neck Surg. 2013; 42:6

[29] Patel MR, Taylor RJ, Hackman TG, et al. Beyond the nasoseptal flap: outcomes and pearls with secondary flaps in endoscopic endonasal skull base reconstruction. Laryngoscope. 2014; 124(4):846–852

[30] Brown JS, Rogers SN, McNally DN, Boyle M. A modified classification for the maxillectomy defect. Head Neck. 2000; 22(1):17–26

[31] Okay DJ, Genden E, Buchbinder D, Urken M. Prosthodontic guidelines for surgical reconstruction of the maxilla: a classification system of defects. J Prosthet Dent. 2001; 86(4):352–363

[32] Cordeiro PG, Santamaria E. A classification system and algorithm for reconstruction of maxillectomy and midfacial defects. Plast Reconstr Surg. 2000; 105(7):2331–2346, discussion 2347–2348

[33] Urken ML, Catalano PJ, Sen C, Post K, Futran N, Biller HF. Free tissue transfer for skull base reconstruction analysis of complications and a classification scheme for defining skull base defects. Arch Otolaryngol Head Neck Surg. 1993; 119(12):1318–1325

# 6 Posttreatment Appearance Following Skull Base Therapy

*Adam A. Dmytriw, John A. Rutka, Arjun Sahgal, Eugene Yu, and Peter Som*

## 6.1 Introduction

Skull base tumors present a treatment challenge due the large number of critical structures that are present in an anatomically dense space. These tumors also require an equally sophisticated approach to intervention and imaging assessment. Single-modality treatment with surgery or radiation is the mainstay for the treatment of early-stage head and neck cancer.[1] In the case of locally advanced disease, a multimodality treatment approach is employed, which combines surgery with adjuvant chemoradiation therapy. In the treatment of skull base cancers, both open craniofacial and endonasal approaches can be used independently or in concert. The postoperative imaging in these cases is notoriously challenging due to the alteration of the normal anatomy, the surgical defects, and any reconstructions. Moreover, a variety of tissue grafts and synthetic materials may be used in these reconstructions. An appreciation of the normally anticipated imaging features after skull base reconstruction lays the cornerstone for recognizing when there is a successful reconstruction as well as when there is the presence of residual disease or the development of a recurrence.

## 6.2 Posttreatment Fundamentals

Current follow-up guidelines from the National Comprehensive Cancer Network allow for a considerable degree of clinician discretion in surveillance practices. It is recommended that imaging and a physical examination be performed every 3 to 4 months for the first 2 years and every 4 to 6 months in years 2 to 5. Following this, follow-up is usually performed annually.[2] This surveillance should not only focus on local recurrent disease, but also be vigilant to identify distant metastases and the development of second primary tumors.

A wide array of imaging modalities is available to contribute to the assessment of the postoperative skull base. These include radiography/fluoroscopy, endoscopy, ultrasonography (US), computed tomography (CT), magnetic resonance imaging (MRI), single photon emission CT (SPECT), and 2-(fluorine 18) fluoro-2-deoxy-D-glucose (FDG) positron emission tomography (PET), with or without CT (PET/CT) or MR (PET/MR). In many centers, CT is often used as the modality of choice for follow-up examinations as CT scanning allows for very good soft-tissue resolution and excellent assessment of bone and readily identifies cervical adenopathy. Rapidity of image acquisition is also a major advantage of CT, which makes it a great modality for scanning patients who are medically unstable or who cannot maintain a still supine position for prolonged periods. It is an ideal test to use in the early perioperative setting to diagnose acute complications. MRI has the advantage of even greater soft-tissue resolution and given that patients with skull base tumors may be at risk for dural invasion or perineural spread, contrast-enhanced MR is the modality of choice. MRI may also help in identifying suspected tumor recurrence. Diffusion-weighted imaging (DWI) MRI may be of particular utility in the early posttreatment period, where other modalities offer false-positive findings.[1] DWI has also been reported to be a useful tool to differentiate tumor recurrence from normal posttreatment changes in the early period after treatment when used in combination with CT and/or MRI.[3]

Many centers also routinely utilize FDG PET/CT as the modality of choice in patient follow-up examinations. However, FDG PET/CT performed within the immediate 12 weeks after treatment may give both false-positive and false-negative results. The false-positive cases are primarily the result of treatment-related inflammation. The false-negative cases are the result of radiation and chemotherapy vascular compromise to the tumor bed and the suppression of glucose transporters in the tumor.[1]

## 6.3 Postsurgical Changes

Distinguishing postsurgical change from tumor recurrence is arguably the most important role that imaging serves following surgery. The challenge in assessment of these images lies in the often-extensive changes to normal anatomy that result from reconstruction, radiation therapy, and scarring. Clinically, recurrence may be asymptomatic and not come to attention until its bulk has caused gross distortion or is distinctly palpable. Imaging is therefore essential in the posttreatment surveillance of head and neck cancer.

Skull base surgery requires intricate reconstructions that are frequently necessary to both maintain negative histopathological margins from a wide local excision and afford the patient minimal morbidity while closing the surgical defect. In this anatomically complex area, various flap reconstructions are used. These include local flaps, pedicle flaps, and free microvascular flap techniques.[4,5] The flaps are intuitively named based on the tissue and vascular supply used. In the local flap technique, neighboring tissue is repositioned geometrically to accommodate the surgical defect. The pedicle flap technique differs in that donor tissue is rotated to fit the defect. The term pedicle denotes the use of the patient's own tissue on its vascular pedicle to close the surgical defect. Finally, free flap techniques may employ either a simple free flap or composite free flap. Either variant requires microvascular anastomosis of the vascular pedicle of the free flap to the local recipient vascular supply in the region of the reconstruction. In the simple variant, only one type of tissue is incorporated into the flap, whereas the term composite belies the use of multiple tissue types. The most common forms of the latter are myocutaneous, fasciocutaneous, free jejunal interposition, and osseous composite flaps.[6]

### 6.3.1 Craniofacial Resection

Craniofacial resection (CFR) of the anterior cranial fossa is a radical surgery performed with the intention of complete tumor extirpation. This procedure is particularly common in the setting of adenocarcinoma (ADC), adenoid cystic carcinoma, chordoma, malignant melanoma, olfactory neuroblastoma, osteosarcoma, and squamous cell carcinoma. Prior to endoscopic surgery, CFR was the sole "gold-standard" procedure for

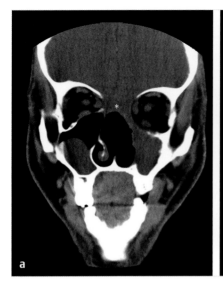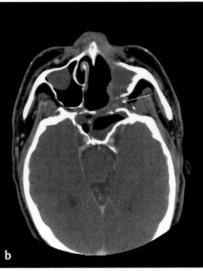

**Fig. 6.1** Coronal **(a)** and axial **(b)** computed tomography images following craniofacial resection of an inverted papilloma. The bony floor of the anterior cranial fossa, the nasal septum, and most of the turbinates have been resected. The reconstructed roof of the nasal cavity appears as a soft-tissue (*asterisk*; **a**) density beneath the frontal lobes. Note the smooth margins along the inferior margin of the flap. Axial image **(b)** also shows soft-tissue density in the left pterygopalatine fossa (*arrow*), which is compatible with scarring that can arise related to the left medial maxillectomy.

tumors that involved the orbital roof, cribriform plate, and fovea ethmoidalis.

The procedure typically begins with a lateral rhinotomy and is frequently followed by a medial maxillectomy, anterior and posterior ethmoidectomy, and sphenoidectomy. A lateral rhinotomy is commonly performed when tumor involves the deep nasal vault, the contiguous anterior paranasal sinuses, and midfacial skeleton. At surgery, the cribriform plate and frontal recesses are exposed along with the lamina papyracea bilaterally. A bicoronal forehead flap and frontal craniotomy are then performed to allow access to disease if it has extended into the anterior cranial fossa. Structures invaded by tumor are removed. The procedure may also require orbital exenteration.

Postoperative imaging will show a craniotomy involving the frontal bone from the level of the glabella inferiorly and to roughly 4 cm above the skull base superiorly. Typically the midpupillary line serves as the lateral craniotomy border.[7] Follow-up imaging will demonstrate resection of the cribriform plate, fovea ethmoidalis, and planum sphenoidale. Partial or near-complete absence of the nasal septum and turbinates may be evident as well as cranialization of the frontal sinuses (▶ Fig. 6.1). Cranialization involves removal of the posterior frontal sinus wall and frontal sinus mucosa. If the procedure is performed in a completely endoscopic manner (i.e., without a bicoronal craniotomy), a Draf III frontal sinusotomy procedure can be performed in place of frontal sinus cranialization. If a medial maxillectomy is performed as part of the resection, the normal fat density or signal in the pterygopalatine fossa will be replaced with a soft-tissue density scar. At our institution, the defect along the floor of the anterior cranial fossa is reconstructed with a synthetic duraplasty inlay graft, an optional intermediate fascia lata onlay graft, and then a vascularized onlay graft (consisting of either a pericranial flap or nasoseptal mucosal flap; ▶ Fig. 6.2). Anterior floor reconstruction will manifest as a soft-tissue density or signal that bridges across the bony defect. Variable degrees of enhancement will be present that may also bulge inferiorly into the nasoethmoid region (▶ Fig. 6.3). Pneumocephalus and extra-axial fluid collection is not uncommon in the early postoperative period. The mass effect and brain displacement secondary to the tumor as well as brain retraction and instrumentation during surgery may result in frontal lobe edema. This seems more pronounced in elderly patients. Accordingly when present, significant frontal lobe edema on MR should not be mistaken for recurrence or progression. A small collection of subdural blood may also be present, which again seems a more common finding in the elderly. With time, encephalomalacia may develop in the frontal lobes and would be manifested as increased T2 signal and volume loss (▶ Fig. 6.4).

Some surgeons interpose fat graft into the reconstruction site. This will manifest as a foci of fat attenuation on CT or as foci of T1 hyperintensity on MRI (▶ Fig. 6.2, ▶ Fig. 6.4).

As anterior skull base tumors may invade or originate from the paranasal sinuses, one specific challenge on follow-up imaging is to distinguish between recurrent or residual tumor and retained secretions. Residual or recurrent tumors manifest as an intermediate signal on T1- and T2-weighted images and demonstrate mild internal enhancement. Secretions may show peripheral enhancement and have low T1 and bright T2 signal. More desiccated or proteinaceous secretions may often demonstrate very bright T1 and/or T2 signal intensities.

Findings suspicious for recurrence would include an enhancing rounded mass along the resection margins and the development of new lesions with or without associated edema (▶ Fig. 6.5, ▶ Fig. 6.6).[8] Tumor recurrence often exerts mass effect locally and appears nodular or infiltrative in nature.

## 6.3.2 Lateral Skull Base Surgery

Lateral approaches to the skull base are most commonly employed in the setting of vestibular schwannomas, paragangliomas, recurrent tumors of the nasopharynx, and primary tumors of the external auditory canal/middle ear. The approaches are varied. Most involve the removal of bone and retraction of brain parenchyma for tumor removal. They can also involve rerouting of the facial nerve and identification of the internal carotid artery. In labyrinthine preservation procedures, the otic capsule is left intact and the labyrinth bypassed. Imaging will commonly show distortion of the normal anatomy

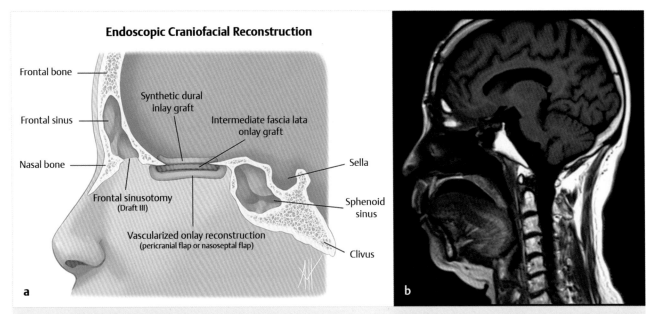

Fig. 6.2 Schematic diagram (a) depicting the complex reconstruction of the floor of the anterior cranial base after an endoscopic craniofacial resection. The defect along the floor of the anterior cranial fossa is reconstructed by use of a synthetic duraplasty inlay graft, an optional intermediate fascia lata onlay graft, and then a vascularized onlay graft (consisting of either a pericranial flap or a nasoseptal flap). (b) A sagittal T1-weighted image showing the corresponding imaging appearance in a patient following resection of an esthesioneuroblastoma. The various layers of the reconstruction manifest as a slightly lobulated intermediate signal soft-tissue bridge along the roof of the nasoethmoid cavity. The two bright foci correspond to interposed fat that was also added for support. The frontal sinuses were resected or cranialized in this instance.

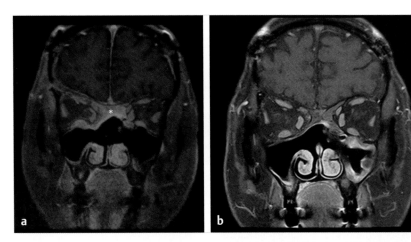

Fig. 6.3 Gadolinium-enhanced T1-weighted imaging with fat saturation post craniofacial resection for a frontal sinus osteosarcoma. (a) A study done as a baseline following surgery. Note the avid enhancement in the reconstructed floor of the cranial fossa (*asterisk*) and the diffuse dural thickening and enhancement. (b) An examination done a few years later. Note that the flap reconstruction now shows much less enhancement and the resolution of dural thickening and enhancement. The cranial and inferior margins of the flap also show very smooth margins.

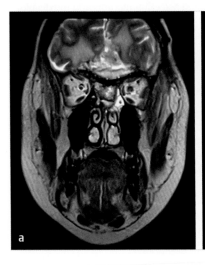 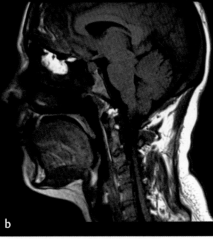

Fig. 6.4 Coronal T2-weighted (a) and sagittal T1-weighted (b) images following resection of a sinonasal undifferentiated carcinoma. Note the bright signal in the bifrontal white matter in keeping with encephalomalacia. The reconstructed floor is also more heterogeneous and lobulated than in the other example (▶ Fig. 6.3) and is causing some mass effect on the frontal brain parenchyma.

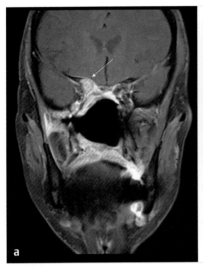
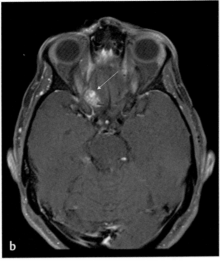

**Fig. 6.5 (a,b)** Coronal and axial enhanced T1-weighted images following craniofacial resection of a mucoepidermoid carcinoma. There is a rounded enhancing focus of recurrent tumor along the resection margins (*arrows*).

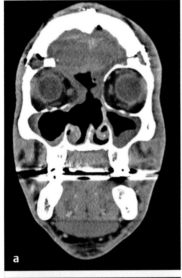
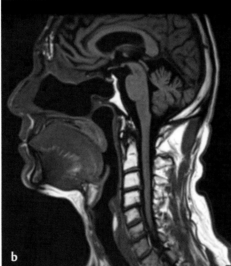
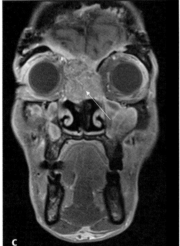
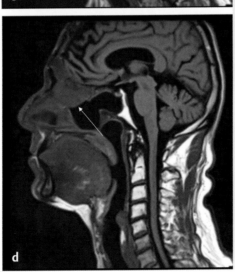

**Fig. 6.6** Coronal computed tomography **(a)** and sagittal T1-weighted **(b)** surveillance image studies showing expected changes following resection of an inverted papilloma with foci of squamous cell carcinoma. Subsequent coronal **(c)** and sagittal **(d)** magnetic resonance imaging shows recurrence in the nasal cavity along the margin of the reconstructed anterior cranial fossa floor (*arrows*).

along the surgical planes of dissection, which is usually transpetrous or transtemporal.

CT is essential in the postoperative period not only for the assessment of a postoperative complication, but also to document the bony anatomy and expected surgical change. Following this, MRI alone is often adequate for further follow-up, although some advocate the use of both modalities especially in the follow-up of petrous cholesteatoma.[9] It is important to note that many variations on these procedures can be performed and that postsurgical findings can vary in terms of the approach and structures removed.

### 6.3.3 Mastoidectomy

A simple (or cortical) mastoidectomy involves removing the lateral wall of the mastoid bone and cortical mastoid air cells with preservation of the external auditory canal. No manipulation of the ossicular chain occurs with this technique. There is no removal of bone in the epitympanum. By comparison, a canal wall-up mastoidectomy (or combined approach technique) involves removal of the mastoid air cells and Koerner's septum (▶ Fig. 6.7). The surgically created mastoid bowl allows for a connection between the antrum and the epitympanum.[10] In both procedures, the external auditory canal is preserved.

A canal wall-down mastoidectomy begins with a canal-up procedure and is then followed by removal of the external auditory canal. This allows for formal communication between the external auditory canal and the mastoid cavity (▶ Fig. 6.8). In a canal wall-down approach, the facial nerve within the mastoid may need to be sacrificed if involved by malignant disease. The procedure may involve a limited lateral temporal bone resection for adequate identification of the facial nerve.[11] The scutum is removed in most cases. If disease involves the ossicular chain, then the ossicles (typically leaving the stapes intact) and tympanic membrane are removed. The facial nerve is skeletonized and may be sacrificed if necessary. The procedure of a radical mastoidectomy typically involves the removal of the tympanic membrane, malleus and incus with preservation of the stapes suprastructure, the external auditory canal, mastoid air cell exenteration, and formal obliteration of the Eustachian tube (▶ Fig. 6.8). In a modified radical mastoidectomy, there is partial ossicular chain preservation (typically the handle of the malleus and the stapes suprastructure [the head of the malleus and incus are typically removed]; ▶ Fig. 6.9). Hearing restoration surgery involving ossicular reconstruction or device implantation can be performed as indicated.

### 6.3.4 Transpetrous Approaches

Transpetrous approach techniques may be employed for many skull base tumors but are frequently performed for the removal of vestibular schwannomas, meningiomas, arachnoid cysts, and intracranial lipomas. The translabyrinthine resection represents a common lateral approach to the petrous apex, internal

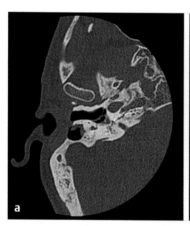
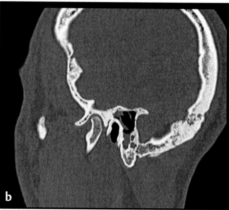

**Fig. 6.7** Axial **(a)** and sagittal **(b)** computed tomography images of a right canal wall-up mastoidectomy. The bony external auditory canal is maintained **(b)**.

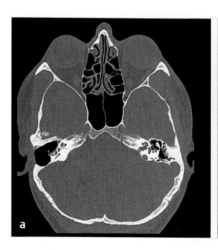
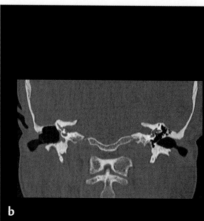

**Fig. 6.8** Axial **(a)** and coronal **(b)** computed tomography shows a canal wall-down mastoidectomy. There is resection of the posterior wall of the external auditory canal. This is also a radical mastoidectomy as the ossicles have been resected.

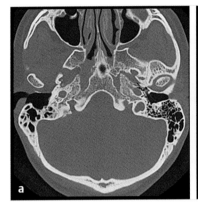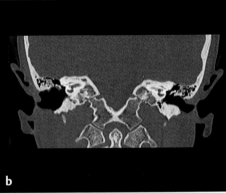

Fig. 6.9 Axial (a) and coronal (b) computed tomography shows a canal wall-down modified radical mastoidectomy.

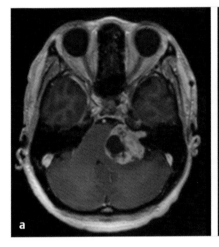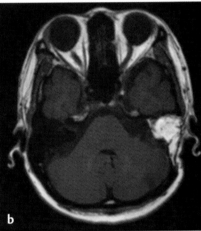

Fig. 6.10 Axial T1-weighted postcontrast image (a) shows a large left vestibular schwannoma. (b) shows the patient following a translabyrinthine resection. The whole petrous bone including the ossicles and vestibular apparatus are removed and a fat graft has been placed into the surgical defect.

auditory canal, and the cerebellopontine (CP) angle. The procedure does not allow for hearing preservation and is often chosen for tumors regardless of size where hearing preservation is not an issue.[12] In this approach, removal of bone around the posterior aspect of the internal auditory canal and petrous apex results in exposure to both petrous apex and CP angle tumors. Further exposure may be gained with the transapical approach where the entire petrous bone is removed superiorly for wider exposure of the anterior CP angle. In addition to the expected absence of bone that is most apparent on CT, obliteration of the defect with fat is commonly seen on MRI (▶ Fig. 6.10). Gliosis in the adjacent cerebellar brain parenchymal from retraction at surgery may also be present.

When large lesions extend into the prepontine cistern, use of a transcochlear approach may be necessary. This technique is indicated most commonly in the setting of anterior-based meningiomas in the CP angle or at the clivus. Similar steps are involved as in a translabyrinthine resection, but the removal of the tympanic and petrous bones up to the clivus is required. The cochlea is removed, allowing for identification of the intrapetrous internal carotid artery as well as both horizontal and vertical segments of the facial nerve in the mastoid which can be transposed anteriorly or posteriorly as required. The external auditory canal is closed in a blind sac fashion and the Eustachian tube formally obliterated. Once again, the cavity is filled with fat and should not be confused with soft tissue representing recurrence.

In summary, the translabyrinthine approach is used for access to the internal auditory canal and CP angle, for access to the trigeminal nerve in Meckel's cave and for lesions involving the jugular foramen. By comparison, the transcochlear approach permits the former but also allows an approach for more anterior and medial lesions involving the clivus, intrapetrous carotid artery, and anterior middle cranial fossa if required. The transcochlear approach typically involves mobilization of the facial nerve with resultant weakness postoperatively being common. There is also greater risk for injury to the internal carotid artery. Surgery tends to be longer in duration.

In a conservative (or retrolabyrinthine) petrosectomy, the posterior fossa dural plate is exposed inferiorly to the level of the jugular bulb preserving the otic capsule. The labyrinth forms the anterior limit of dissection. With this approach, the facial nerve is usually skeletonized and preserved in its vertical segment. Surgical exposure is slightly more limited but does allow for access to both posterior and middle cranial fossa dural plates. It is often combined with a temporal craniotomy that allows for retraction of the temporal lobe. Further exposure to the posterior fossa dura occurs with removal of bone posterior to the sigmoid sinus in the retrosigmoid (or suboccipital) area. In a lateral subtotal petrosectomy, the external auditory canal, tympanic membrane, malleus, and incus are removed. The ear canal skin is closed in a blind sac fashion and the Eustachian tube is formally obliterated. The term "lateral" in this context denotes that bone removal stops at but does not include the labyrinth. Hearing and labyrinthine function is preserved although the individual would have a maximum conductive hearing loss on the operated side. A total petrosectomy extends the dissection to the petrous apex as indicated for carcinoma involving the temporal bone. The goal would be to perform an en bloc resection if possible in order to avoid tumor spillage at surgery. The labyrinth, cochlea, and facial nerve would be removed. The surgical plane medially would traverse the internal auditory canal. Care would be taken not to injure the intrapetrous carotid artery.

The infratemporal approach is used to expose the inferior part of the temporal bone including the parapharyngeal space internal carotid artery and internal jugular vein/jugular bulb. This approach allows for the removal of lesions from the CP angle to both the parapharyngeal and the jugulo-carotid spaces. Anterior transposition of the facial nerve is again required for direct surgical access in addition to an extension of the dissection into the neck for great vessel and lower cranial nerve identification. Depending on tumor extension, the infralabyrinthine portion of the petrous bone is removed and usually the external auditory canal. There is a known predisposition for cerebrospinal fluid (CSF) leakage, which is often offset by staging the surgery over two sessions.[13]

As previously mentioned a conservative (retrolabyrinthine) petrosectomy may be combined with a suboccipital craniotomy to afford a greater posterolateral approach to the CP angle, upper neck, and jugular foramen. The external auditory canal is kept intact along with the otic capsule. In addition, the parapharyngeal space will be seen to communicate through an inferior mastoid approach. A fat plug can usually be seen postoperatively, which is placed during the intra-extradural closure. Careful assessment of the postoperative internal carotid is imperative although it is unclear whether the limited carotid manipulation from this approach predisposes it to injury or whether this technique is chosen in cases where intrapetrous carotid canal involvement appears more likely.[14]

## 6.3.5 Transtemporal and Retrosigmoid Approaches

To visualize the anterior and posterior aspects of the petrous bone, a total transtemporal approach may be employed. Employing a sizable (6 × 5 mm) temporal craniotomy, bone is removed above the petrous bone revealing the temporal lobe dura. At surgery, the dura is elevated along posterior to anterior along the petrous bone. A transtentorial dural opening in addition to splitting of the tentorium cerebelli (and additional splitting of the tentorium cerebelli) can be performed if required to further elevate the temporal lobe for greater exposure.

Alternatively, another direct approach to the CP angle can be made through a retrosigmoid (suboccipital or paracerebellar) craniotomy. This is typically recommended for tumors such as vestibular schwannomas or meningiomas which do not involve the distal end of the internal auditory canal or impinge the brainstem in those with serviceable hearing. Retrosigmoid bone is removed and the dura is opened to allow access to the posterior aspect of the temporal bone and CP angle. Retrolabyrinthine surgery is indicated as a hearing preservation procedure. Removal of the posterior bony portion of the porus acusticus

allows for visualization of the intracanalicular facial, cochlear, and superior and inferior vestibular nerves. Hearing preservation rates may be present in 50 to 70% of carefully selected cases and are both tumor and extent dependent in the internal auditory canal.[15] Despite cochlear nerve preservation, hearing is often lost from vascular injury to the labyrinthine arteries in the internal auditory canal. Though all techniques discussed will demonstrate expected patterns of bone removal, tissue seals around the internal auditory canal and cerebellar edema not infrequently seen following surgical retraction. The retrosigmoid approach has been well documented to have varying degrees of cerebellar edema and gliosis from surgical retraction not related to tumor pathology (► Fig. 6.11).

Dedicated T1-weighted MR, angled perpendicular to the dorsal aspect of the brainstem, can be used to visualize the facial nerve when detailed follow-up is required. The precise course of a transposed nerve can be followed or its sacrifice documented on this sequence. Facial nerve transposition is favorable to its surgical sacrifice for anatomic exposure whenever possible. On high-resolution T2-weighted MR or constructive interference in steady-state (CISS) sequences, the normal nerve can be seen as a hypointense linear structure extending from the brainstem to the internal auditory canal. It is normally surrounded by CSF and lies anterior to the vestibulocochlear nerve complex.[16] Gadolinium is necessary to best visualize its tympanic and mastoid segments as well as the geniculate ganglion. While enhancement of these segments can reflect neoplastic involvement, caution is advised as postsurgical inflammation may impart the same appearance. In facial nerve reanimation surgery, a graft (often a sural or greater auricular nerve interposition graft) may be present for reconstruction of the nerve. Reanimated nerves may also enhance in the segments where the facial nerve does not typically do and should not be mistaken for recurrence.

## 6.3.6 Endoscopic Surgery

With careful patient selection, an increasing number of patients with sinonasal and anterior cranial fossa tumors are successfully being managed with a total endoscopic approach that spares the patient a lateral rhinotomy and the craniotomy portion of an open CFR.[17] In such cases, margins of the mucosa, periorbital, and dura should be microscopically clear to ensure local control on par with traditional combined approaches.

One method of reconstructing a skull base defect employs the Hadad–Bassagasteguy technique. In this technique, a nasoseptal mucoperiosteal flap supported by a nasoseptal vascular pedicle is used to seal the skull base defect (► Fig. 6.12). On T1- and T2-weighted imaging, these nasoseptal flaps appear isointense to brain. Immediately following surgery, a minority of these flaps may not enhance, but most do so. Most flaps also decrease in thickness on follow-up at 6 months. A small minority, however, increase in thickness. Neither characteristic can be used to predict flap failure, and the significance of these findings remains unknown. Enhancement on follow-up is likely the greatest predictor of flap viability with the caveat that some flaps may not enhance on early postoperative imaging but still remain viable.[18,19] Free fat may be also noted between the defect and sinonasal cavity if placed intraoperatively.

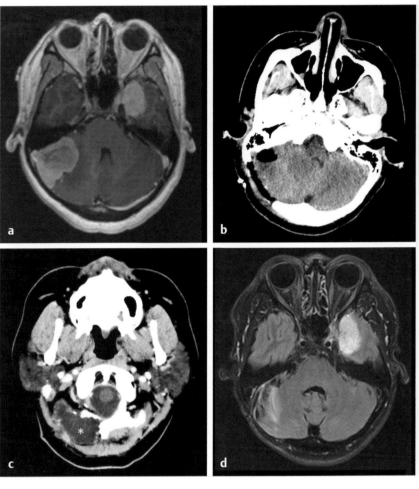

**Fig. 6.11** Axial T1-weighted postcontrast image **(a)** shows a large right posterior fossa meningioma. Note the presence of a second meningioma in the left middle cranial fossa. **(b,c)** Immediate postoperative CT scans after a retrosigmoid craniectomy and resection of the posterior fossa mass. There is the expected presence of pneumocephalus along the surgical margins. In addition, a pseudomeningocele (*asterisk*; **c**) is also present along the posterior neck. FLAIR (fluid-attenuated inversion recovery) image **(d)** is a long-term follow-up showing gliosis in the right cerebellum. The pseudomeningocele is also resolved (not shown).

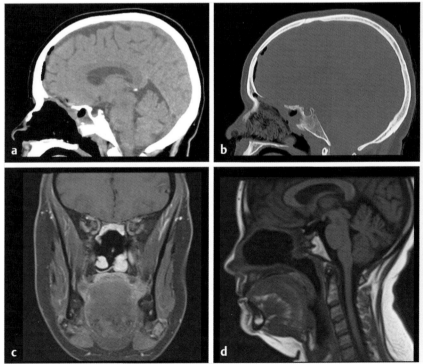

**Fig. 6.12** Immediate postoperative sagittal computed tomography images **(a,b)** following a pure endoscopic resection of ethmoid sinus carcinoma. The reconstruction involved a fascia lata and nasoseptal reconstruction. A Draf III frontal sinusotomy was also performed. A small amount of expected pneumocephalus is evident. Later surveillance imaging consisting of coronal contrast-enhanced T1-weighted **(c)** and sagittal unenhanced T1-weighted **(d)** images shows the floor reconstruction as thin smooth-enhancing soft tissue holding up the cranial contents.

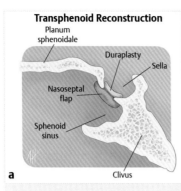
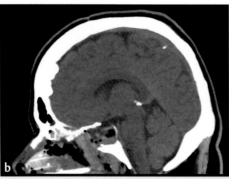
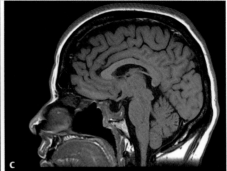

**Fig. 6.13** **(a)** Sagittal graphic diagram shows the posttranssphenoidal floor reconstruction in the setting of associated cerebrospinal fluid leak. **(b)** An early postoperative sagittal computed tomography image following transsphenoidal resection of a pituitary adenoma. The reconstructed floor is quite bulky and heterogeneous. This is intermixed foci of air and blood present among a nasoseptal flap. A dark focus corresponds to fat graft. **(c)** A later sagittal T1-weighted magnetic resonance shows the appearance once the region has had time to settle. The reconstruction appears as smooth soft tissue that parallels the expanded sellar floor.

Endoscopic transsphenoidal surgery to gain access to the sellar contents involves removal of the sphenoid rostrum and anterior sinus wall of the sphenoid. A defect in the floor of the sphenoid bone is expected with variable absence of the septum and turbinates. Reconstruction includes the use of varying combinations of absorbable gelatin powder, hemostatic cellulose polymers, fibrin sealants, and fat grafts. During the surgical resection if a CSF leak becomes evident, a more complex reconstruction is employed. The bony and dural defects are first covered with a lyophilized dural substitute used as an inlay graft. Fibrin sealant as well as absorbable gelatin sponge material is also often used, followed by a pedicled nasoseptal flap as a final layer. The postoperative appearance of the reconstruction may appear quite heterogeneous (▶ Fig. 6.13). CT imaging would typically show plaquelike or lobulated soft tissue bridging the defect. MRI would show the same soft tissue, but the signal intensity can be quite variable reflecting the presence of blood product, fibrosis in addition to the reconstruction flap itself. Extensive signal change in the remaining sphenoid may also be present.

## 6.4 External Beam Radiation

Radiation therapy imparts its own set of surveillance challenges by causing considerable edema, inflammation, and fibrosis. In order to distinguish treatment effects from tumor recurrence, the interpretation of postradiation imaging requires a familiarity with the expected common postradiation tissue changes. The most common method of delivering radiotherapy is by external beam radiation. This is usually delivered using photons from a linear accelerator. Less commonly employed but increasing available is proton therapy and its role in skull base and head and neck cancers is currently being evaluated in prospective randomized trials. The potential benefit of proton therapy is that it delivers its dose to a precise field with any radiation effects on adjacent tissues being minimal, that is there is less collateral damage beyond the high-dose target volume and, therefore, the late effect profile of radiation therapy may be better. However, to date there is no proven outcome advantage of proton therapy over conventional external beam therapy. Intensity-modulated radiotherapy (IMRT) was a major advance in

delivering external beam radiation, as it allowed for molding of the radiation field to avoid critical structures such as the brain and eyes. IMRT allows the radiation beam to modulate while being delivered, and effectively differentially dose within the treatment field. In the case of skull base tumors with several adjacent critical dose-limiting organs at risk (OAR), IMRT allows higher doses within the tumor while simultaneously modulating the intensity to reduce dose to the OAR. The overall exposure to the healthy normal tissues is also minimized, and significantly reduced as compared to the prior approach of three-dimensional conformal radiation therapy (3DCRT). Nowadays 3DCRT is used only for noncomplex cases where the dose prescribed to the tumor is one that is also tolerable to the OAR and, hence, modulation is not required.

Brachytherapy is a method of delivering focal radiation to a tumor by either implanting radiation pellets in the tumor bed or implanting temporary catheters in the tumor to deliver the radiation. This method has been used in the past for skull base tumors and it is the best technique for delivering high radiation doses to a localized tumor bed. However, it is limited only to accessible sites such as the tongue or nasopharynx. It is also technically demanding, requires significant expertise, and has the potential for serious adverse effects if critical structures are damaged. Given the advances with dose conformity achieved by IMRT, the use of brachytherapy in the skull base is diminishing.

Stereotactic radiosurgery (SRS) refers to a single high dose of radiation delivered to an immobilized patient (in the past, use of an invasive head frame was common) to ablate gross tumor. It is not intended to be the primary therapy for malignant tumors as the exposure is subtherapeutic to the margin of surrounding tissue that may be harboring microscopic disease. It is an excellent tool for small benign intracranial tumors such as vestibular schwannomas, meningiomas, or even metastases. As the technology of external beam radiation has evolved to a high precision as a result of image guidance and the integration of robotic technology, SRS has been developed for body sites, known as stereotactic body radiotherapy (SBRT). The radiation is delivered in one to five fractions of high doses with the intent to ablate gross tumor.

A typical curative course of external beam radiotherapy usually consists of 60 to 70 Gy delivered over 7 weeks at

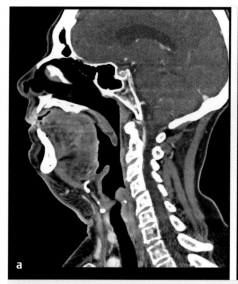
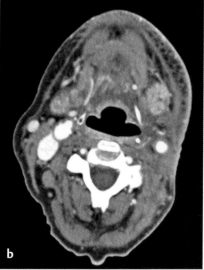
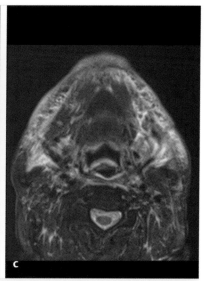

**Fig. 6.14** Sagittal **(a)** and axial **(b)** computed tomography (CT) images in the same patient following radiation therapy demonstrate skin thickening, haziness, and reticulation in the subcutaneous fat in the neck. There is also edema involving the epiglottis and preepiglottic space fat. The axial CT image also shows thickening of the platysma muscle and changes related to a left neck dissection—absence of the left internal jugular vein and generalized soft-tissue volume loss. Axial T2-weighted image with fat saturation **(c)** in another patient shows diffuse high-signal edema and reticulation within the tissues of the face bilaterally.

approximately 10 Gy per week. The current standard for head and neck curative radiation requires immobilization of the head in a thermoplastic mask to maximize reproducing the precise delivery of the radiation dose, thin slice CT (1–3 mm) encompassing the entire radiation field for dose calculation, possible fusion with MR images for optimal contouring of the tumor and adjacent structures, typically 4 to 7 beams of radiation equally spaced in a coplanar arrangement (e.g., every 30–40 degrees), a linear accelerator equipped with a multileaf collimator that allows for IMRT, and image guidance. This new paradigm is a major advance as it allows for a maximal tumor dose with limited dosing to adjacent healthy tissues. This minimizes the typical side effect of prior radiation therapy such as xerostomia, dysphagia, fibrosis, and brain necrosis. As a result of these advances in delivering radiation therapy, it is now often utilized as the primary treatment modality for many head and neck cancers.

### 6.4.1 Postradiation Changes

The reactions caused by radiation therapy can be divided into early or late changes. Early reactions occur within 90 days of radiation treatment[20,21] and most of these are reversible. These reactions include skin reddening/erythema, skin desquamation, and a mucositis, which are present in almost all patients. The late reactions may appear months to years following treatment and these include vascular complications, soft tissue and osteoradionecrosis, xerostomia and related dental caries, and dysphagia. In rare cases, a secondary radiation-induced neoplasm may occur.[20]

As expected, both the duration and extent of radiation reactions are dependent on the target volume and dose of radiation, though it is not clear if the relationship is strictly linear and evaluations of individual susceptibility to radiosensitivity are

ongoing. Beyond inherent sensitivity, it has been shown that alcohol and smoking likely have a negative effect on radiosensitivity.[22] The incidence of early reactions appears to increase with the administration of neoadjuvant chemotherapy.[23]

Common CT and MRI findings of early reactions include local cutaneous and platysma thickening, and subcutaneous fat reticulation caused by obstructed venolymphatic capillaries (▶ Fig. 6.14). Retropharyngeal edema as well as edema mainly of the oropharynx, hypopharynx, and supraglottic larynx is also common (▶ Fig. 6.15). On contrast-enhanced studies, thickening and enhancement of the pharyngeal mucosa can be seen with a mucositis and increased density in the parotid and less often the submandibular glands may be found with radiation-induced sialadenitis (▶ Fig. 6.16, ▶ Fig. 6.17).

## 6.5 Disease Recurrence

Following surgery, even substantial tumor recurrence may be clinically silent and thus imaging plays a key role in its detection. This is particularly true in the skull base where meaningful palpation is commonly not an option. As noted, the surgical bed and margins are most often where disease recurs[24] and most recurrences develop within the first 2 years after treatment. However, it should be noted that uncommonly, a rapid recurrence may develop within weeks of the end of treatment.

On CT imaging, tumor has a similar attenuation to that of skeletal muscle and differentiation from granulation tissue may be impossible. Any mass occurring in the primary tumor bed should raise concern for a tumor recurrence (▶ Fig. 6.18).[25] If a region has a lower attenuation than muscle, it likely represents edema.[26] Any progressive enlargement of an area on serial imaging also should raise concern for tumor recurrence and suggest the need for a biopsy. Recurrent tumor may be well defined or show peripheral ill definition. Bone destruction may

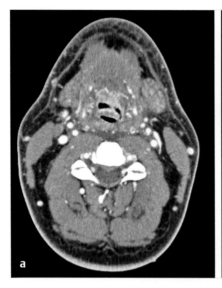
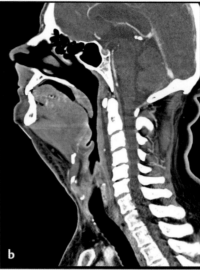

**Fig. 6.15** Axial (a) and sagittal (b) enhanced computed tomography images show skin and subcutaneous changes in the lower face and neck related to edema and obstructed venolymphatic structures. Both images also show low attenuation fluid in the retropharyngeal space.

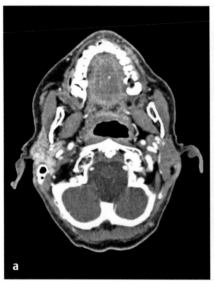
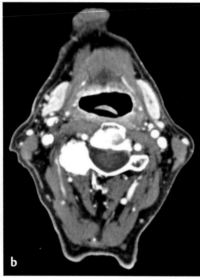

**Fig. 6.16** (a,b) Axial contrast-enhanced computed tomography images show increased signal in the right parotid and both submandibular glands following radiation to the neck reflecting secondary sialadenitis.

also be present. On MRI, tumor usually has intermediate T1-weighted signal intensity and slightly higher T2-weighted signal intensity and demonstrates enhancement on T1-weighted, post contrast fat-suppressed images. Low T2-weighted signal intensity usually indicates a highly cellular area and may indicate granulation tissue, fibrosis, or an aggressive neoplasm. In these cases, often biopsy is indicated.

Although posttreatment scarring and granulation tissue may mimic a tumor recurrence, serial imaging usually shows retraction of the fibrosis and granulation tissue and growth of the tumor.[27]

If DWI is used, high intensity with a corresponding low ADC is worrisome for recurrence.[3,28] Vandecaveye et al report that low ADC in the context of squamous cell carcinoma has a sensitivity of 94.6%, specificity of 95.9%, and accuracy of 95.5% in the differentiation of recurrence from nontumoral tissue, presumably due to the marked hypercellularity of the former. Postsurgical changes such as fibrosis and necrosis, inflammation, and edema are inherently less dense in nature and exhibit a higher

ADC. On T1-weighted MR, squamous cell carcinoma recurrence usually appears as an enhancing mass with low-intermediate signal intensity, and high DWI signal, and low ADC values.

## 6.6 Postoperative Complications

The majority of complications in skull base reconstruction occur in the immediate postoperative period. Included in these are seroma/fluid retention, fistula formation, infection/abscess, and flap necrosis. A myriad patient-related factors that increase the risk of complication have been reported, including age, regular alcohol or tobacco consumption, anemia, malnutrition, and postoperative medical complications.[29] In addition, duration of surgery, flap choice, and primary tumor stage are significant risk factors. Patients at greatest risk for complication following skull base reconstruction usually have undergone either dural resection or pretreatment chemoradiotherapy, or both. Dural resection cases have been reported to have a complication rate

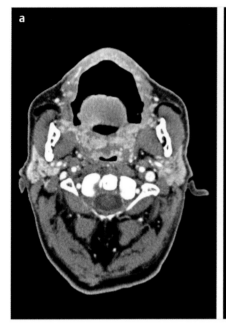
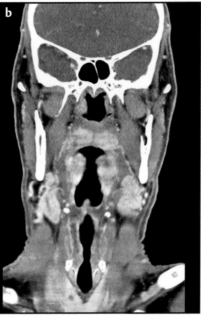

Fig. 6.17 Axial (a) and coronal (b) contrast-enhanced images show prominence and avid enhancement of the pharyngeal mucosa in the oropharynx compatible with postradiation mucositis. Note the presence of bilateral sialadenitis involving the parotid and submandibular glands.

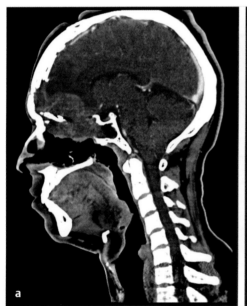
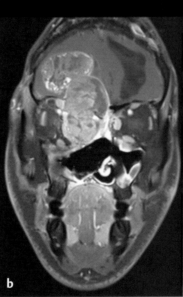
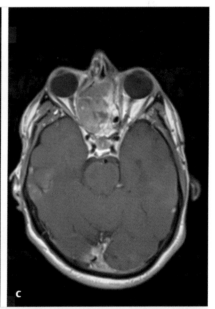

Fig. 6.18 Sagittal computed tomography (a) and coronal (b) and axial (c) T1-weighted gadolinium-enhanced images depict massive recurrence of ADC along the reconstructed anterior cranial fossa floor. The heterogeneously enhancing mass bulges superiorly to elevate and possibly invade the frontal lobe parenchyma.

as high as 81%.[30] Complication rates following chemoradiation therapy may be as high as 52% compared to 11% in patients with no prior intervention. Naturally, cases that require chemoradiation therapy tend also to involve those with more extensive disease. Despite this, however, the disparity suggests these interventions are independent risk factors.

## 6.6.1 Collections and Fistula Formation

Fluid collections following surgery are not necessarily a cause for concern and large seromata may spontaneously resolve.

Two important distinctions that need to be made are in identifying a CSF leak and a chylous fistula. While the latter is rare at the skull base, it is reported to occur in 2% of accompanying neck dissections.[31] Given that the thoracic duct is usually involved, a chylous leak is most likely to be seen in the inferior lower left neck (▶ Fig. 6.19). Thus, scrutiny of a benign-appearing fluid collection in this region is essential. Unfortunately, many surgical complications may present similarly on imaging. Thus, on CT and MRI, a peripherally enhancing fluid collection may represent a chylous leak, a hematoma, an abscess or a seroma.

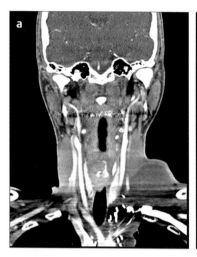
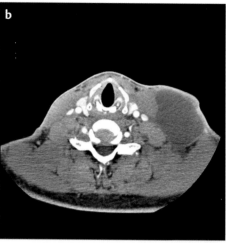

Fig. 6.19 Contrast-enhanced coronal (a) and axial (b) images of a chylous leak. These appear as a uniform, thin-walled, low attenuation fluid collection located in the base of the left neck.

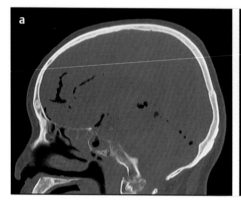
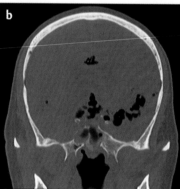

Fig. 6.20 Sagittal (a) and coronal (b) bone window images in a patient who developed severe headache and cerebrospinal fluid (CSF) rhinorrhea several years after radiation therapy for nasopharyngeal carcinoma. The images reveal diffuse intracranial air and a CSF fluid level in the sphenoid sinus. Patchy areas of bone loss in the sella turcica and along the lateral wall of the right sphenoid sinus are present compatible with radiation-related bony necrosis. The bony defects were confirmed at the time of endoscopic exploration and repair.

The presence of pain, cellulitis and an elevated white count may suggest an abscess, and diffusion restriction on MRI increases the likelihood of an infected collection provided this is no superimposed hemorrhage. Although the seroma is the least likely to have rim enhancement, such enhancement can occur. However, even the presence of enhancement does not completely rule out this possibility.

## 6.6.2 Cerebrospinal Fluid Leak, Meningoencephalocele

Given the complex and extensive nature of skull base surgery and radiation, the development of a CSF leak is a real potential complication. A CSF leak may either be detected incidentally on imaging or the patient may present with clear rhinorrhea and/ or otorrhea, which is often exacerbated on a Valsalva maneuver. In the latter case, the standard of care is obtaining an assay for $\beta_2$-transferrin content on a sample of collected fluid. The identification of a CSF leak is critical in order to avoid the possibility of intracranial hypotension and herniation, but also meningitis risk and rebound intracranial hypertension.[32] When a CSF leak is suspected, imaging is necessary to confirm the diagnosis, identify the specific osteodural defect, and rule out an associated meningoencephalocele. Given that CSF leak can now be reliably repaired endoscopically, there is a need for precisely localizing the anatomical defect. Radionuclide and CT cisternog-

raphy were the standard for leak assessment for decades, but the trend toward intrathecal contrast injection is decreasing in an era where better-tolerated less invasive techniques are available.[33] Modern CT, MR, and MR cisternography are not contraindicated in patients with secondary meningitis and do not rely on active CSF leakage at the time of assessment.

With its excellent bone resolution, CT is heavily relied upon to identify any potential skull base defects with a sensitivity as high as 92%, and with a specificity of 100% even in the absence of active leak.[34] At the site of a suspected skull base defect, an air-fluid level or opacification of the contiguous mastoid, middle ear or upper nasal cavity or paranasal sinus may be present. Accompanying occasionally may be pneumocephalus with or without associated tension (▶ Fig. 6.20).[35] Once a potential site of a CSF leak is identified, it is imperative that the search for additional sites should continue. The entire skull base, middle ear, and mastoid must be carefully scrutinized. CT may overestimate the size of a bony defect and the fact that the bony defect may not correspond with the site of a corresponding dural defect.[36] A common point of confusion is the presence of Pacchionian granulations, as they may mimic postsurgical bony defects. However, these granulations do not impart mass effect. MR is indicated in situations where fluid or soft tissue is subjacent to a bony defect and it cannot be reliably distinguished or identified on CT. Thus, on CT, granulation tissue, a cholesteatoma, or a cholesterol granuloma may not be distinguished from temporal lobe herniation on CT in the postoperative

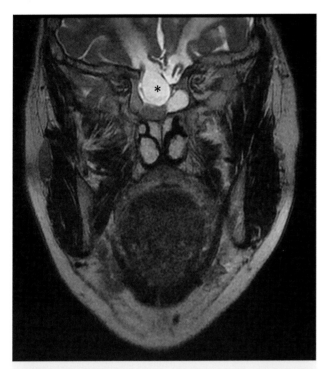

**Fig. 6.21** Coronal T2-weighted image shows a meningocele (*asterisk*) that has herniated down through a defect in the base of skull following an endoscopic skull base resection and repair.

setting. However, T2-weighted imaging complemented by fast imaging employing steady-state acquisition (FIESTA) sequence allows a more actuate assessment of the herniation contents and usually resolves any issue. FIESTA sequences will usually clearly depict gyri and CSF, thus identifying meningoencephalocele or herniation as well as CSF sacculation.[37]

Employing heavily T2-weighted multiplanar sequences combined with subtraction of non-CSF signal, MR cisternography allows for maximum-intensity projection (MIP) measures of flow with excellent anatomical detail. A CSF leak can be seen as a hyperintense tract from the subarachnoid space into the paranasal sinuses. In addition, a meningocele and a meningoencephalocele are clearly visible with this technique as well as on conventional T2 sequences (▶ Fig. 6.21). It is possible to visualize potential involvement of a meningoencephalocele with vascular or optic structures, and to distinguish signal intensity changes related to gliosis.[38] Pooling CSF is occasionally difficult to distinguish from mucosal secretions; however, the latter may demonstrate T1 hyperintensity depending on the degree of inspissation and protein content. With the addition of gadolinium, the dural stalk of a meningoencephalocele can be distinguished from mucosal thickening in equivocal cases.[39] The sensitivity and specificity of MR cisternography may be lower than that of CT, and should be reserved for challenging cases. When used in concert, the combined sensitivity and specificity are reported to be 95 and 100%.[40] The notion of these modalities complementing each other for planning of leak repair is an important one. While MR cisternography can depict the CSF column and associated conditions well, the precise bony detail obtained with CT with or without 3D reconstruction is often still needed.

## 6.6.3 Reconstruction Ischemia and Necrosis

Reconstruction ischemia and necrosis is often first questioned when a flap fails bedside vascular testing. While this complication is rare, missing a nonviable flap is devastating, and any concerns regarding flap perfusion should prompt immediate investigation.[41,42] Risk factors for this complication include age, regular alcohol or tobacco consumption, anemia, malnutrition, and postoperative as well as any pre-existing medical complications such as sickle cell trait/disease, polycythemia vera, or any thrombophilia. On imaging, whether a flap reconstruction enhances avidly or poorly does not reliably predict necrosis. One of the most reliable signs is venous thrombosis, which most commonly occurs within 1 to 5 days following surgery.[43] At the skull base, this is particularly significant as extension of thrombosis can involve critical tributaries. Dedicated vascular studies to exclude both arterial and venous thrombosis are merited in the setting of suspected reconstruction necrosis. A common pitfall in the assessment of flaps is T2 hyperintensity, which was once thought to suggest a nonviable reconstruction. While it is a positive finding, it reflects muscular inflammation and early denervation.[44]

## 6.6.4 Mucosal Necrosis

Despite refinements in targeted radiotherapy for skull base neoplasia, mucosal necrosis remains a possible late reaction, usually occurring within 6 to 12 months after treatment. When present, it can seriously affect patient quality of life due to its impact on deglutition and mastication.[45] However, spontaneous recovery occurs in the vast majority of cases.[46] Mucosal necrosis should be distinguished from mucositis whenever possible. In contrast to necrosis, mucositis is an acute inflammatory process that exhibits not only sloughing of mucosal cells but also their rapid replenishment.[20] Thus, the temporal difference of mucositis and necrosis should allow differentiation in most cases. It is important to note that as an inflammatory process, mucositis is a hyperemic process that promotes vascular tissue supply. By comparison, with necrosis, severe ongoing inflammation gradually begets fibrosis and lymphovascular flow impedance. Ultimately, the result is hypoperfused mucosa, which ulcerates as anoxia progresses. Unenhanced studies may simulate necrosis by revealing gas formation from opportunistic organisms and tissue breakdown. This is more clearly delineated on CT than MR.

On enhanced CT and MR, necrotic mucosa enhances poorly, or not at all, and frank ulcerations may be seen (▶ Fig. 6.22).[45] A significant challenge arises in the context of mixed ulcerated and enhancing tissue. While it is reasonable to expect that this heterogeneity might be present in hypoperfused mucosa, the picture may also be that of recurrent disease. Vexingly, both of these phenomena declare themselves in the late posttreatment period. Whenever possible, doubt should be resolved with clinical and endoscopic examination and tissue sampling. Furthermore, patients with mucosal necrosis may well proceed to develop a recurrence. Thus even in established cases of tissue necrosis, close surveillance is necessary.

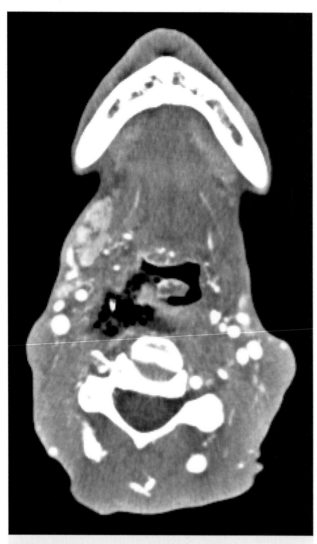

Fig. 6.22 Axial computed tomography image shows an area of deep soft-tissue loss and ulceration in the right oropharynx. Retained secretions are noted in the ulcer crater. The patient had previously received radiation for a hypopharyngeal carcinoma. Panendoscopy and biopsy were negative for tumor recurrence.

## 6.7 Long-Term Complications

### 6.7.1 Osteoradionecrosis

Osteoradionecrosis (or radiation osteonecrosis) is the result of vascular compromise and the involved bone appears demineralized, with cortical sequestrations and then disruption of the medullary cavity.[47] As each sequestrum is extruded, the patient usually experiences pain. Exposed bone or sequestrations are likely to be seen at endoscopy. The incidence of osteoradionecrosis has been reported to be as high at 22% in the head and neck literature, though much of this involves the mandible. It is estimated the radiation osteonecrosis occurs in the skull base with an incidence of 3%.[48] Most of these cases received re-irradiation for recurrent disease.

The development of osteoradionecrosis is a late reaction, which is usually seen anywhere from 12 to 36 months following therapeutic radiation. For reasons that are not fully understood, recent prior surgical intervention is a major risk factor for this complication. It is generally felt that the threshold for osteoradionecrosis is a fractionated dose of 50 Gy, and that vigilance for this complication should be heightened for these patients. However, this complication has been seen at the skull base after a dose of 45 Gy as well.[43] The physical location of tumor relative to the affected bone is also a major risk factor. Other risk factors include tumor stage, as well as field size, dose and energy of treatment. Notably, coexistent infection appears to accelerate the process of osteoradionecrosis.[49]

Patients with skull base osteoradionecrosis usually come to clinical attention because of chronic dull pain, epistaxis, halitosis, and soft-tissue swelling, and occasionally causing facial deformity not related to ant surgery. Owing to the fact that this process may fistulize with the adjacent mucosa, odynophagia, dysphagia, and drainage may be present.

As noted, the imaging features of osteoradionecrosis include osteopenia, cortical bone loss, sequestration, and permeative erosion within the marrow. Periosteal bone formation as the bone attempts to heal may also be evident (▶ Fig. 6.23), as can variable degrees of adjacent soft-tissue edema. The presence of air gas formation within the marrow space may also be seen and is a diagnostic finding (▶ Fig. 6.24, ▶ Fig. 6.25). The most

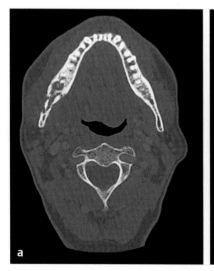
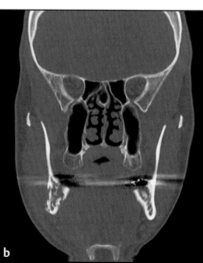

Fig. 6.23 Axial (a) and coronal (b) computed tomography images in a patient with right mandibular osteoradionecrosis following radiation for tonsillar carcinoma. There is frank cortical erosion and internal marrow lytic change. Internal foci of bony sequestra are also noted.

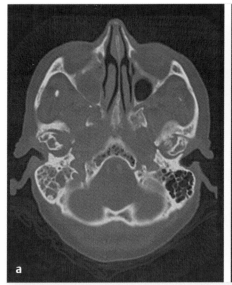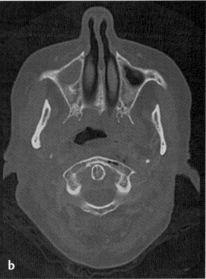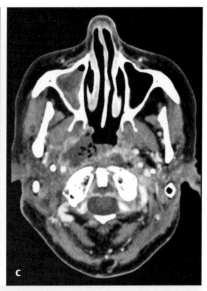

Fig. 6.24 Axial bone window (a,b) and soft-tissue window (c) computed tomography images in a patient with prior radiation for nasopharyngeal carcinoma. There is longstanding ulcerative soft-tissue necrosis in the right nasopharynx. The patient developed headache and visual symptoms, and imaging revealed the presence of air lucency within the clivus and anterior arch of C1. A new collection in the left prevertebral with contiguous extension into the periodontoid space was also present. The findings were compatible with skull base osteonecrosis and secondary abscess formation.

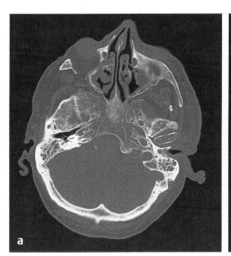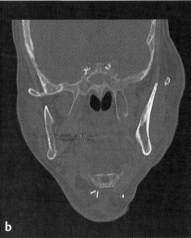

Fig. 6.25 Axial (a) and coronal (b) bone window computed tomography images in a patient who had undergone two prior rounds of radiation for facial skin carcinoma. Note the diffuse osteopenia and permeative change involving the bony central skull base compatible with early osteoradionecrosis.

common locations for radiation osteonecrosis to occur in the skull base include the temporal bone, the carotid canal, the sphenoid bone, and the clivus.

The most sensitive finding of osteoradionecrosis on MR is a change in marrow signal intensity, which may be associated with soft-tissue thickening. On T1-weighted MR, this is manifested as a hypointense area that, on T2-weighted MR, has a heterogeneous hyperintensity in the affected marrow. Coronal CT reconstructions may be helpful in better delineating the extent of osteoradionecrosis.

Importantly, bony destruction and associated soft-tissue fullness are also potentially indicative of a tumor recurrence. In equivocal cases, it is imperative that an accompanying soft-tissue mass is evaluated, as this finding favors a tumor recurrence (▸ Fig. 6.26). 99Tcm-sestamibi SPECT/CT may also be of utility, where 99Tcm-MDP and FDG tracer positivity suggests chronic inflammation and negativity of 9Tcm-sestamibi is highly sugges-

tive of the absence of recurrence.[50] Additionally, a logical approach to the site of osteoradionecrosis is needed. When cortical destruction is noted at a site distant from the location of the original tumor or reconstruction, the suspicion for a recurrence can be lessened.[26]

## 6.7.2 Radiation Vasculopathy

The majority of patients who experience radiation vasculopathy have a pre-existing vascular disease secondary to smoking, dyslipidemia, hypertension, or diabetes mellitus. Nevertheless, intimal disease, venous thrombosis, and progression of atherosclerosis are known complications of radiation therapy and they can affect any postradiation patient.[51]

Even with the reassurance that mucosal necrosis spontaneously resolves in 95% of patients, cases must be scrutinized as accompanying infection or pseudoaneurysm formation may

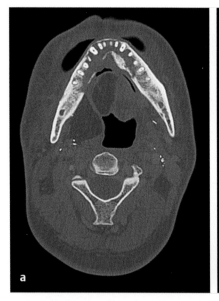
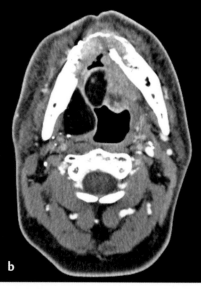

**Fig. 6.26** Axial bone **(a)** and soft-tissue **(b)** window images in a patient who had undergone prior right hemiglossectomy and radiation for a tongue carcinoma. There is extensive lytic change involving the cortex and marrow of the anterior mandible. The presence of overt soft-tissue density within the areas of bony lysis is worrisome for tumor recurrence. Tissue sampling revealed recurrent carcinoma.

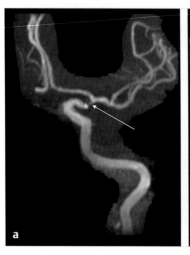
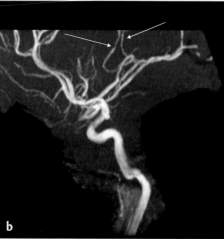

**Fig. 6.27** Two magnetic resonance angiography maximum-intensity projection images of the carotid and intracranial vasculature showing radiation-related vasculopathy. Areas of vessel narrowing are shown by the *arrows*. The first patient **(a)** received intracranial radiation for an astrocytoma, while the second patient **(b)** received intracranial radiation for an ependymoma.

occur. The latter may have particularly disastrous consequences, such as massive hemorrhage or reconstruction ischemia.[45] The imaging options include MR and CT angiography. Digital subtraction angiography (DSA) can be considered, particularly if embolization or a covered stent placement is planned.[52] Osteoradionecrosis can be associated with significant vascular injury at the skull base due to the proximity of vital structures. The most significant of these are carotid blowout and/or aneurysm formation, which carry with them a high mortality rate.[53]

Pure radiation-induced vasculopathy is thought to involve primarily intimal damage with subsequent proliferation, and was first demonstrated in literature pertaining to breast radiation.[54] Primarily affecting patients that receive doses of 50 Gy or greater, its latency period appears to be extremely variable, being on the order of months to decades following treatment.[51] The histopathologic changes of radiation-induced vasculopathy are intimal proliferation, thrombosis, and accelerated atherosclerosis. Field-dependent vasculopathy is often bilateral, and it may be safer to assume that this may occur when assessing these patients.[46] MR and CT angiography may demonstrate gross thickening of the vessel wall, and areas of vessel narrow-

ing (▶ Fig. 6.27). Secondary ischemic foci may also develop in the brain if the intracranial vessels are involved. DSA remains the gold standard for characterization of vasculopathy and collateral networks.[55] In addition, DSA offers the benefit of same-session intervention as needed. Radiation vasculopathy may also result in SMART (strokelike migraine attacks after radiation therapy) syndrome, and MRI during an attack typically shows cortical thickening and contrast enhancement. This may mimic leptomeningeal enhancement or ischemic disease.

### 6.7.3 Cerebral Necrosis

In the realm of head and neck cancer radiation therapy, skull base treatment carries the most pronounced risk of incidental cerebral injury. Although 80% of cases of focal brain necrosis occur within 3 years of treatment, such necrosis may present as late as 10 years after treatment.[56] Of particular concern is temporal lobe necrosis, which may be as high at 3% following treatment for nasopharyngeal carcinoma.[57] Expectedly, this was more common with previous radiation techniques involving wider areas of radiation and parallel-opposed lateral field tech-

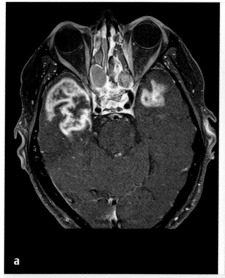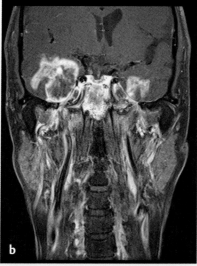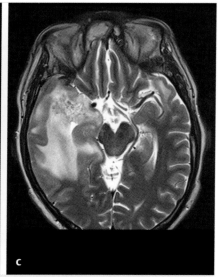

**Fig. 6.28** Postgadolinium-enhanced axial (**a**) and coronal (**b**) images show bilateral areas of heterogeneous enhancement in the right and left temporal lobes. Axial T2-weighted image (**c**) shows associated mass effect and high signal edema bilaterally. The patient had received radiation for treatment of nasopharyngeal carcinoma.

niques. With the advent of dynamic arc intensity modulation, comparatively generous sparing of normal tissue can be achieved. In addition, targeted doses can now be delivered at sub-60-Gy levels.

A ring-enhancing parenchymal mass within a radiation field on CT or MR is highly suggestive of cerebral necrosis (▶ Fig. 6.28).[58] The degree of edema associated with this is highly variable but is likely to be cytotoxic in nature, owing to an increase in urokinase plasminogen activator and a simultaneous decrease in tissue plasminogen activator. Vasogenic edema from direct endothelial damage is also likely present. As with any ring-enhancing cerebral mass, abscess, glioma, and metastasis are all difficult to exclude. To this end, DWI and molecular imaging are important problem-solving modalities.[59] On DWI, necrotic brain tissue exhibits markedly low signal with elevated ADC values, as might be expected from evolving necrosis of any kind. Normal cortex and most tumors will have lower ADC values by comparison.[60] This may be corroborated by low *N*-acetylaspartate and elevated lactate levels on MR spectroscopy, though its use is not a standard element of posttreatment investigation at this time. As with osteoradionecrosis, necrotic brain is not expected to be FDG avid due to its nonviable state, particularly compared with recurrence or metastasis. As a consequence, PET/CT is also a useful problem-solving tool for the differentiation of necrosis from tumor.[61] Simultaneous comparison of DWI and metabolic data with PET/MR has begun to show promise in streamlining this investigation.[62] In temporal lobe necrosis, patient symptoms are myriad and often nonspecific. Such symptoms include nausea, headache, seizures, and memory loss. T2-weighted MR will typically show substantial edema surrounding a mass, while on postcontrast CT or MR, this mass usually demonstrates ring enhancement.

Special note should be made in the setting of patients who undergo SRS rather than IMRT. Patients who receive SRS commonly, if not invariably, experience transient blood–brain barrier changes. As a result, tumor may appear to enlarge and may also be hyper-enhancing any time between 3 and 12 months following treatment. This phenomenon may persist for an additional 6 months from its onset.[63] Marked vasogenic edema will also be appreciated on MR. Unfortunately; the findings associated with recurrence are similar and represent a significant challenge. On postcontrast studies, it has been suggested that recurrence is more likely to retain central enhancement than treated tumor.[64] On MR, it is important to make comparisons with careful temporal correlation. On postcontrast T1 images, lesions will commonly appear to increase in size at 3 to 12 months, and subsequently reduce in size at 12 to 16 months. Some practices advocate the calculation of a lesion quotient, which is arrived at by dividing the hypointense T2 nodule cross-sectional area by that same area as seen on postcontrast T1. Units can vary as long as like units are compared. Patients with recurrence possessed quotients of 0.6 or higher, and those with necrosis 0.3 or lower. Simplified, this implies that a cellular tumor is hypointense on T2, as is an enhancing nodule, and both these findings are more likely to represent recurrence than necrosis.[65]

## 6.7.4 Spinal and Cranial Neuropathy

Cervical cord and brainstem injury may result from radiation therapy at the skull base in a minority of patients, despite advances in IMRT and shielding techniques. Cord edema appears as hyperintense signal on T2-weighted MRI, with corresponding hypointensity on T1-weighted sequences (▶ Fig. 6.29). In the acute and subacute phase, this can be accompanied by significant contrast enhancement. This may be an incidental finding, though the typical presentation is paraparesis, sensation of electric shock in the neck radiating to the upper limbs (Lhermitte's sign) or paresthesia at 3 to 6 months.[66] Beyond this phase, necrosis or atrophy with deformity may result in the years following radiation therapy.

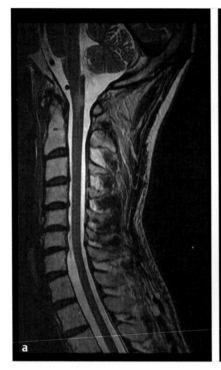 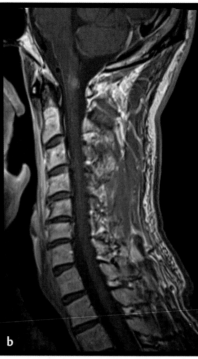

**Fig. 6.29** Sagittal T2-weighted (**a**) and postgadolinium-enhanced T1-weighted (**b**) images in a patient who received radiation therapy for a tonsillar carcinoma. The patient subsequently developed a region of elevated T2 signal with corresponding vague enhancement in the cervicomedullary junction suggestive of spinal cord edema and myelomalacia.

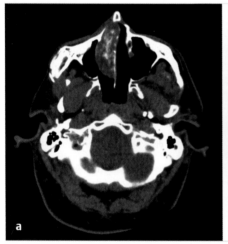 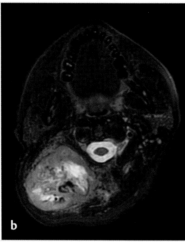

**Fig. 6.30** Two different patients with radiation-induced malignancies arising after a latency period of over 40 years. Both were treated for retinoblastoma as infants. The axial computed tomography (**a**) shows a right nasal cavity osteosarcoma. Note the internal ossified matrix. The axial fat-saturated T2 image (**b**) shows an angiosarcoma in the posterolateral neck. Note the presence of multiple irregular low-signal vascular flow voids.

When cranial nerves such as the hypoglossal, vagus, or spinal accessory nerve are affected, sequelae of muscle denervation such as edema and eventual fat infiltration may be seen. This process is commonly insidious, and may present over the source of a decade with palatal elevation, gag reflex, uvular deviation, and trapezius weakness. The optic nerves and chiasm can be involved when the anterior skull base is irradiated. Transverse myelitis may also be seen in the postradiation patient, and is usually irreversible.[48]

## 6.8 Neoplasm Induction

Direct induction of neoplasm by radiation therapy is an extremely rare but significant event. Postradiation osteosarcoma arising within the bony skull base,[67] mandible, and maxilla[68] occurs rarely, but any structure within the radiation field can be affected. One study of 426 patients undergoing radiation therapy for nasopharyngeal carcinoma found an incidence rate of approximately 0.037%, which the authors also concluded conferred a poorer prognosis than other sites.[69]

To confidently diagnose post-irradiation neoplasm, the lesion in question must be centered in or near the tissue of the original radiation field. Though the latency is felt to be a minimum of 4 years, caution dictates that the suspicion be raised when a lesion is seen even at 3 years following treatment. In the case of radiation-induced osteosarcoma, the tumor mass is situated within the radiation field; however, the tumor appearance may or may not demonstrate an obvious osteoblastic matrix. When an osteoblastic matrix is present, CT demonstrates a mass lesion with associated aggressive spiculated or sunburst bone formation (▶ Fig. 6.30). Additional more detailed imaging with MRI is often done to further define the lesion extent.

Fat-saturated T1-weighted MR images usually show a heterogeneously enhancing mass with bony destruction. In addition to osteosarcoma, other sarcomas, meningioma, and anaplastic ependymoma have been reported (▶ Fig. 6.30).[70] Benign and anaplastic meningiomas appear as enhancing extra-axial lesions. The latter may show more associated underlying brain edema, internal heterogeneity, and a higher likelihood of adjacent brain and bony invasion.

# 6.9 Conclusion

In the posttreatment skull base, imaging changes correspond with the nature of the interventions applied. Thus, knowledge of the normal appearance of open and endoscopic surgical reconstruction, as well as external beam and stereotactic radiation therapy is essential to correctly identify complication or a recurrence. An appreciation for the latencies involving tumor recurrence and early versus late complications at the skull base also helps bolster a logical approach to equivocal findings. Finally, command of the strengths and drawbacks of various imaging modalities will allow for troubleshooting of challenging cases and avoid unnecessary over-investigation.

# References

[1] Mukherji SK, Wolf GT. Evaluation of head and neck squamous cell carcinoma after treatment. AJNR Am J Neuroradiol. 2003; 24(9):1743–1746

[2] Pfister DG, Spencer S, Brizel DM, et al. National Comprehensive Cancer Network. Head and neck cancers, Version 2.2014. Clinical practice guidelines in oncology. J Natl Compr Canc Netw. 2014; 12(10):1454–1487

[3] Vandecaveye V, De Keyzer F, Dirix P, Lambrecht M, Nuyts S, Hermans R. Applications of diffusion-weighted magnetic resonance imaging in head and neck squamous cell carcinoma. Neuroradiology. 2010; 52(9):773–784

[4] Wehage IC, Fansa H. Complex reconstructions in head and neck cancer surgery: decision making. Head Neck Oncol. 2011; 3:14

[5] Hudgins PA. Flap reconstruction in the head and neck: expected appearance, complications, and recurrent disease. Eur J Radiol. 2002; 44(2):130–138

[6] Tomura N, Watanabe O, Hirano Y, Kato K, Takahashi S, Watarai J. MR imaging of recurrent head and neck tumours following flap reconstructive surgery. Clin Radiol. 2002; 57(2):109–113

[7] Abu-Ghanem S, Fliss DM. Surgical approaches to resection of anterior skull base and paranasal sinuses tumors. Balkan Med J. 2013; 30(2):136–141

[8] Raut AA, Naphade PS, Chawla A. Imaging of skull base: pictorial essay. Indian J Radiol Imaging. 2012; 22(4):305–316

[9] Sanna M, Pandya Y, Mancini F, Sequino G, Piccirillo E. Petrous bone cholesteatoma: classification, management and review of the literature. Audiol Neurootol. 2011; 16(2):124–136

[10] Mukherji SK, Mancuso AA, Kotzur IM, et al. CT of the temporal bone: findings after mastoidectomy, ossicular reconstruction, and cochlear implantation. AJR Am J Roentgenol. 1994; 163(6):1467–1471

[11] Munir N, Tandon S, Brown JS, Lesser TH. Trans-mastoid facial nerve localisation for malignant neoplasms confined to the parotid gland. Br J Oral Maxillofac Surg. 2012; 50(8):736–738

[12] Chamoun R, MacDonald J, Shelton C, Couldwell WT. Surgical approaches for resection of vestibular schwannomas: translabyrinthine, retrosigmoid, and middle fossa approaches. Neurosurg Focus. 2012; 33(3):E9

[13] Zanoletti E, Martini A, Emanuelli E, Mazzoni A. Lateral approaches to the skull base. Acta Otorhinolaryngol Ital. 2012; 32(5):281–287

[14] Sanna M, Bacciu A, Falcioni M, Taibah A, Piazza P. Surgical management of jugular foramen meningiomas: a series of 13 cases and review of the literature. Laryngoscope. 2007; 117(10):1710–1719

[15] Yamakami I, Uchino Y, Kobayashi E, Yamaura A, Oka N. Removal of large acoustic neurinomas (vestibular schwannomas) by the retrosigmoid approach with no mortality and minimal morbidity. J Neurol Neurosurg Psychiatry. 2004; 75(3):453–458

[16] Gupta S, Mends F, Hagiwara M, Fatterpekar G, Roehm PC. Imaging the facial nerve: a contemporary review. Radiol Res Pract. 2013; 2013:248039

[17] Dmytriw AA, Witterick IJ, Yu E, et al. Endoscopic resection of malignant sinonasal tumours: current trends and imaging workup. OA Minimally Invasive Surgery. 2013; 1(1):3

[18] Kang MD, Escott E, Thomas AJ, et al. The MR imaging appearance of the vascular pedicle nasoseptal flap. AJNR Am J Neuroradiol. 2009; 30(4):781–786

[19] Learned KO, Adappa ND, Lee JY, Newman JG, Palmer JN, Loevner LA. MR imaging evolution of endoscopic cranial defect reconstructions using nasoseptal flaps and their distinction from neoplasm. AJNR Am J Neuroradiol. 2014; 35(6):1182–1189

[20] Stone HB, Coleman CN, Anscher MS, McBride WH. Effects of radiation on normal tissue: consequences and mechanisms. Lancet Oncol. 2003; 4(9):529–536

[21] Trotti A. Toxicity in head and neck cancer: a review of trends and issues. Int J Radiat Oncol Biol Phys. 2000; 47(1):1–12

[22] Rugg T, Saunders MI, Dische S. Smoking and mucosal reactions to radiotherapy. Br J Radiol. 1990; 63(751):554–556

[23] Trotti A, Bellm LA, Epstein JB, et al. Mucositis incidence, severity and associated outcomes in patients with head and neck cancer receiving radiotherapy with or without chemotherapy: a systematic literature review. Radiother Oncol. 2003; 66(3):253–262

[24] Pedicini P, Caivano R, Fiorentino A, Strigari L. Clinical radiobiology of head and neck cancer: the hypothesis of stem cell activation. Clin Transl Oncol. 2015; 17(6):469–476

[25] Lell M, Baum U, Greess H, et al. Head and neck tumors: imaging recurrent tumor and post-therapeutic changes with CT and MRI. Eur J Radiol. 2000; 33(3):239–247

[26] Hermans R. Posttreatment imaging in head and neck cancer. Eur J Radiol. 2008; 66(3):501–511

[27] Saito N, Nadgir RN, Nakahira M, et al. Posttreatment CT and MR imaging in head and neck cancer: what the radiologist needs to know. Radiographics. 2012; 32(5):1261–1282, discussion 1282–1284

[28] Vandecaveye V, De Keyzer F, Nuyts S, et al. Detection of head and neck squamous cell carcinoma with diffusion weighted MRI after (chemo)radiotherapy: correlation between radiologic and histopathologic findings. Int J Radiat Oncol Biol Phys. 2007; 67(4):960–971

[29] Sakai A, Okami K, Onuki J, Miyasaka M, Furuya H, Iida M. Statistical analysis of post-operative complications after head and neck surgery. Tokai J Exp Clin Med. 2008; 33(3):105–109

[30] Sakashita T, Oridate N, Homma A, et al. Complications of skull base surgery: an analysis of 30 cases. Skull Base. 2009; 19(2):127–132

[31] Balm AJ, Lohuis PJ, Copper MP. Surgical technique–unwrapping the neck node levels around a sternocleidomastoid muscle bar: a systematic way of performing (modified) radical neck dissection. Eur J Surg Oncol. 2005; 31(10):1216–1221

[32] Horowitz G, Fliss DM, Margalit N, Wasserzug O, Gil Z. Association between cerebrospinal fluid leak and meningitis after skull base surgery. Otolaryngol Head Neck Surg. 2011; 145(5):689–693

[33] Zapalac JS, Marple BF, Schwade ND. Skull base cerebrospinal fluid fistulas: a comprehensive diagnostic algorithm. Otolaryngol Head Neck Surg. 2002; 126(6):669–676

[34] Connor SE. Imaging of skull-base cephalocoeles and cerebrospinal fluid leaks. Clin Radiol. 2010; 65(10):832–841

[35] Mammis A, Agarwal N, Eloy JA, Liu JK. Intraventricular tension pneumocephalus after endoscopic skull base surgery. J Neurol Surg A Cent Eur Neurosurg. 2013; 74 Suppl 1:e96–e99

[36] La Fata V, McLean N, Wise SK, DelGaudio JM, Hudgins PA. CSF leaks: correlation of high-resolution CT and multiplanar reformations with intraoperative endoscopic findings. AJNR Am J Neuroradiol. 2008; 29(3):536–541

[37] Lloyd KM, DelGaudio JM, Hudgins PA. Imaging of skull base cerebrospinal fluid leaks in adults. Radiology. 2008; 248(3):725–736

[38] Sillers MJ, Morgan CE, el Gammal T. Magnetic resonance cisternography and thin coronal computerized tomography in the evaluation of cerebrospinal fluid rhinorrhea. Am J Rhinol. 1997; 11(5):387–392

[39] Alonso RC, de la Peña MJ, Caicoya AG, Rodriguez MR, Moreno EA, de Vega Fernandez VM. Spontaneous skull base meningoencephaloceles and cerebrospinal fluid fistulas. Radiographics. 2013; 33(2):553–570

[40] Shetty PG, Shroff MM, Fatterpekar GM, Sahani DV, Kirtane MV. A retrospective analysis of spontaneous sphenoid sinus fistula: MR and CT findings. AJNR Am J Neuroradiol. 2000; 21(2):337–342

[41] Pusic AL, Chen CM, Patel S, Cordeiro PG, Shah JP. Microvascular reconstruction of the skull base: a clinical approach to surgical defect classification and flap selection. Skull Base. 2007; 17(1):5–15

[42] El-Sayed IH, Roediger FC, Goldberg AN, Parsa AT, McDermott MW. Endoscopic reconstruction of skull base defects with the nasal septal flap. Skull Base. 2008; 18(6):385–394

[43] Hanna EY, DeMonte F. Comprehensive Management of Skull Base Tumors. Boca Raton, FL: CRC Press; 2008

[44] Chong VF. Post treatment imaging in head and neck tumours. Cancer Imaging. 2005; 5:8–10

[45] Debnam JM, Garden AS, Ginsberg LE. Benign ulceration as a manifestation of soft tissue radiation necrosis: imaging findings. AJNR Am J Neuroradiol. 2008; 29(3):558–562

[46] Becker M, Schroth G, Zbären P, et al. Long-term changes induced by high-dose irradiation of the head and neck region: imaging findings. Radiographics. 1997; 17(1):5–26

[47] Huang XM, Zheng YQ, Zhang XM, et al. Diagnosis and management of skull base osteoradionecrosis after radiotherapy for nasopharyngeal carcinoma. Laryngoscope. 2006; 116(9):1626–1631

[48] Sataloff RT, Hartnick CJ. Sataloff's Comprehensive Textbook of Otolaryngology: Head & Neck Surgery: Pediatric Otolaryngology. New Delhi: Jaypee Brothers, Medical Publishers Pvt. Limited; 2015

[49] Gunderson LL, Willett CG, Calvo FA, Harrison LB. Intraoperative Irradiation: Techniques and Results. New York, NY: Humana Press; 2011

[50] Tan AE, Ng DC. Differentiating osteoradionecrosis from nasopharyngeal carcinoma tumour recurrence using 99Tcm-sestamibi SPECT/CT. Br J Radiol. 2011; 84(1005):e172–e175

[51] Rabin BM, Meyer JR, Berlin JW, Marymount MH, Palka PS, Russell EJ. Radiation-induced changes in the central nervous system and head and neck. Radiographics. 1996; 16(5):1055–1072

[52] Low YM, Goh YH. Endovascular treatment of epistaxis in patients irradiated for nasopharyngeal carcinoma. Clin Otolaryngol Allied Sci. 2003; 28(3):244–247

[53] Lam HC, Abdullah VJ, Wormald PJ, Van Hasselt CA. Internal carotid artery hemorrhage after irradiation and osteoradionecrosis of the skull base. Otolaryngol Head Neck Surg. 2001; 125(5):522–527

[54] Yi A, Kim HH, Shin HJ, Huh MO, Ahn SD, Seo BK. Radiation-induced complications after breast cancer radiation therapy: a pictorial review of multimodality imaging findings. Korean J Radiol. 2009; 10(5):496–507

[55] Zou WX, Leung TW, Yu SC, et al. Angiographic features, collaterals, and infarct topography of symptomatic occlusive radiation vasculopathy: a case-referent study. Stroke. 2013; 44(2):401–406

[56] Chan YL, Leung SF, King AD, Choi PH, Metreweli C. Late radiation injury to the temporal lobes: morphologic evaluation at MR imaging. Radiology. 1999; 213 (3):800–807

[57] Dassarath M, Yin Z, Chen J, Liu H, Yang K, Wu G. Temporal lobe necrosis: a dwindling entity in a patient with nasopharyngeal cancer after radiation therapy. Head Neck Oncol. 2011; 3:8

[58] Chong VF, Rumpel H, Fan YF, Mukherji SK. Temporal lobe changes following radiation therapy: imaging and proton MR spectroscopic findings. Eur Radiol. 2001; 11(2):317–324

[59] Chan YL, Yeung DK, Leung SF, Chan PN. Diffusion-weighted magnetic resonance imaging in radiation-induced cerebral necrosis. Apparent diffusion coefficient in lesion components. J Comput Assist Tomogr. 2003; 27(5):674–680

[60] Asao C, Korogi Y, Kitajima M, et al. Diffusion-weighted imaging of radiation-induced brain injury for differentiation from tumor recurrence. AJNR Am J Neuroradiol. 2005; 26(6):1455–1460

[61] Verma N, Cowperthwaite MC, Burnett MG, Markey MK. Differentiating tumor recurrence from treatment necrosis: a review of neuro-oncologic imaging strategies. Neuro-oncol. 2013; 15(5):515–534

[62] Varoquaux A, Rager O, Dulguerov P, Burkhardt K, Ailianou A, Becker M. Diffusion-weighted and PET/MR imaging after radiation therapy for malignant head and neck tumors. Radiographics. 2015; 35(5):1502–1527

[63] Shah R, Vattoth S, Jacob R, et al. Radiation necrosis in the brain: imaging features and differentiation from tumor recurrence. Radiographics. 2012; 32(5):1343–1359

[64] Friedman DP, Morales RE, Goldman HW. MR imaging findings after stereotactic radiosurgery using the gamma knife. AJR Am J Roentgenol. 2001; 176(6):1589–1595

[65] Dequesada IM, Quisling RG, Yachnis A, Friedman WA. Can standard magnetic resonance imaging reliably distinguish recurrent tumor from radiation necrosis after radiosurgery for brain metastases? A radiographic-pathological study. Neurosurgery. 2008; 63(5):898–903, discussion 904

[66] Flemming KD, Jones LK. Mayo Clinic Neurology Board Review: Clinical Neurology for Initial Certification and MOC. Oxford: Oxford University Press; 2015

[67] Hansen MR, Moffat JC. Osteosarcoma of the skull base after radiation therapy in a patient with McCune-Albright syndrome: case report. Skull Base. 2003; 13(2):79–83

[68] Chabchoub I, Gharbi O, Remadi S, et al. Postirradiation osteosarcoma of the maxilla: a case report and current review of literature. J Oncol. 2009; 2009:876138

[69] Wei-Wei L, Qiu-Liang W, Guo-Hao W, Zhi-Hua C, Zong-Yuan Z. Clinicopathologic features, treatment, and prognosis of postirradiation osteosarcoma in patients with nasopharyngeal cancer. Laryngoscope. 2005; 115(9):1574–1579

[70] Spallone A, Marchione P, DI Capua M, Belvisi D. Radiation-induced anaplastic ependymoma mimicking a skull base meningioma: a case report. Exp Ther Med. 2016; 11(2):455–457

# 7 Neuroendovascular Procedures for Skull Base Neoplasia

*Adam A. Dmytriw and Aditya Bharatha*

## 7.1 Introduction

Neuroendovascular procedures in the setting of skull base neoplasia are typically performed to achieve preoperative tumor embolization. They are also occasionally performed to treat emergent complications arising from tumor pathology or treatment. The primary skull base tumors that most commonly benefit most from angioembolization are meningioma, juvenile angiofibroma, and paraganglioma.[1] However, other hypervascular tumors may also benefit (hemangiopericytoma, chordoma, plasmacytoma, olfactory neuroblastoma, and metastasis especially renal and thyroid carcinoma). The goal of tumor embolization is to reduce the tumor vascularity.[2] A variety of embolic agents have been used. The most common agents include temporary or semi-permanent agents like polyvinyl alcohol (PVA) and gelfoam and permanent liquid embolic agents such as n-butyl-cyanoacrylate (NBCA), ethylene vinyl alcohol copolymer (Onyx), and, in certain cases, coils.[3] Following preoperative embolization, it is recommended that surgery be performed within 72 hours of the procedure in order to maximize the effect before collaterals and tumor neoangiogenesis can reperfuse the tumor. The goal of preoperative embolization is to increase the safety of subsequent surgical procedures by limiting intraoperative hemorrhage, reduce the need for blood transfusion, increase visibility in the surgical field, and shorten hospitalization length.

Embolization sessions typically begin with angiography to document the tumor supply and assess vascular collaterals. Thereafter, dedicated angiography of the vessel to be embolized is performed to exclude the presence of dangerous anastomoses. Upon discovery of such an anastomosis, the channel can be closed with coils and embolization may then proceed safely, or the pedicle can be abandoned. Once a safe approach has been established, the embolic material of choice is injected under fluoroscopic control. In situations where there is encasement of large arteries like the internal carotid artery (ICA) or vertebral, where inadvertent or deliberate sacrifice may be anticipated, preoperative balloon test occlusions may be performed.

Neuroendovascular embolization is also of utility in the setting of spontaneous hemorrhage from skull base neoplasia (e.g., epistaxis) or posttherapeutic vascular injuries such as carotid blowout/large artery laceration. There is a high morbidity associated with open surgical exploration and vessel coagulation/ligation in these situations. Hence, where feasible, endovascular techniques are now the preferred modality to address such problems.

This chapter will discuss the clinical and radiological issues as they pertain to preoperative embolization of the commonly treated primary skull base tumors (meningioma, juvenile angiofibroma, paraganglioma) and then detail the general neurointerventional procedural protocol which can be applied to other tumors.

## 7.2 Meningioma

Meningiomas are extra-axial tumors that commonly occur as derivatives from arachnoid cell degeneration and dural fibroblasts. Their origin from arachnoid cells leads to their common occurrence intradurally[4]; however, they can also occur at the skull base, or rarely in the neck along the carotid sheath. Meningiomas are generally benign lesions, frequently identified incidentally on autopsy, and possess small likelihood of becoming malignant over time. As the most common benign intracranial neoplasms, they represent about 15% of central nervous system (CNS) neoplasms, with a slight female predominance (2:1), partially attributable to the presence of estrogen and/or progesterone receptors.[5] There is an established genetic correlation with neurofibromatosis (NF) type 2 in which case they may be associated with bilateral acoustic neuromas and schwannomas in an autosomal-dominant pattern of inheritance. They can also be familial and independent of NF-2. Meningiomas generally present in middle-aged patients ranging from ages 25 to 65 years, peaking in incidence at age 45 years. Multiple meningiomas occur far less frequently, in 1 to 2% of cases, predominantly affecting the central form of NF. Meningiomas have been seen up to 25 years after cranial radiation therapy, and these present more aggressively and in greater numbers with higher recurrence.

These typically indolent tumors do not usually invade local structures in the brain, but are able to cause compressive symptoms including vision changes, headaches, seizures, and hormonal deregulation if the pituitary is involved. They may encase and narrow vessels. Malignant meningioma is a rare but aggressive variant, with the capability of invading the brain and producing distant metastasis. Meningiomatosis is a subtype that is multifocal with an atypically early and aggressive presentation. Hemangiopericytomas are another variant with angiomatous characteristics, though current thinking is that they may belong in the solitary fibrous tumor spectrum of disease. En plaque meningiomas have a high incidence in females and are characteristically osteogenic with minimal compressive symptoms.

Meningiomas can occur in many locations including the convexity dura, dural sinus, anterior cranial fossa, parasellar, sphenoid wing, cavernous sinus, and posterior fossa. Intraventricular meningiomas are exceedingly rare, and when present are often located in the lateral ventricles. Orbital meningiomas usually involve the optic nerve sheath and can result in decreasing visual acuity, optic atrophy/paresis, and exophthalmos.

Meningiomas of the central skull base and cavernous sinus deserve special mention as they can be difficult to manage due to the encasement of critical structures such as cranial nerves III, IV, V, VI, the ICA, the sellar contents, and the optic apparatus.

Tumors in this location are often fed not only by external carotid artery (ECA) branches, but also by direct meningeal tributary arteries from the ICA, including the inferolateral trunk and the meningohypophyseal trunk. While the ECA supply can be embolized, embolization of ICA feeders is less safe because direct selection of these small dural feeders is often not possible, and there is risk of reflux of embolic material into the ICA. Occasionally, a balloon may be inflated in the cavernous sinus distal to these branches to redirect particles into the tumor, but the risk-to-benefit ratio of such maneuvers is questionable.

Ischemic complications can occur if there is unintentional migration of embolic material into branches supplying the brain parenchyma or cranial nerves, resulting in neurological deficits. Ischemic necrosis from occlusion of arteries supplying the skin of the face or scalp can also occur. It should be noted that ischemia to cranial nerves and scalp necrosis is probably more common with liquid embolics such as onyx or NBCA, which have the ability to penetrate deeper into the microvasculature, as compared to particles.

A preoperative occlusion test may be performed if there is the anticipated possibility of occlusion or laceration of the ICA during surgery. In patients who pass the test, intentional removal en bloc with either preoperative endovascular or intraoperative surgical sacrifice of the ICA may be preferable to trying to dissect the tumor off the artery. If the preoperative test occlusion fails, a subtotal resection with a cuff of tumor being intentionally left along with the vessel can be done. Alternatively, a vessel sacrifice and bypass type procedure can be contemplated (albeit with higher morbidity).

Postembolization tumor swelling and intratumoral hemorrhage are also known possible complications, due to excessive intralesional ischemic necrosis.[6] The rate of complication from meningioma devascularization has been reported between 2.5 and 6.4%.[7] The complications include excessive ischemic necrosis leading to postoperative hemorrhage, and migratory embolization commonly through arterial anastomosis between dural and nonparenchymal structures, leading to neuroparenchymal or extracranial ischemia.[8] Hemorrhagic complications are usually due to venous obstruction from embolic material or edema, or rupture of frail feeding vessels.

An outline of the expected common feeder vessels for various anatomic locations of meningioma is noted in ▶ Table 7.1.

The benefits of preoperative embolization of meningiomas are heavily contingent on their anatomic location, which in turn influences their vascular supply. The goal of embolization is a reduction in perioperative blood loss. The majority of convexity meningiomas do not require embolization due to their superficial and thereby readily, surgically accessible blood supply (e.g., superficial temporal, occipital, middle meningeal, posterior meningeal arteries).[9] The goals with preoperative embolization of meningiomas overlap with skull base neoplasms in general, including but not limited to reduction of tumor vasculature,

minimizing blood loss, improved surgical field of view, and attenuation of tumor dimensions. PVA particles are usually favored for initial use, starting with smaller 50 to 150 microparticles if there is a low risk of collateral occlusion and necrosis and increasing in size if there is high flow shunting into veins. The embolization of vessels that are inaccessible surgically are especially useful when possible (▶ Fig. 7.1).

A particular concern when managing petrous branches of the middle meningeal artery (MMA) arises due to the anastomoses with the vasa nervosum of the facial nerve (CN VII). Similar concerns arise when embolization is performed in the neuromeningeal trunk of the ascending pharyngeal artery, which supplies the vasa nervosum of lower cranial nerves. It is important to avoid smaller microparticles and liquid embolic agents in these instances. Particles greater than 150 μm are suggested in such pedicles.

Large-scale studies involving embolization of meningiomas reveal complication rates in the range of less than 2%.[8] Brain ischemia (nontarget embolization) is the most feared complication and is rare. The degree of devascularization and therefore surgical benefit endowed by embolization may be dependent on tumor size. Previous studies have shown skull base meningiomas less than 6 cm that underwent embolization had significantly reduced blood loss, while those less than 6 cm showed less significant differences. This may be attributable to the abundant collateral blood supply with larger tumors.[10] However, as skull base meningiomas are often supplied by branches of the ICA and vertebrobasilar system, inability to safely embolize these pedicles may have hindered successful devascularization, and account for the less effective devascularization occurring with larger meningiomas.

In more aggressive or advanced cases where tumor resection is not feasible or would inflict an unjustifiable degree of complications, an aggressive embolization strategy may be appropriate. If a safe vascular pedicle is readily accessible, significant tumor necrosis can be induced by embolization with alcohol or NBCA. Sometimes this can even eliminate the necessity of surgical intervention; however, there is very limited data on the safety or effectiveness of this approach.

Radiofrequency and cryoablative techniques have also shown promise in patients who are either poor surgical candidates or fail surgical attempt at cure and subsequent chemoradiotherapy. Other types of minimally invasive ablative therapies have been entertained such as MR-guided laser ablation, laser interstitial thermal therapy,[11] and chemoembolization. Some of these techniques have been applied to other tumor types as well.[12]

## 7.3 Juvenile Nasopharyngeal Angiofibroma

Juvenile nasopharyngeal angiofibromas (JNAs) are rare benign tumors of the head and neck.[13] They most commonly affect adolescent males aged 7 to 29 years, peaking in incidence at ages 14 to 17 years.[14] Current literature does not indicate an ethnic or geographic predisposition, and cases involving females or older male patients should include a broader differential diagnosis.

JNAs are comprised of irregular blood vessels with distorted architecture set in a fibrous stroma. JNAs are benign but can

**Table 7.1** Meningioma vascular supply by anatomical region

| Meningioma location | Predicted main vascular supply |
|---|---|
| Convexity | Middle meningeal artery (MMA) |
| Parasagittal | MMA |
| Olfactory groove | Internal carotid artery (ICA) dural branches, ophthalmic artery, and ethmoidal branches |
| Tentorium and clivus | Cavernous ICA, MMA, tentorial artery, artery of Davidoff/Schecter |
| Posteromedial posterior fossa | Meningeal branches of occipital artery, ascending pharyngeal artery |
| Lateral posterior fossa | MMA, falcotentorial branches |
| Falcine | Terminal MMA branches, anterior falx artery branches |
| Intraventricular | Choroidal arteries |
| Sphenoid wing and clinoid | MMA |

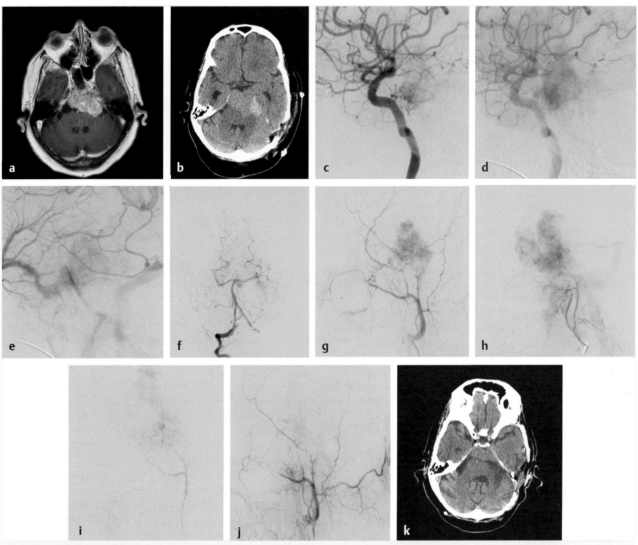

**Fig. 7.1** Preoperative embolization of skull base meningioma. **(a)** Axial T1 postgadolinium shows a large petroclival meningioma involving the left cavernous sinus and Meckel's cave presenting with symptomatic brainstem compression. **(b)** Initial staged resection was performed and the tumor was found to be highly vascular. Postoperative noncontrast computed tomography (CT) shows hemorrhage in the surgical bed with similar tumor bulk. The patient was referred for embolization in advance of further resection. **(c–e)** Early and late arterial and venous phase of a left internal carotid artery (ICA) angiogram shows supply to the tumor from dural (meningohypophyseal and clival) branches of the ICA. Note early arterial blush with late persistence into the venous phase, typical for meningioma (the "in-law sign"... comes early, stays late!). These branches are too small for superselective catheterization. Embolization with particles could be performed with a balloon inflated distally in the cavernous ICA followed by robust aspiration prior to balloon deflation; however, this is not without risk of inadvertent embolization. **(f)** Right vertebral artery injection shows minimal supply to tumor from tiny branches parasitized from the basilar and posterior cerebral artery (PCA; not amenable to embolization). **(g)** Left external carotid artery (ECA) injection shows robust supply to the tumor from the middle meningeal artery (MMA) and distal ECA branches. **(h)** Left ascending pharyngeal arterial injection shows additional robust supply to tumor. **(i)** Superselective microcatheter angiography of a tumor feeder from the ascending pharyngeal artery prior to embolization with polyvinyl alcohol (PVA) particles and gelfoam pledgets. Embolization subsequently performed in the MMA and distal ECA (not shown). **(j)** Final global left ECA run shows marked devascularization of tumor supply from this pedicle. **(k)** Postoperative CT shows significant debulking of tumor.

exhibit locally aggressive behavior. Tumors that have not undergone radiation show exceedingly rare transition into malignancy. Their source of origin remains controversial, but these tumors mostly originate from the posterior nasal cavity, in close proximity to the sphenopalatine foramen. Rather than direct invasion of adjacent bone, gradual remodeling occurs. Typical extension is laterally through the sphenopalatine fossa, pterygomaxillary fossa, and retroantral infratemporal region resulting in the characteristic "antral bowing." As the tumor grows,

local invasion into the oropharynx, nasal cavity, maxillary or ethmoid sinuses, and orbit may occur. Similarly, superior extension into the sphenoid sinus, sella, cavernous sinus, and middle cranial fossa are possible. Orbital extension is typically extraconal and intracranial extension is typically extradural.

Axial and coronal CT images with bone window images will nicely depict the extent to which bone remodeling and erosion is present. Enhanced MRI is helpful in assessing the vascularity and local extension of tumor.[15] JNAs are typically well circumscribed

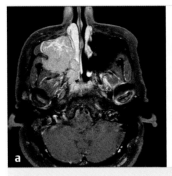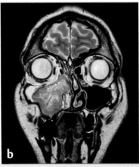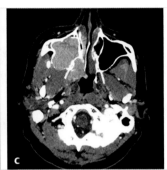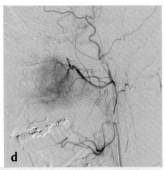

**Fig. 7.2** Malignant sinonasal tumor mimicking juvenile nasopharyngeal angiofibroma (JNA). A 37-year-old male with recurrent epistaxis, **(a)** T1 postgadolinium, **(b)** coronal T2, and **(c)** axial computed tomography angiogram images show a large avidly enhancing mass involving the nasal cavity, nasopharynx, and maxillary antrum with extension into the retroantral space. However, the age and lack of antral bowing are atypical. **(d)** Right external carotid artery injection in preparation for embolization shows much less vascularity than expected for JNA. Embolization was nevertheless performed. Pathological diagnosis was EBV (Epstein-Barr virus) positive plasmablastic lymphoma.

despite the propensity for local extension, avidly enhancing, and may demonstrate vascular flow voids. Angiography commonly illustrates the tumor as a high-flow lesion with dense capillary filling and shunting into prominent veins. At times, malignant sinonasal tumor may mimic a JNA or other benign masses. Careful scrutiny, often involving both CT and MRI, is required for challenging cases. Typically speaking, aggressive lesions possess ill-defined margins, and demonstrate invasion of adjacent tissue and bony destruction, whereas benign masses remodel and expand bone (▶ Fig. 7.2).[16]

Clinically, JNAs will often appear highly vascular and may present with recurrent (classically unilateral) epistaxis. Due to the vascularity of JNA and risk of catastrophic hemorrhage, image-guided biopsy is to be avoided when the diagnosis is entertained.[17] It should be noted that other sinonasal cancers like squamous cell and vascular metastatic disease can simulate the clinical presentation of a JNA through recurrent epistaxis and compressive symptoms.

The blood supply for JNAs typically originates from branches of the internal maxillary artery, namely the sphenopalatine and descending palatine arteries, as well as the ascending pharyngeal arteries and facial arteries. Additional supply can be parasitized from dural branches of the ICA including the meningohypophyseal and inferolateral trunk, and ethmoidal branches off the ophthalmic artery.

Preoperative embolization has the same objective as the other tumors described in this chapter. The goal is reduction of intraoperative bleeding, which may facilitate more comprehensive tumor resection, and shorter recovery. Radiation is another adjunct in circumstances where complete resection is deemed too risky, but has been reported to increase the risk of malignant transformation.

In general, superselective microcatheter embolization of the individual tumor feeders is preferred to arbitrary embolization from a more proximal position even if the latter would encompass all vessels in close proximity to the tumor. In addition to improving the penetration of embolic material into the tumor capillary bed (important for effective embolization), and reducing the chance of inadvertent nontarget embolization through anastomoses, it must be noted that in these tumors, extensive reconstruction of the posterior nasal cavity is frequently required. The superficial temporal and deep temporal arteries

provide important vascular supply to the healing soft tissues and to the temporalis muscle flaps which may be used in the reconstruction. Unnecessary embolization of these branches (which might be acceptable in other embolization procedures such as for idiopathic epistaxis) may predispose the patient to suboptimal wound healing or tissue necrosis especially when liquid embolics are used.

Preoperative embolization can shorten operation time, increase intraoperative visibility, and reduce complication rates. Previous systematic analyses have illustrated this point, by estimating the decrease in endoscopic surgical resection blood loss from greater than 800 to around 400 mL after embolization. A similar effect was seen with open surgery, which showed a reduction from greater than 1,900 to less than 700 mL after preoperative devascularization.[13] Due to extensive collateral supply to these tumors, there can still be significant residual vascularity despite embolization of the safe pedicles.[18] While this may portend more intraoperative bleeding, overaggressive embolization may put the patient at risk of stroke from migration of the embolic agent into the intracranial circulation via the collateral network, and cranial nerve palsies due to unintended occlusion of the vasa nervorum with embolic material.[8] This must be weighed against the adjunctive nature of the embolization procedure.

▶ Fig. 7.3 depicts the pre- and postembolization appearance of a JNA involving the left nasal cavity and masticator space prior to surgical resection. Embolization of PVA particles and gelfoam into the left distal internal maxillary artery resulted in a marked reduction in tumor vascularity.

Where satisfactory transarterial embolization is not feasible for technical reasons, direct puncture techniques followed by injection of liquid agents like NBCA and Onyx have been reported. Ultrasound or CT guidance can be used for more accurate placement of the needle within the tumor while avoiding critical structures.[19] The injection is then performed under fluoroscopic or sometimes CT control.

## 7.4 Paraganglioma

Paraganglioma (PGL), also known as glomus tumor, chemodectoma, and nonchromaffin PGL, originate from neural crest tissue and secrete vasoactive substances including catecholamines

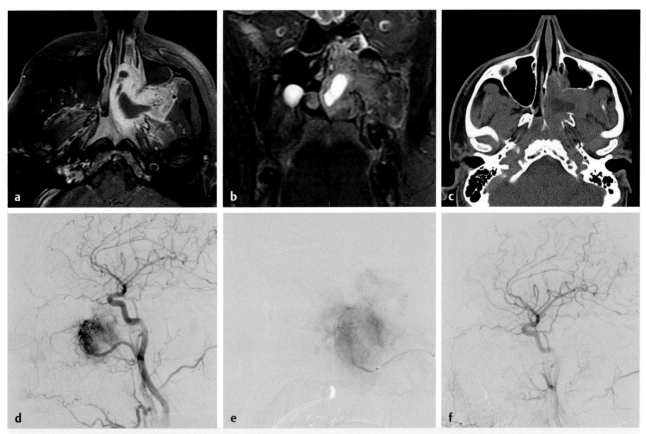

**Fig. 7.3** Embolization of juvenile nasopharyngeal angiofibroma. An 18-year-old man with recurrent epistaxis. Axial T1 **(a)** fat-saturated postgadolinium, **(b)** coronal T2 fat-saturated and **(c)** axial computed tomography images show an avidly enhancing, partially solid and cystic mass centered in the posterior nasal cavity with extension into the nasopharynx and laterally through the widened sphenopalatine foramen into the infratemporal fossa with remodeling of the posterior maxillary wall ("antral bowing"). **(d)** Marked hypervascularity is seen on a left common carotid artery (LCCA) angiogram. **(e)** Microcatheter angiogram in the distal internal maxillary artery prior to embolization with polyvinyl alcohol (PVA) particles and gelfoam pledgets. **(f)** Final LCCA angiogram showing devascularization of tumor. Surgery was uneventful.

and serotonin. They account for 0.6% of all head and neck tumors.[20] Adrenergic symptoms should be investigated with urinary VMA and 5-HIAA to test for catecholamines and serotonin, respectively. In general, they present as tumors within the carotid body (at the carotid bifurcation), the jugulotympanic region, or less frequently as vagal tumors or in other locations such as the orbit, nasal cavity, thyroid gland, and sympathetic trunk.[21] The most common locations for presentation, in decreasing order are carotid, tympanic, jugular, vagal, laryngeal, orbital, and nasopharyngeal. Some group tympanic and jugular as unified entities termed jugulotympanic or temporal paragangliomas.[22] Location is highly correlated with the likelihood of malignant transformation, which has been reported at a range from 2 to 19%.[23] Malignant potential is most easily recalled as occurring in the opposite order from rareness, with nasopharyngeal tumors exhibiting the highest likelihood. Many subtypes show equal distribution between males and females; however, the tympanic, jugular, vagal, and nasopharyngeal tumors are more common in females. PGLs have also been associated with other tumors of the amine precursor uptake and decarboxylation (APUD) system such as pituitary adenomas, thyroid carcinomas, and pheochromocytomas. These tumors are typically inherited in an autosomal-dominant fashion with variable expression. Approximately 30% of cases are multicen-

tric diseases, predominantly involving two (84%), followed by three (13%), and four (2%) tumors. Those that have secretory actions and are multicentric have been more closely correlated with a likelihood of malignancy.

Tympanic paragangliomas often present with pulsatile tinnitus. Conductive hearing loss, bleeding, facial nerve (CN VII) palsy, and discoloration of the tympanic membrane are also common presentations. Unchallenged growth into the mastoid may present as retroauricular discomfort.[24]

Jugular variants may present early on with isolated tongue spasms related to CN IX, and accompanying hypoglossal neuralgia with or without intermittent tinnitus.[8] Later presentation includes paralysis affecting CNs IX, X, and XI causing hoarseness, soft palate deviation, dysphagia, and weakness of the trapezius as well as sternocleidomastoid muscle (Vernet's syndrome). With continuous growth, cranial nerves VII and XII may become involved, resulting in paralysis of the ipsilateral facial muscles and tongue, in addition to loss of taste on the anterior two-thirds of the tongue. Progression into the tympanic cavity can present with symptoms that overlap with tympanic paragangliomas. They can also grow causing compression of the internal jugular vein, although this is generally asymptomatic. PGLs in the jugulotympanic region are the second most common head and neck paragangliomas, second to carotid subtypes.[25]

Carotid body tumors present as palpable pulsatile masses that may grow to involve the oral cavity, larynx, or parapharyngeal space. Symptoms range from pain, dysphagia, hoarseness, CN XII deficit, Horner's syndrome, and syncope. Carotid body tumors represent the most common location for head and neck paragangliomas estimated to represent at least 60% of all lesions.[20]

Vagal paragangliomas often present as cervical or pharyngeal masses, impacting cranial nerves in approximately 30% of patients. The nerves commonly compressed in decreasing sequence include CNs X, XII, IX, and XI, and symptoms occur rapidly in the intravagal subtype, which are located at or below the ganglion nodosa.[22] Later presentation of symptoms suggests an extravagal subtype that is extending intracranially or to the skull base, which by definition arises from the other surrounding paraganglia.[26]

On CT or MR images, paragangliomas are usually seen as an avidly enhancing mass along the carotid sheath, displacing adjacent structures. The carotid body tumor is centered at the carotid bifurcation. Jugulotympanic lesions are situated higher up and involve the jugular foramen and commonly cause a permeative widening or erosion of foramen and adjacent bone. They also extend into the middle ear cavity. MR classically shows a "salt and pepper" appearance on T1, referring to the appearance of blood products situated adjacent to flow voids on T1-weighted images.[27]

Diagnosis is usually made in correlation with serum/urine catecholamines or metanephrines. If there is still doubt, such as in an asymptomatic patient or one on anticholinergic medication (e.g., tricyclic antidepressants), an MIBG (metaiodobenzylguanidine) or octreotide scan may be considered. Percutaneous biopsy should be avoided where the diagnosis is entertained due to the risk of bleeding. Digital subtraction angiography is used to elucidate the vascular supply of the tumor, for embolization and surgical planning. A vascular tumor blush is invariably seen, with the most common prominent feeder being the ascending pharyngeal artery; however, there is often supply from multiple additional ECA branches and occasionally ICA or vertebral artery supply. Image-guided biopsy is contraindicated, and may precipitate catecholamine crisis.

There is some debate as to whether intravenous contrast medium itself can cause catecholamine crisis, though this has been difficult to reliably delineate. During angioembolization procedures, anesthesia support and availability of appropriate medications for hemodynamic support and alpha blockade are recommended.

Preoperative embolization of hypervascular tumors involves either direct intratumoral injection with polymerizing agent or superselective catheterization of the feeding branches with transarterial embolization (▶ Fig. 7.4). The dominant feeder is usually the ascending pharyngeal. The neuromeningeal branch of

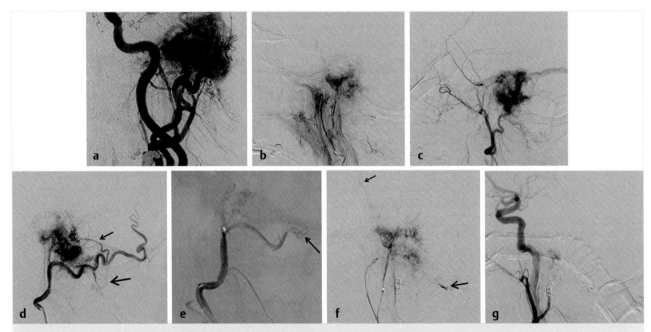

**Fig. 7.4** Embolization of glomus jugulare. Depiction of dangerous anastomoses during embolization of glomus jugulare tumor. **(a)** Left common carotid artery (LCCA) injection shows a hypervascular skull base tumor. **(b)** Ascending pharyngeal supply. **(c)** Posterior auricular supply. **(d)** Occipital artery supply. *Large arrow* shows C1 occipital–vertebral anastomosis. Proximal embolization would be of high risk. Therefore, polyvinyl alcohol embolization was performed with the microcatheter placed distally within the small branch labeled by the *small arrow*. **(e)** Then the occipital artery was coil occluded (*arrow*) proximal to the takeoff of the occipital–vertebral anastomosis. Now further particle embolization can be safely performed without risk of particles embolizing into the vertebral artery. The parent occipital artery was then closed with coils (not shown) on the way out to occlude the remaining small feeders from below. **(f)** The posterior auricular supply was embolized uneventfully (not shown). Next the ascending pharyngeal artery was selected with a microcatheter. After partial embolization with 150-μm particles, the operator decided to do a run. Anastomoses to the internal carotid artery (*small arrow*) and vertebral artery (*large arrow*) were now visible with flash filling. The embolization procedure was terminated at this point. The importance of periodic angiography to look for the appearance of dangerous anastomoses during embolization of high-risk pedicles cannot be overemphasized. Looking back, they are faintly visible on the original angiogram **(b)**, but became more apparent as the embolization progressed and competitive flow into other vessels was reduced. Further or aggressive injection of particles in this pedicle would be high risk for ischemic complication. **(g)** Final CCA angiogram showed satisfactory devascularization with some residual filling mainly from the partially embolized ascending pharyngeal pedicle. The patient awoke with no new neurological deficit.

the ascending pharyngeal artery supplies CNs IX to XII; hence, it is strongly preferred to use larger particles (at least > 150 µm) rather than small particles or liquid embolics when embolizing in this pedicle.

For circumstances where there are small tributary vessels that arise from the internal carotid or vertebral arteries which cannot be directly accessed for catheterization, direct intratumor injection and embolization may be preferred.[20] Percutaneous tumor ablation with ethylene vinyl alcohol copolymer (onyx) has been successful in small series, but remains to be compared with traditional methods.[3,28]

# 7.5 Technical Aspects of Neuroendovascular Therapy for Skull Base Tumors

## 7.5.1 Preembolization Imaging

It is very common for patients with skull base tumors being evaluated for possible surgery and/or embolization to undergo both CT and MRI. CT provides optimal delineation of bone anatomy and when combined with CT angiography (CTA) can delineate the vascular anatomy and any potential vascular access challenges (tortuosity, stenosis) preoperatively. CTA is very useful for judging the amount of arterial phase enhancement which typically correlates very well with angiography. MRI provides superior soft-tissue definition and better depicts local extension of the tumor. In follow-up, MRI can delineate areas of tumor necrosis. It is also more sensitive for imaging of complications such as tumor swelling, mass effect, and intracranial complications of embolization such as ischemic stroke.

## 7.5.2 Decision to Perform Embolization

Tumor hypervascularity by itself does necessitate embolization. If the tumor is small, the major blood supplies are superficial or easily accessible, and if the anticipated blood loss is manageable and expected to be well tolerated, then embolization may not be necessary. Conversely, if significant bleeding is anticipated without embolization that may jeopardize prognosis or survival, or if the tumor is a larger tumor situated in a precarious anatomic location surrounded by critical neurovascular structures, and supplied with numerous deep, surgically inaccessible tributaries, then embolization should be performed.

The decision to perform preoperative embolization must include consideration of the benefits outlined previously in this chapter weighed against the risks. The most significant risk is that of stroke due to thromboembolic complication. This can result in temporary or permanent neurological deficit, vision loss, or even death. Other important risks are cranial nerve injury, tissue necrosis, access vessel injury (dissection, pseudoaneurysm, and groin hematoma), infection, allergic reaction, anesthetic reaction, and treatment failure (unsuccessful embolization or significant bleeding despite embolization).

The following criteria should be contemplated before a decision is made[7]:

- Lesion size, location, vascularity, edema.
- Surgical accessibility of arterial feeders.
- Endovascular accessibility of arterial feeders.
- Proximity of important vessels at risk during embolization.
- Dangerous vascular collaterals and anastomoses.
- Flow dynamics within lesions.
- Atherosclerosis and vessel tortuosity.
- General medical condition, anesthetic risk.
- Open surgical plan and associated risk.
- Patient preference.

## 7.5.3 Procedural Details of Embolization

Transfemoral access is typically used although radial or brachial approaches are also acceptable.

Initial diagnostic angiography of the internal and external carotid arteries and vertebral arteries is typically performed but can be individualized based on the location of the tumor. Assessment of venous invasion by catheter angiography was historically important, but now MR venography and CT venography provide superior depiction of tumor invasion of the dural sinuses or the jugular bulbs.[7,8]

Once a decision is made to proceed with transarterial embolization, the patient is usually put to sleep. Unless there is an easily accessible single target for embolization, and a highly cooperative patient, general anesthesia is recommended for patient safety and comfort and to ensure adequate depiction of vascular anatomy free of motion degradation.

The patient should be heparinized to an ACT of 250 to 350 to reduce the risk of thromboembolic complication from the presence of an indwelling guide catheter. The diagnostic catheter is replaced by a guiding catheter through which a microcatheter is advanced for selection of the tumor feeders. Microcatheters of .021 or larger are recommended for particle or gelfoam pledget embolization to prevent catheter clogging (smaller catheters can be used with liquid embolics). Each branch supplying the tumor is carefully catheterized and a microcatheter angiogram is performed to confirm tumor supply and to ensure no filing of dangerous anastomoses to the intracranial circulation. It is desirable to navigate past nontumor branches to minimize nontarget embolization in the soft tissues. Once a satisfactory position is achieved, injection of embolic material (e.g., most commonly PVA particles mixed with contrast, embolic microspheres are also used by some operators) is performed under fluoroscopic control looking for reflux or nontarget embolization. A "blank" subtracted roadmap image is commonly used to improve visibility. Once persistent reflux is seen, the injection is terminated. If a dangerous anastomosis is encountered, it may be possible to navigate distal or occlude the connecting channel with coils and then proceed with embolization. If not, injection into the pedicle is terminated.

The goal is to achieve distal embolization into the microvasculature of the tumor, as this provides the most effective devascularization. As a general guiding principle, smaller particles (e.g., < 150 μm PVA) permit more successful penetration and result in longer and more extensive devascularization. This induces central necrosis and softening of the tumor for removal, a phenomenon which can be visualized on contrast-enhanced MRI. This trade-off occurs at the cost of a greater risk of tissue necrosis, migration into collateral channels, and injury to the vasa nervorum in certain pedicles. Vice versa, larger particles (150–500 μm) are often associated with reduced tissue necrosis and reduced neuropathy from damage to the vasa nervorum, at the expense of reduced target embolization. Intermediate size particles (150–350 μm) often provide the satisfactory penetration into the tumor while being of a size considered unlikely to embolize into the small angiographically occult dangerous anastomoses or vasa nervorum. Large particles are recommended in situations involving arteriovenous shunting in order to reduce pulmonary embolization. Gelfoam pledgets may be used at the end of the embolization to temporarily occlude the parent feeder. Coils are occasionally used to close off channels to unwanted vessels or anastomoses as noted earlier, but are not ideal for tumor embolization as they produce a proximal ligation, which is typically ineffective.

An alternative to particles is to use liquid embolics like NBCA and Onyx. NBCA can be mixed with lipiodol to produce different viscosities individualized to the tumor angioarchitecture. Tantalum is added to improve visibility at higher glue concentrations. Use of liquid embolics results in a greater degree of vessel occlusion than PVA or microspheres. However, these agents will irreversibly close the parent artery during injection. Therefore, if early reflux occurs there may be minimal tumor penetration. They are also small enough to embolize into angiographically imperceptible anastomotic channels and hence are associated with greater risk of nontarget embolic complications, cranial nerve injury, and tissue necrosis compared to particles.

There is an important balance between aggressive management with preoperative embolization in order to obtain as close to complete devascularization as possible and simultaneously minimizing the likelihood of complications. When the focus is on complication avoidance, the following guiding principles should govern the approach of the interventionalist:

- Microcatheter angiography should be performed prior to commencing embolization and periodically during embolization to identify vascular anomalies or anastomoses, or normal collateral branches that may be visible at the outset or which may only appear during the embolization once flow into the larger feeders has been occluded (▶ Fig. 7.4).[29]
- *Example*: When considering devascularization of the MMA, pretherapeutic angiography of the ICA is mandatory to document ophthalmic artery anatomy and choroidal blush and identify anatomic variant origins. Prior to and during embolization, magnified runs are performed to look for meningolacrimal arterial connection to the ophthalmic artery that may threaten vision.
- *Example*: Before injecting into the occipital artery, both occipital and vertebral runs should be interrogated for flash filling of the occipital–vertebral anastomoses and even when not seen, they should be assumed to be present even if not visualized and steps should be taken to mitigate risk.

- The interventionalist should be familiar with the vasa nervorum and arteries supplying cranial nerves (most importantly petrosal branch of MMA; stylomastoid branch of posterior auricular or occipital; ascending pharyngeal; accessory meningeal), and recognize that smaller particulate or liquid embolic agents in these pedicles may cause cranial nerve palsy.[29]
- The microcatheter must be securely positioned so the force of injection during occlusion will not dislodge the catheter and result in nontarget embolization. This should be tested with variable force injections of contrast prior to injection of embolic material. Resultant dislodging or reflux of embolic material can lead to inadvertent embolization of critical vessels.
- A modern biplane DSA angiography unit is strongly preferred for visibility and safety.

## 7.5.4 Direct Percutaneous Puncture

Direct percutaneous image-guided access can be used to biopsy tumors where a pathological diagnosis is preferred prior to definitive treatment, or can be used as an alternative access to the tumor for injection of embolic material. Most often performed with 16- to 20-gauge needles, CT, US, or fluoroscopy-guided angiography may be used to direct needle placement and avoid vital structures. Liquid agents such as NBCA, Onyx, or alcohol can be employed for intralesional ablation. The risks for these procedures are similar to those of transarterial embolization. During the injection, it is critical to ensure that there is no unintended extratumoral intravascular embolization via intratumoral vessels or leakage into paratumoral tissues. Hemorrhage along the tract can rarely occur, and thus transfusion products should be available. PGLs in particular appear to respond well to a direct puncture and injection of a liquid polymerizing agent.[30] PGLs that are limited to the neck without involvement of the skull base are embolized via a percutaneous lateral cervical approach.[30] Those involving the skull base and posterior fossa are managed with a retropetrosal approach, most commonly through the jugular foramen. Careful monitoring (anesthesiologist) and premedication with an alpha-blockading agent should be considered prior to intervention.

## 7.5.5 Follow-Up and Monitoring

After transarterial embolization, the groin access site is typically closed with direct compression following reversal of heparin with protamine or using a closure device. The patient should be carefully examined after extubation with a neurological exam to assess for ischemic complications and cranial nerve injury. In many centers, patients are admitted to an intensive care unit (ICU) or step-down unit for observation for 24 to 48 hours post embolization or in the interval before surgery. Localized pain and fever are commonly noted.[31] Analgesics will often be required. Corticosteroids (e.g., dexamethasone) may be prescribed to mitigate postembolization tumor swelling. Surgery should ideally be performed within 72 hours of the preoperative embolization procedure. Postprocedural imaging is generally geared toward following the treated lesion.

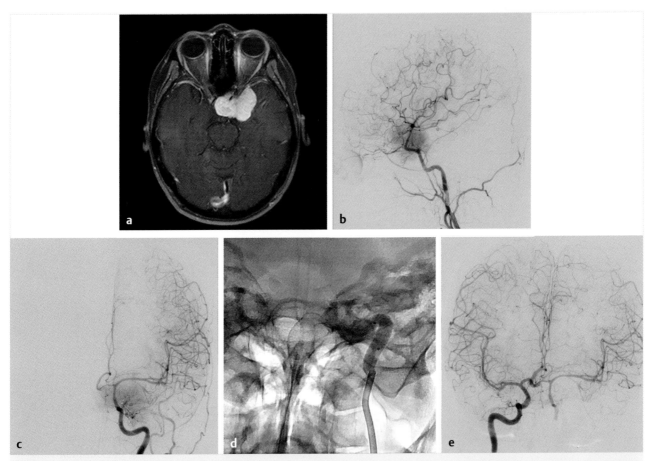

**Fig. 7.5** Left internal carotid artery (ICA) test occlusion. **(a)** Axial T1 fat-saturated postgadolinium image shows a large left paraclinoid meningioma encasing and mildly narrowing the ICA flow void. **(b,c)** Left ICA angiogram shows narrowing of paraclinoid ICA, elevation of the M1 and A1 vessels, and tumor blush. **(d,e)** Contralateral right ICA injection with balloon inflated in the left ICA shows robust cross-flow across the anterior communicating artery with nearly symmetric venous phase (not shown) and no clinical deterioration. This is a clinical and angiographic pass.

## 7.6 Balloon Test Occlusion and Management of Iatrogenic Vessel Injury

Balloon test occlusion (BTO) is an important diagnostic tool in patients with skull base tumors that are in close proximity to, or encase, the carotid or vertebral arteries. The procedure is performed with the patient awake. Bilateral groin access is obtained. Under systemic heparinization, a temporary occlusion balloon is navigated through a guide catheter into the vessel being studied and inflated distal to the point of proposed sacrifice. This will simulate as closely as possible the level of the planned occlusion. Through the other groin, diagnostic angiography of the remaining cervical vessels is performed to assess the angiographic collaterals (▶ Fig. 7.5). The patient is assessed clinically for signs of ischemia in the territory being tested. If there are signs of clinical ischemia, the balloon is deflated and the procedure terminated (test fail). Some groups administer adjunctive testing such as hypotensive challenge, perfusion imaging with a first pass nuclear medicine perfusion tracer (e.g., Tc-99 m ethyl cysteinate dimer [Tc-99 m ECD]) for subsequent brain single-photon emission computed tomography (SPECT) perfusion imaging, or Xenon-enhanced computed tomography (XE-CT) or computer tomographic perfusion with the balloon inflated. After 30 minutes, the balloon is deflated. Patients who pass on clinical, angiographic with or without adjunctive test criteria are thought to have a low risk of infarction following vessel sacrifice (< 5%). However, recent reports have suggested there may be a higher rate of immediate or

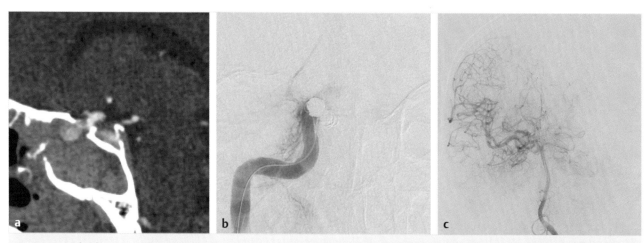

**Fig. 7.6** Carotid siphon injury following transsphenoidal surgery. The patient presented with massive hemorrhage during attempted transsphenoidal resection of a pituitary adenoma. The sinonasal cavity was packed and patient sent for a computed tomography (CT) angiogram while actively bleeding. **(a)** Sagittal CT shows laceration of the carotid anterior genu with pseudoaneurysm formation within the blood-filled sphenoid antrum. **(b)** Endovascular treatment with occlusion of the aneurysm and sacrifice of the parent internal carotid artery (ICA) following angiographically passed balloon test occlusion (not shown). **(c)** The right middle cerebral artery territory perfused through the vertebral circulation via the posterior communicating artery and right anterior cerebral artery filling through the left ICA via the anterior communicating artery. No further hemorrhage when packing removed. Uneventful clinical recovery.

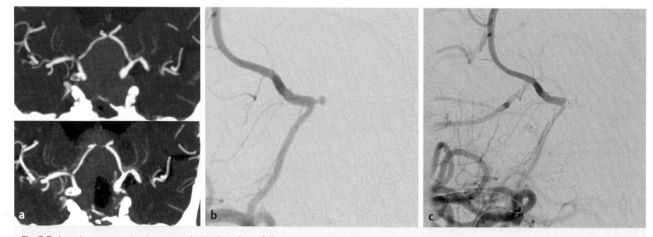

**Fig. 7.7** Anterior communicating artery (ACOM) avulsion following transsphenoidal surgery. **(a)** Preoperative (*top*) and postoperative (*bottom*) computed tomography angiogram following transsphenoidal debulking of pituitary adenoma complicated by postoperative subarachnoid hemorrhage. Splaying of the ACOM is seen (presumed avulsive injury). **(b)** Right internal carotid artery injection confirms pseudoaneurysm. **(c)** Successful endovascular repair with coiling.

delayed ipsilateral stroke than previously thought (in the range of 10–15%.[32]) There is a small risk of complication including stroke from the BTO itself, in the range of 2 to 4%.[33]

Large artery vascular injury is an uncommon complication following skull base surgery. Management options include BTO followed by vessel sacrifice (▶ Fig. 7.6), surgical repair or bypass, and reconstructive endovascular approaches using coils (▶ Fig. 7.7), stent-supported coiling, and flow diverting stents.[32,34,35]

## 7.7 Summary

Neurointerventional procedures can play an important role in the management of skull base neoplasms. The spectrum of procedures performed includes transarterial and percutaneous tumor embolization, biopsy, preoperative artery test occlusion and sacrifice, and endovascular management of hemorrhagic and vascular complications related to the tumor and tumor therapy.

# References

[1] Sekhar LN, Biswas A, Hallam D, Kim LJ, Douglas J, Ghodke B. Neuroendovascular management of tumors and vascular malformations of the head and neck. Neurosurg Clin N Am. 2009; 20(4):453–485

[2] Dmytriw AA, Ter Brugge KG, Krings T, Agid R. Endovascular treatment of head and neck arteriovenous malformations. Neuroradiology. 2014; 56(3): 227–236

[3] Quadros RS, Gallas S, Delcourt C, Dehoux E, Scherperel B, Pierot L. Preoperative embolization of a cervicodorsal paraganglioma by direct percutaneous injection of onyx and endovascular delivery of particles. AJNR Am J Neuroradiol. 2006; 27(9):1907–1909

[4] Nagashima G, Fujimoto T, Suzuki R, Asai J, Itokawa H, Noda M. Dural invasion of meningioma: a histological and immunohistochemical study. Brain Tumor Pathol. 2006; 23(1):13–17

[5] Iplikcioglu AC, Hatiboglu MA, Ozek E, Ozcan D. Is progesteron receptor status really a prognostic factor for intracranial meningiomas? Clin Neurol Neurosurg. 2014; 124:119–122

[6] Hishikawa T, Sugiu K, Hiramatsu M, et al. Nationwide survey of the nature and risk factors of complications in embolization of meningiomas and other intracranial tumors: Japanese Registry of NeuroEndovascular Therapy 2 (JR-NET2). Neuroradiology. 2014; 56(2):139–144

[7] Morris P. Interventional and Endovascular Therapy of the Nervous System: A Practical Guide. New York, NY: Springer; 2001

[8] Connors JJ, Wojak JC. Interventional Neuroradiology: Strategies and Practical Techniques. Philadelphia, PA: Saunders; 1999

[9] James RF, Kramer DR, Page PS, Gaughen JR, Jr, Martin LB, Mack WJ. Strategic and technical considerations for the endovascular embolization of intracranial meningiomas. Neurosurg Clin N Am. 2016; 27(2):155–166

[10] Oka H, Kurata A, Kawano N, et al. Preoperative superselective embolization of skull-base meningiomas: indications and limitations. J Neurooncol. 1998; 40 (1):67–71

[11] Passacantilli E, Antonelli M, D'Amico A, et al. Neurosurgical applications of the 2-μm thulium laser: histological evaluation of meningiomas in comparison to bipolar forceps and an ultrasonic aspirator. Photomed Laser Surg. 2012; 30(5):286–292

[12] Owen RP, Ravikumar TS, Silver CE, Beitler J, Wadler S, Bello J. Radiofrequency ablation of head and neck tumors: dramatic results from application of a new technology. Head Neck. 2002; 24(8):754–758

[13] Boghani Z, Husain Q, Kanumuri VV, et al. Juvenile nasopharyngeal angiofibroma: a systematic review and comparison of endoscopic, endoscopic-assisted, and open resection in 1047 cases. Laryngoscope. 2013; 123(4):859–869

[14] Pellitteri PK, McCaffrey TV. Endocrine Surgery of the Head and Neck. Clifton Park, NY: Thomson Delmar Learning; 2003

[15] Gupta S, Gupta S, Ghosh S, Narang P. Juvenile nasopharyngeal angiofibroma: case report with review on role of imaging in diagnosis. Contemp Clin Dent. 2015; 6(1):98–102

[16] Eggesbø HB. Imaging of sinonasal tumours. Cancer Imaging. 2012; 12:136–152

[17] Lutz J, Holtmannspötter M, Flatz W, et al. Preoperative embolization to improve the surgical management and outcome of juvenile nasopharyngeal

[18] angiofibroma (JNA) in a single center: 10-year experience. Clin Neuroradiol. 2016; 26(4):405–413

[18] Parikh V, Hennemeyer C. Microspheres embolization of juvenile nasopharyngeal angiofibroma in an adult. Int J Surg Case Rep. 2014; 5(12):1203–1206

[19] Hurst RW, Rosenwasser RH. Neurointerventional Management: Diagnosis and Treatment. 2nd ed. Boca Raton, FL: Taylor & Francis; 2012

[20] Moore MG, Netterville JL, Mendenhall WM, Isaacson B, Nussenbaum B. Head and neck paragangliomas: an update on evaluation and management. Otolaryngol Head Neck Surg. 2016; 154(4):597–605

[21] Papaspyrou K, Mann WJ, Amedee RG. Management of head and neck paragangliomas: review of 120 patients. Head Neck. 2009; 31(3):381–387

[22] Berenstein A, Lasjaunias P, Brugge KG. Paragangliomas. Surgical Neuroangiography. Vol 2: Clinical and Endovascular Treatment Aspects in Adults. Berlin, Germany: Springer; 2004:227–264

[23] Burnichon N, Buffet A, Gimenez-Roquuplo AP. Pheochromocytoma and paraganglioma: molecular testing and personalized medicine. Curr Opin Oncol. 2016; 28(1):5–10

[24] Offergeld C, Brase C, Yaremchuk S, et al. Head and neck paragangliomas: clinical and molecular genetic classification. Clinics (Sao Paulo). 2012; 67 Suppl 1:19–28

[25] Karaman E, Yilmaz M, Isildak H, et al. Management of jugular paragangliomas in otolaryngology practice. J Craniofac Surg. 2010; 21(1):117–120

[26] Makeieff M, Thariat J, Reyt E, Righini CA. Treatment of cervical paragangliomas. Eur Ann Otorhinolaryngol Head Neck Dis. 2012; 129(6):308–314

[27] Lee KY, Oh YW, Noh HJ, et al. Extraadrenal paragangliomas of the body: imaging features. AJR Am J Roentgenol. 2006; 187(2):492–504

[28] Martínez-Galdámez M, Saura P, Cenjor C, Pérez Higueras A. Percutaneous onyx embolization of cervical paragangliomas. J Vasc Interv Radiol. 2011; 22 (9):1271–1274

[29] Geibprasert S, Pongpech S, Armstrong D, Krings T. Dangerous extracranial-intracranial anastomoses and supply to the cranial nerves: vessels the neurointerventionalist needs to know. AJNR Am J Neuroradiol. 2009; 30(8):1459–1468

[30] Ozyer U, Harman A, Yildirim E, Aytekin C, Akay TH, Boyvat F. Devascularization of head and neck paragangliomas by direct percutaneous embolization. Cardiovasc Intervent Radiol. 2010; 33(5):967–975

[31] Borg A, Ekanayake J, Mair R, et al. Preoperative particle and glue embolization of meningiomas: indications, results and lessons learned from 117 consecutive patients. Neurosurgery. 2013; 73(2 Suppl Operative):244–251;–discussion, 252

[32] Whisenant JT, Kadkhodayan Y, Cross DT, III, Moran CJ, Derdeyn CP. Incidence and mechanisms of stroke after permanent carotid artery occlusion following temporary occlusion testing. J Neurointerv Surg. 2015; 7(6):395–401

[33] Mathis JM, Barr JD, Jungreis CA, et al. Temporary balloon test occlusion of the internal carotid artery: experience in 500 cases. AJNR Am J Neuroradiol. 1995; 16(4):749–754

[34] Sylvester PT, Moran CJ, Derdeyn CP, et al. Endovascular management of internal carotid artery injuries secondary to endonasal surgery: case series and review of the literature. J Neurosurg. 2016; 125(5):1256–1276

[35] Mathis JM, Barr JD, Horton JA. Therapeutic occlusion of major vessels, test occlusion and techniques. Neurosurg Clin N Am. 1994; 5(3):393–401

# 8 Cross-Sectional Computed Tomography and Magnetic Resonance Imaging Atlas of the Skull Base

*Almudena Perez-Lara, Eugene Yu, and Reza Forghani*

## 8.1 Introduction

Optimal diagnostic evaluation and treatment planning for skull base pathology is contingent on accurate detection and determination of the anatomic extent of the lesion. Cross-sectional imaging techniques such as computed tomography (CT) and magnetic resonance imaging (MRI) enable detailed visualization of the intricate normal anatomy and disease spread at the skull base and play a central role in the diagnostic evaluation and surveillance of patients with skull base pathology. Skull base anatomy is complex consisting of different bones, soft tissues, and air-containing cavities. There are also complex anatomical relationships and potential pathways of disease spread. As a result, familiarity with the detailed anatomy of this area is a prerequisite for optimal diagnostic evaluation, and, frequently, a combination of different techniques such as CT and MRI is required for proper diagnosis and treatment planning.

CT scans have a very high spatial resolution and can be acquired with short scan times. In addition to evaluation of soft tissues, CT enables excellent visualization of fine bone detail and anatomy. With modern high-resolution CT scans, the major skull base foramina and a wide array of anatomic structures and variations can be visualized with a high level of detail and confidence. CT is also the test of choice for visualization and determination of important anatomic variations in the paranasal sinuses that help guide endoscopic sinus surgery and help avoid complications. MRI examinations are longer to acquire than CT scans but have excellent soft-tissue contrast. These scans enable detailed evaluation of skull base anatomy and pathology, and in particular are excellent for characterization of soft-tissue abnormalities, intracranial spread of disease, and spread of disease across different spaces and along the major neural pathways.

The purpose of this atlas is to provide an overview of the imaging anatomy of the skull base on CT and MRI. In preparing this atlas, our hope is to provide both basic and essential information for the less familiar reader as well as more detailed and intricate anatomical information for advanced interpretation in an easily accessible atlas format that can be used as an educational tool or as a reference in clinical practice. In this atlas, CT is mainly used for demonstration of detailed bone anatomy and related important anatomical relationships, whereas MRI is used to demonstrate the normal soft-tissue anatomy in adjacent structures and spaces such as the sella, cavernous sinus, major foramina, and posterior fossa.

## 8.2 Atlas of Osseous Anatomy of the Skull Base

### 8.2.1 Axial Image Set

#### Axial Computed Tomography (No Contrast)

Axial high-resolution CT image(s) without contrast (▶ Fig. 8.1, ▶ Fig. 8.2, ▶ Fig. 8.3, ▶ Fig. 8.4). The skull base and paranasal

sinuses are formed by the fusion of multiple bones, as shown. The anterior skull base can be broadly described as constituting the floor of the anterior cranial fossa and the roof of the nose, ethmoid air cells, and orbits. These anatomic relationships are important and constitute different potential pathways of spread of pathology. Some of the key anatomic structures are constant, but others, such as paranasal sinuses, can have significant variations in their detailed anatomy. In the case of frontal sinuses, there is typically an inter-sinus septum that may be midline or paramedian in location. In addition, there can be intra-sinus septa within the frontal sinuses.

Axial high-resolution CT image(s) without contrast (▶ Fig. 8.5, ▶ Fig. 8.6, ▶ Fig. 8.7, ▶ Fig. 8.8). The skull base and paranasal sinuses are formed by the fusion of multiple bones, as shown. In the region of the anterior skull base, different compartments including the intracranial compartment, orbits, nasal cavity, and paranasal sinuses partly abut one another. These anatomic relationships are important and constitute different potential pathways of spread of pathology. CT is excellent for the evaluation of detailed skull base bone anatomy including major foramina and fissures. In this case, the superior orbital fissure is seen. This fissure or cleft is located between the lesser and greater wings of the sphenoid through which cranial nerves (III, IV, V1, VI) and the superior ophthalmic vein are transmitted to the orbit.

Axial high-resolution CT image(s) without contrast (▶ Fig. 8.9, ▶ Fig. 8.10, ▶ Fig. 8.11, ▶ Fig. 8.12). The skull base and paranasal sinuses are formed by the fusion of multiple bones, as shown. In the region of the anterior skull base, different compartments including the intracranial compartment, orbits, nasal cavity, and paranasal sinuses partly abut one another. These anatomic relationships are important and constitute different potential pathways of spread of pathology. CT is excellent for the evaluation of detailed skull base bone anatomy including major foramina and fissures. The superior orbital fissure is a cleft between the lesser and greater wings of the sphenoid through which cranial nerves (III, IV, V1, VI) and the superior ophthalmic vein traverse into the orbit. The optic nerve and ophthalmic artery pass through the optic canal. Variations such as pneumatization of the anterior clinoid process have an increased association with optic nerve exposure and dehiscence and are considered an indicator of optic nerve vulnerability during endoscopic sinus surgery.

Axial high-resolution CT image(s) without contrast (▶ Fig. 8.13, ▶ Fig. 8.14, ▶ Fig. 8.15, ▶ Fig. 8.16). CT is excellent for the evaluation of detailed skull base bone anatomy including major foramina and fissures. The superior orbital fissure is a cleft between the lesser and greater wings of the sphenoid through which cranial nerves (III, IV, V1, VI) and the superior ophthalmic vein traverse into the orbit. The inferior orbital fissure transmits the zygomatic branch of V2 (maxillary division of trigeminal nerve) and the inferior ophthalmic vein. The inferior orbital fissure is also in continuity with the superior aspect of the pterygopalatine fossa (PPF), an important site of anatomic convergence of multiple neural pathways. Anatomic variations of the paranasal

(*text continued on page 195*)

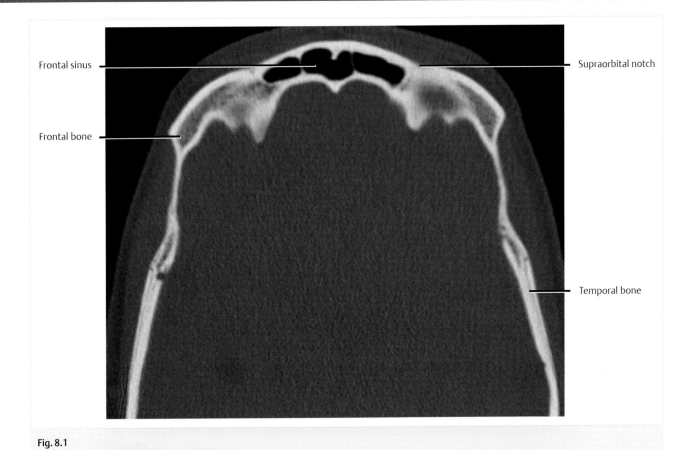

Frontal sinus

Supraorbital notch

Frontal bone

Temporal bone

**Fig. 8.1**

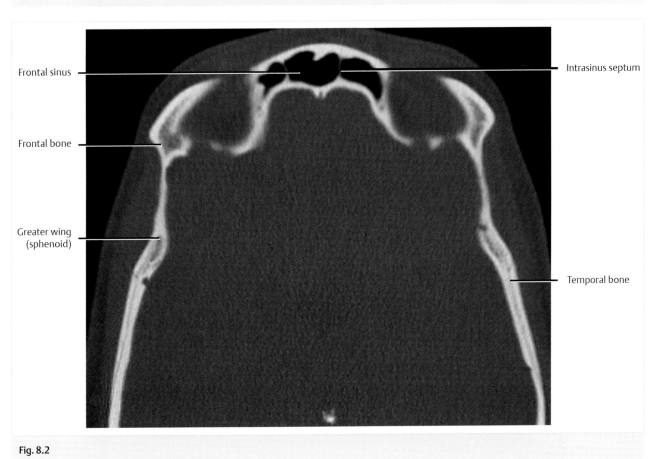

Frontal sinus

Intrasinus septum

Frontal bone

Greater wing
(sphenoid)

Temporal bone

**Fig. 8.2**

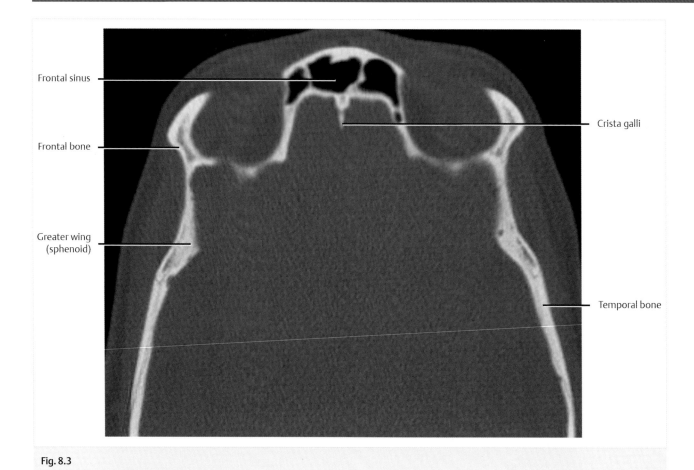

Frontal sinus

Crista galli

Frontal bone

Greater wing
(sphenoid)

Temporal bone

Fig. 8.3

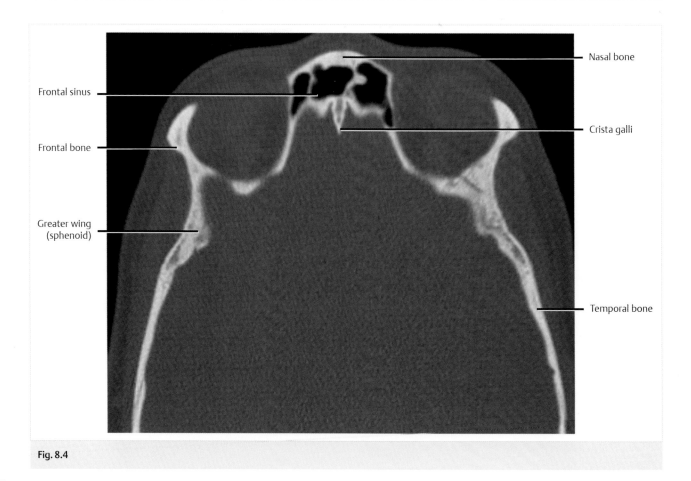

Nasal bone

Frontal sinus

Crista galli

Frontal bone

Greater wing
(sphenoid)

Temporal bone

Fig. 8.4

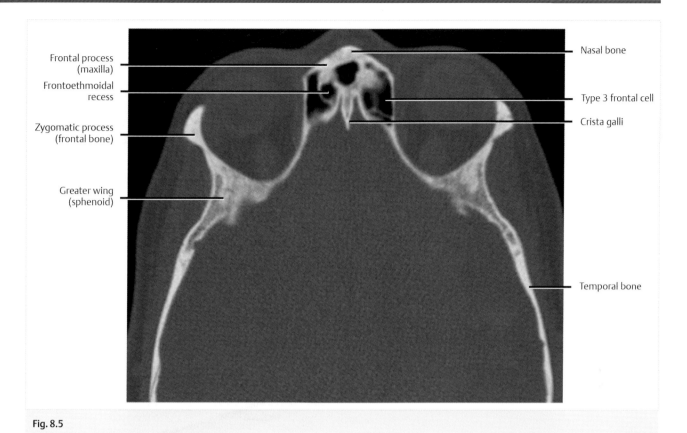

Frontal process (maxilla)

Frontoethmoidal recess

Zygomatic process (frontal bone)

Greater wing (sphenoid)

Nasal bone

Type 3 frontal cell

Crista galli

Temporal bone

Fig. 8.5

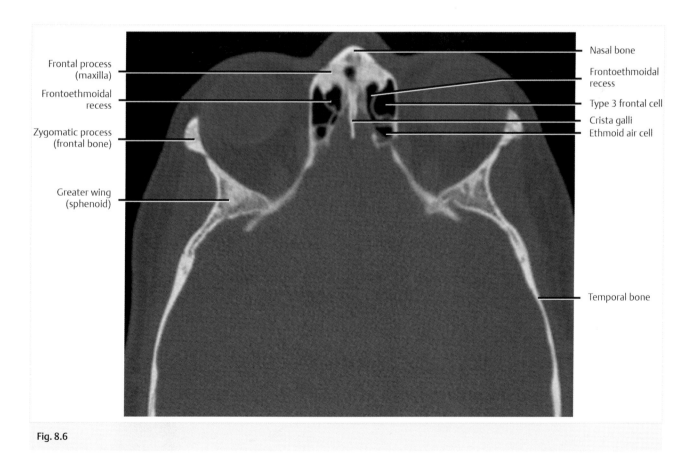

Frontal process (maxilla)

Frontoethmoidal recess

Zygomatic process (frontal bone)

Greater wing (sphenoid)

Nasal bone

Frontoethmoidal recess

Type 3 frontal cell

Crista galli

Ethmoid air cell

Temporal bone

Fig. 8.6

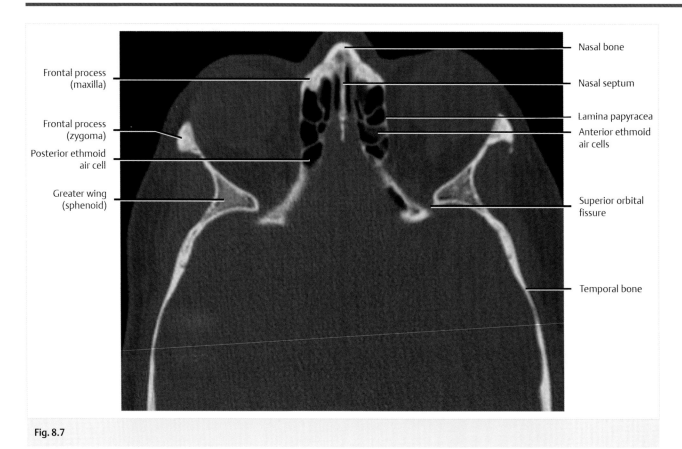

Frontal process (maxilla)

Frontal process (zygoma)

Posterior ethmoid air cell

Greater wing (sphenoid)

Nasal bone

Nasal septum

Lamina papyracea

Anterior ethmoid air cells

Superior orbital fissure

Temporal bone

Fig. 8.7

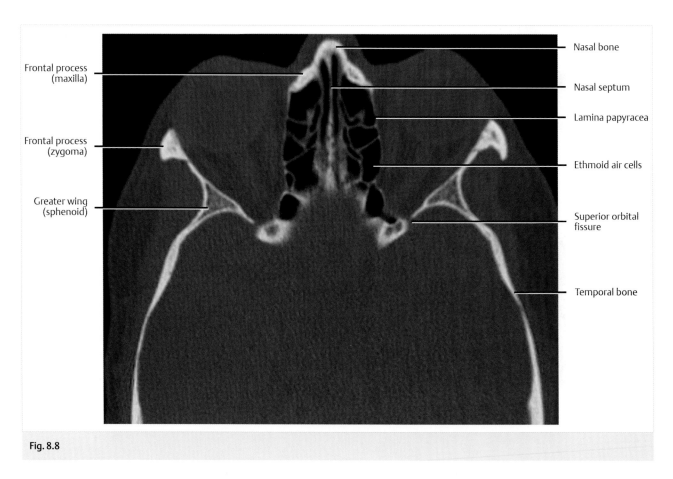

Frontal process (maxilla)

Frontal process (zygoma)

Greater wing (sphenoid)

Nasal bone

Nasal septum

Lamina papyracea

Ethmoid air cells

Superior orbital fissure

Temporal bone

Fig. 8.8

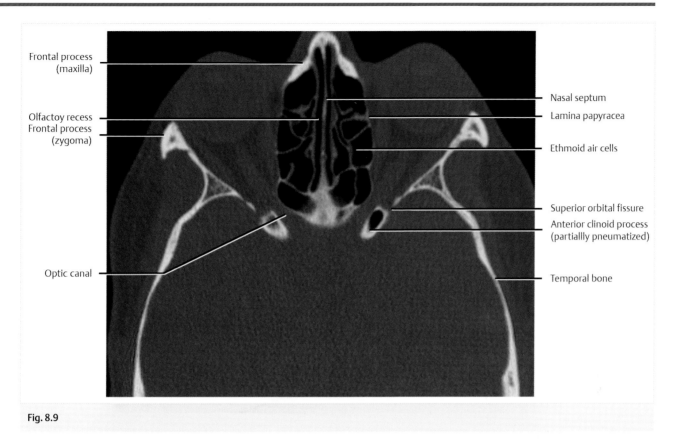

Frontal process (maxilla)

Olfactoy recess
Frontal process (zygoma)

Optic canal

Nasal septum

Lamina papyracea

Ethmoid air cells

Superior orbital fissure
Anterior clinoid process (partiallly pneumatized)

Temporal bone

**Fig. 8.9**

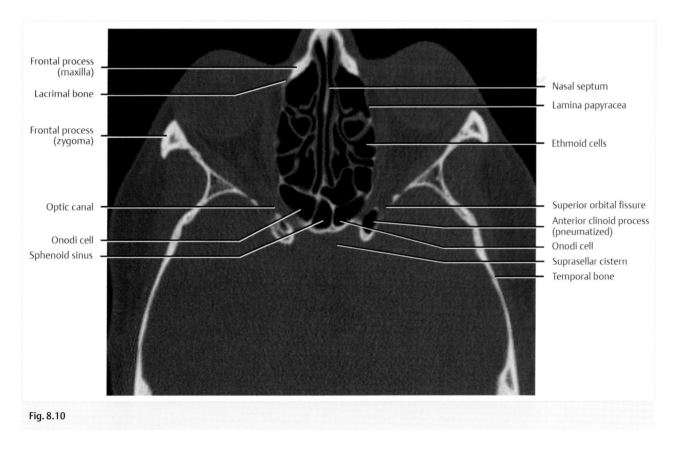

Frontal process (maxilla)

Lacrimal bone

Frontal process (zygoma)

Optic canal

Onodi cell
Sphenoid sinus

Nasal septum

Lamina papyracea

Ethmoid cells

Superior orbital fissure
Anterior clinoid process (pneumatized)

Onodi cell

Suprasellar cistern
Temporal bone

**Fig. 8.10**

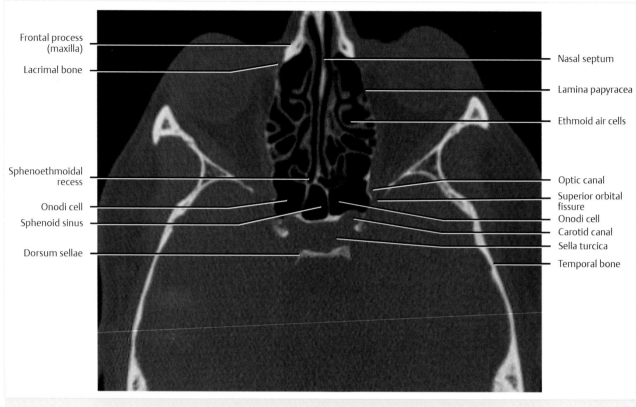

Frontal process (maxilla)
Lacrimal bone
Sphenoethmoidal recess
Onodi cell
Sphenoid sinus
Dorsum sellae

Nasal septum
Lamina papyracea
Ethmoid air cells
Optic canal
Superior orbital fissure
Onodi cell
Carotid canal
Sella turcica
Temporal bone

**Fig. 8.11**

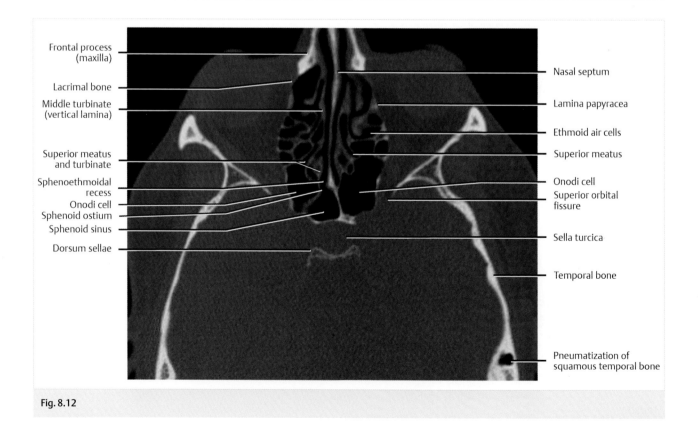

Frontal process (maxilla)
Lacrimal bone
Middle turbinate (vertical lamina)
Superior meatus and turbinate
Sphenoethmoidal recess
Onodi cell
Sphenoid ostium
Sphenoid sinus
Dorsum sellae

Nasal septum
Lamina papyracea
Ethmoid air cells
Superior meatus
Onodi cell
Superior orbital fissure
Sella turcica
Temporal bone
Pneumatization of squamous temporal bone

**Fig. 8.12**

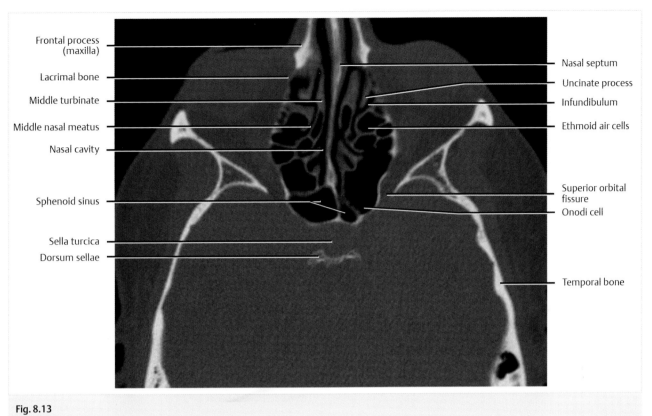

Frontal process (maxilla)
Lacrimal bone
Middle turbinate
Middle nasal meatus
Nasal cavity
Sphenoid sinus
Sella turcica
Dorsum sellae

Nasal septum
Uncinate process
Infundibulum
Ethmoid air cells
Superior orbital fissure
Onodi cell
Temporal bone

Fig. 8.13

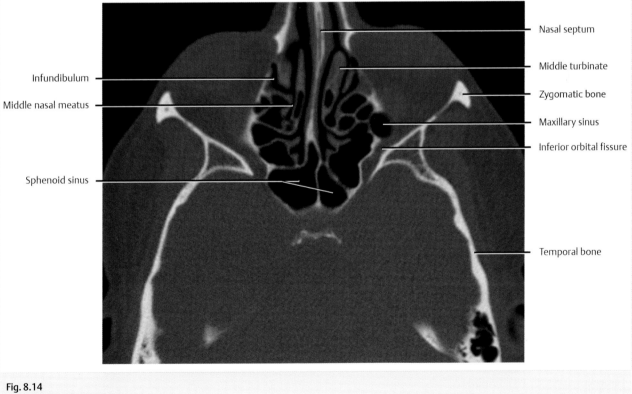

Infundibulum
Middle nasal meatus
Sphenoid sinus

Nasal septum
Middle turbinate
Zygomatic bone
Maxillary sinus
Inferior orbital fissure
Temporal bone

Fig. 8.14

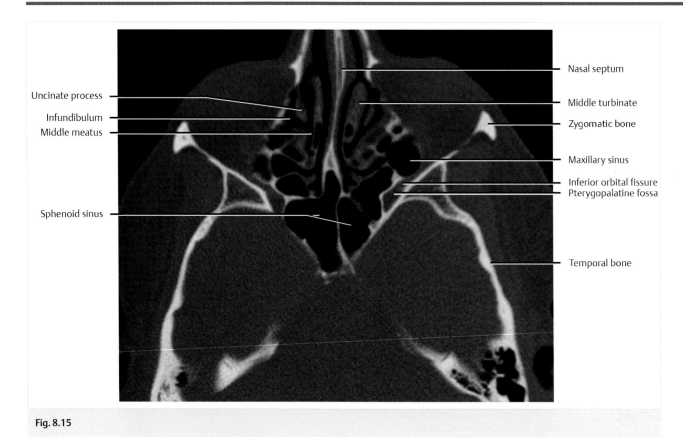

Uncinate process

Infundibulum

Middle meatus

Sphenoid sinus

Nasal septum

Middle turbinate

Zygomatic bone

Maxillary sinus

Inferior orbital fissure
Pterygopalatine fossa

Temporal bone

Fig. 8.15

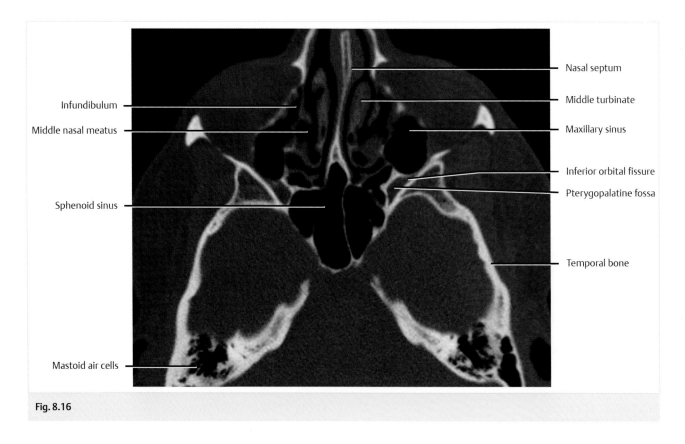

Infundibulum

Middle nasal meatus

Sphenoid sinus

Mastoid air cells

Nasal septum

Middle turbinate

Maxillary sinus

Inferior orbital fissure

Pterygopalatine fossa

Temporal bone

Fig. 8.16

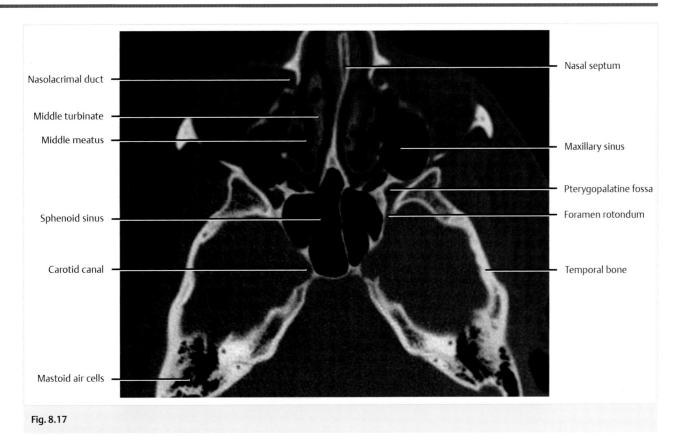

Nasolacrimal duct

Middle turbinate

Middle meatus

Sphenoid sinus

Carotid canal

Mastoid air cells

Nasal septum

Maxillary sinus

Pterygopalatine fossa

Foramen rotondum

Temporal bone

**Fig. 8.17**

sinuses such as Onodi cells (well seen on coronal reformats) are important to recognize because there is potential for misidentification during endoscopic surgery that would put closely related critical structures, in particular the optic nerves, at risk for inadvertent surgical injury.

Axial high-resolution CT image(s) without contrast (▶ Fig. 8.17, ▶ Fig. 8.18, ▶ Fig. 8.19, ▶ Fig. 8.20). CT is excellent for the evaluation of detailed skull base bone anatomy including major foramina and fissures. The PPF is an important elongated, vertically oriented, predominantly fat-filled region located lateral to the posterior aspect of the nasal cavity that has an important relationship to the skull base and paranasal sinuses. The PPF is an important site of anatomic convergence of multiple neural pathways, and familiarity with this area is critical, particularly for evaluation of tumors where there is potential for perineural spread of tumor affecting treatment planning and management. At the lateral boundary of the PPF, there is an opening referred to as the pterygomaxillary fissure, an elongated vertical communication with the infratemporal fossa. The superior aspect of PPF is in continuity with the inferior orbital fissure and inferiorly, the PPF tapers into the greater palatine canal ultimately leading to the greater and lesser palatine foramina. Medially, the sphenopalatine foramen opens just posterior to the superior or middle meatus where the foramen is covered by mucosa. Posteriorly, the foramen rotundum communicates with the middle cranial fossa, transmitting the maxillary (V2) branch of the trigeminal nerve, artery of foramen rotundum, and emissary veins.

Axial high-resolution CT image(s) without contrast (▶ Fig. 8.21, ▶ Fig. 8.22, ▶ Fig. 8.23, ▶ Fig. 8.24). CT is excellent for the evaluation of detailed skull base bone anatomy including

major foramina and fissures. The PPF is an important elongated, vertically oriented, predominantly fat-filled region located lateral to the posterior aspect of the nasal cavity that has an important relationship to the skull base and paranasal sinuses. The PPF is an important site of anatomic convergence of multiple neural pathways, and familiarity with this area is critical, particularly for evaluation of tumors where there is potential for perineural spread of tumor affecting treatment planning and management. At the lateral boundary of the PPF, there is an opening referred to as the pterygomaxillary fissure, an elongated vertical communication with the infratemporal fossa. The superior aspect of PPF is in continuity with the inferior orbital fissure and inferiorly, the PPF tapers into the greater palatine canal, ultimately leading to the greater and lesser palatine foramina. Medially, the sphenopalatine foramen opens just posterior to the superior or middle meatus where the foramen is covered by mucosa. Posteriorly, the foramen rotundum communicates with the middle cranial fossa, transmitting the maxillary (V2) branch of the trigeminal nerve, artery of foramen rotundum, and emissary veins. The Vidian (pterygoid) canal is also located posteriorly and extends to the foramen lacerum, transmitting the Vidian nerve. More posteriorly in the central skull base, another important foramen, foramen ovale, transmits the mandibular (V3) branch of the trigeminal nerve, lesser petrosal nerve, accessory meningeal branch of maxillary artery, and emissary vein, and provides a direct communication between the cranial cavity and the masticator space.

Axial high-resolution CT image(s) without contrast (▶ Fig. 8.25, ▶ Fig. 8.26, ▶ Fig. 8.27, ▶ Fig. 8.28). CT is excellent for the evaluation of detailed skull base bone anatomy including major foramina and fissures. Inferiorly, the PPF tapers into the greater

(*text continued on page 201*)

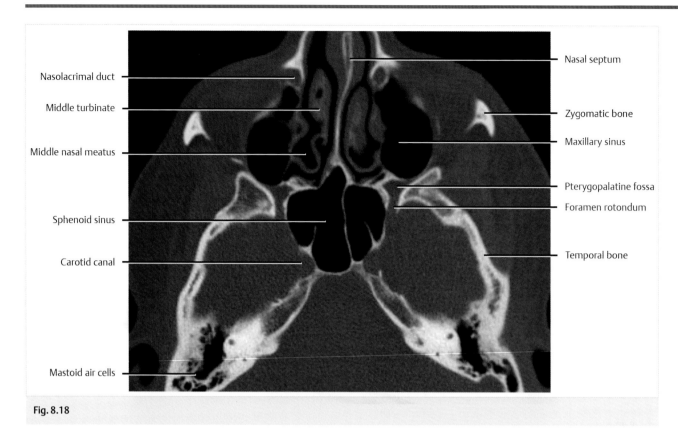

Nasolacrimal duct

Middle turbinate

Middle nasal meatus

Sphenoid sinus

Carotid canal

Mastoid air cells

Nasal septum

Zygomatic bone

Maxillary sinus

Pterygopalatine fossa

Foramen rotondum

Temporal bone

**Fig. 8.18**

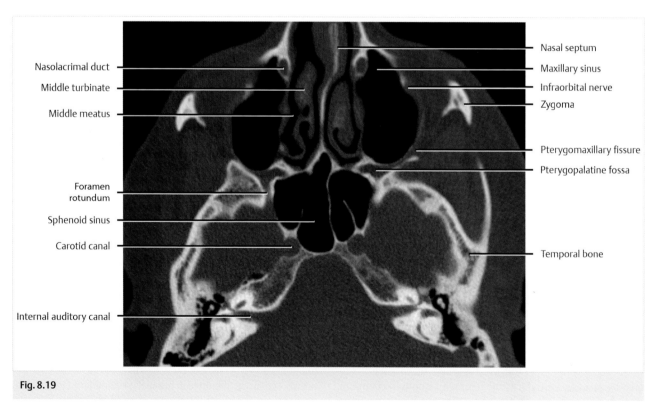

Nasolacrimal duct

Middle turbinate

Middle meatus

Foramen rotundum

Sphenoid sinus

Carotid canal

Internal auditory canal

Nasal septum

Maxillary sinus

Infraorbital nerve

Zygoma

Pterygomaxillary fissure

Pterygopalatine fossa

Temporal bone

**Fig. 8.19**

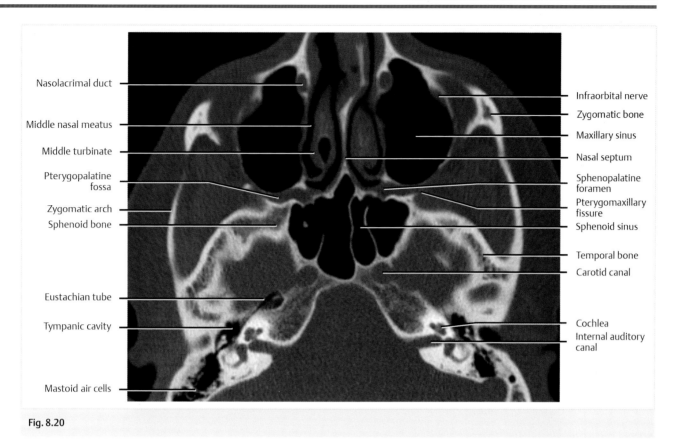

Nasolacrimal duct

Middle nasal meatus

Middle turbinate

Pterygopalatine fossa

Zygomatic arch

Sphenoid bone

Eustachian tube

Tympanic cavity

Mastoid air cells

Infraorbital nerve

Zygomatic bone

Maxillary sinus

Nasal septum

Sphenopalatine foramen

Pterygomaxillary fissure

Sphenoid sinus

Temporal bone

Carotid canal

Cochlea

Internal auditory canal

Fig. 8.20

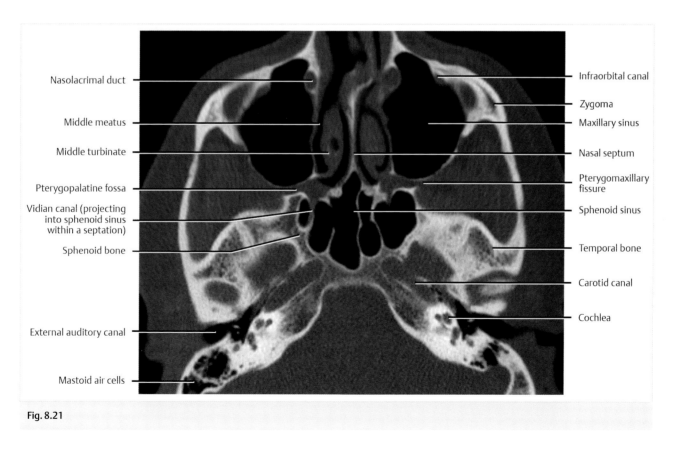

Nasolacrimal duct

Middle meatus

Middle turbinate

Pterygopalatine fossa

Vidian canal (projecting into sphenoid sinus within a septation)

Sphenoid bone

External auditory canal

Mastoid air cells

Infraorbital canal

Zygoma

Maxillary sinus

Nasal septum

Pterygomaxillary fissure

Sphenoid sinus

Temporal bone

Carotid canal

Cochlea

Fig. 8.21

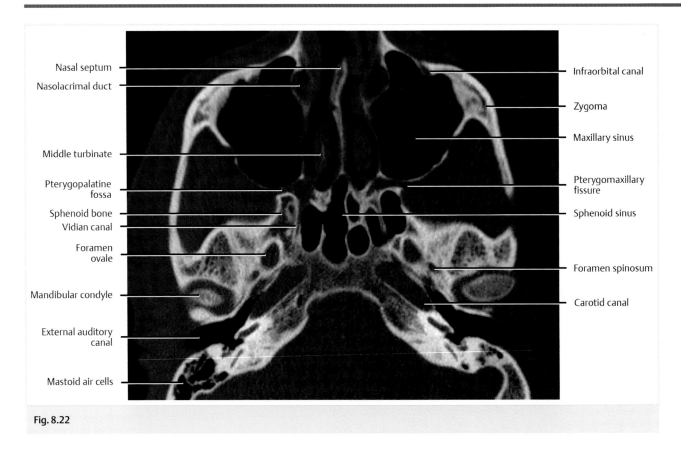

Nasal septum

Nasolacrimal duct

Middle turbinate

Pterygopalatine fossa

Sphenoid bone
Vidian canal

Foramen ovale

Mandibular condyle

External auditory canal

Mastoid air cells

Infraorbital canal

Zygoma

Maxillary sinus

Pterygomaxillary fissure

Sphenoid sinus

Foramen spinosum

Carotid canal

**Fig. 8.22**

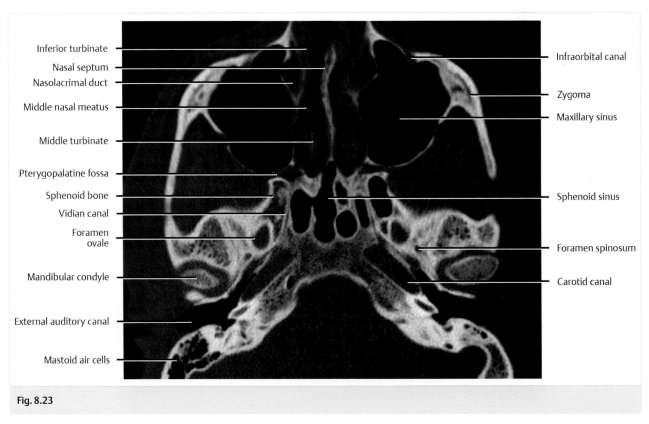

Inferior turbinate

Nasal septum

Nasolacrimal duct

Middle nasal meatus

Middle turbinate

Pterygopalatine fossa

Sphenoid bone

Vidian canal

Foramen ovale

Mandibular condyle

External auditory canal

Mastoid air cells

Infraorbital canal

Zygoma

Maxillary sinus

Sphenoid sinus

Foramen spinosum

Carotid canal

**Fig. 8.23**

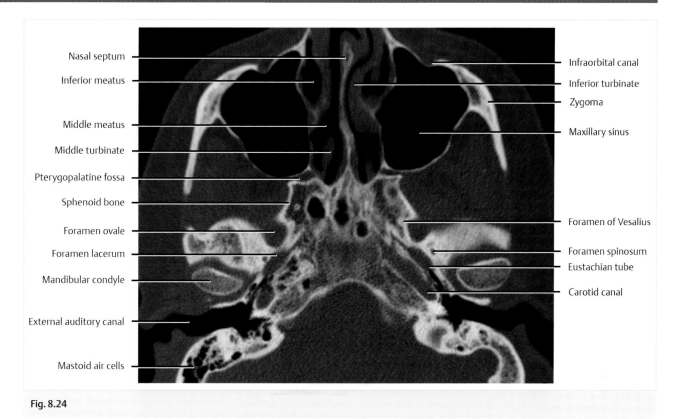

Nasal septum

Inferior meatus

Middle meatus

Middle turbinate

Pterygopalatine fossa

Sphenoid bone

Foramen ovale

Foramen lacerum

Mandibular condyle

External auditory canal

Mastoid air cells

Infraorbital canal

Inferior turbinate

Zygoma

Maxillary sinus

Foramen of Vesalius

Foramen spinosum

Eustachian tube

Carotid canal

Fig. 8.24

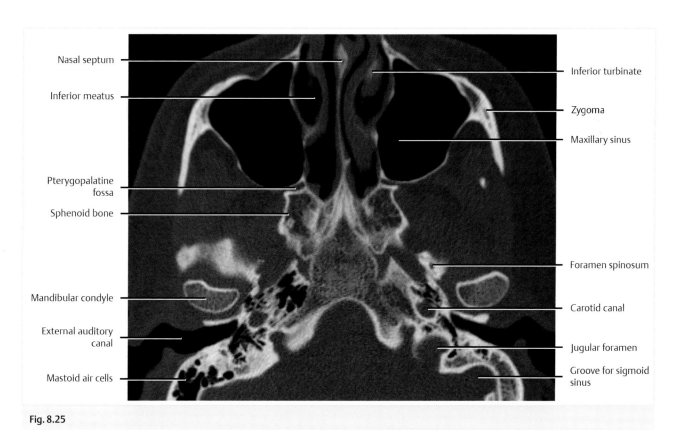

Nasal septum

Inferior meatus

Pterygopalatine fossa

Sphenoid bone

Mandibular condyle

External auditory canal

Mastoid air cells

Inferior turbinate

Zygoma

Maxillary sinus

Foramen spinosum

Carotid canal

Jugular foramen

Groove for sigmoid sinus

Fig. 8.25

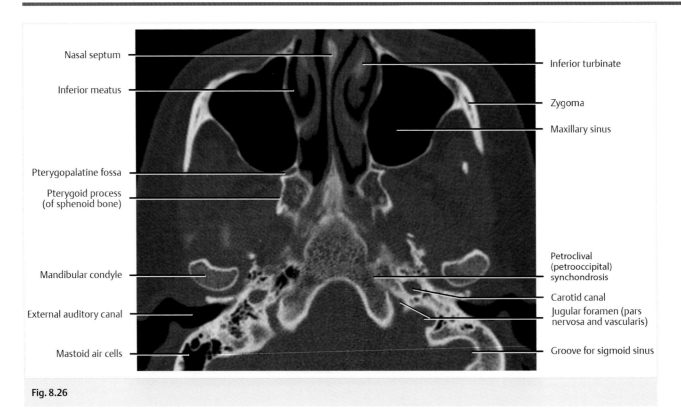

Nasal septum

Inferior meatus

Pterygopalatine fossa

Pterygoid process
(of sphenoid bone)

Mandibular condyle

External auditory canal

Mastoid air cells

Inferior turbinate

Zygoma

Maxillary sinus

Petroclival
(petrooccipital)
synchondrosis

Carotid canal

Jugular foramen (pars
nervosa and vascularis)

Groove for sigmoid sinus

Fig. 8.26

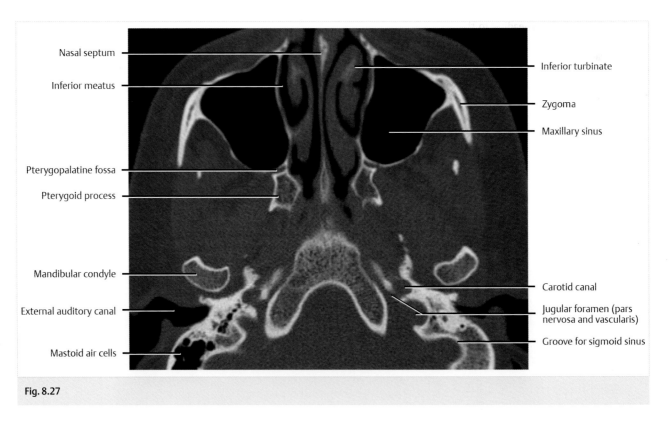

Nasal septum

Inferior meatus

Pterygopalatine fossa

Pterygoid process

Mandibular condyle

External auditory canal

Mastoid air cells

Inferior turbinate

Zygoma

Maxillary sinus

Carotid canal

Jugular foramen (pars
nervosa and vascularis)

Groove for sigmoid sinus

Fig. 8.27

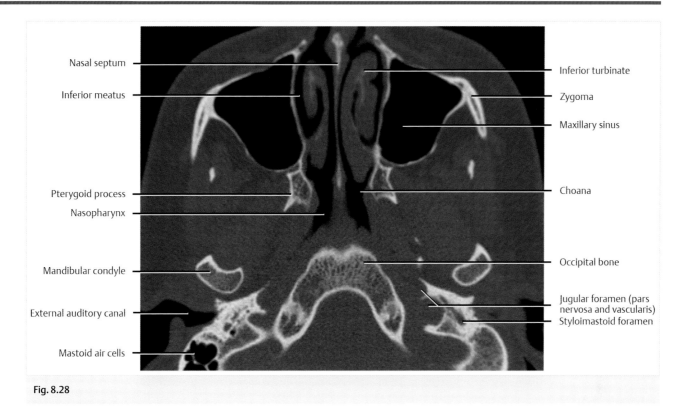

Nasal septum

Inferior meatus

Pterygoid process

Nasopharynx

Mandibular condyle

External auditory canal

Mastoid air cells

Inferior turbinate

Zygoma

Maxillary sinus

Choana

Occipital bone

Jugular foramen (pars nervosa and vascularis)
Styloimastoid foramen

**Fig. 8.28**

palatine canal, ultimately leading to the greater and lesser pala-tine foramina. More posteriorly in the posterior skull base, the jugular foramen has two parts, the pars nervosa and pars vascu-laris, which are partly divided by the jugular spine. Medially and anteriorly, the pars nervosa contains cranial nerve IX, Jacobson nerve, and inferior petrosal sinus. Laterally and more posteriorly, the larger pars vascularis contains cranial nerves X and XI, Arnold nerve, jugular bulb, and posterior meningeal artery. The stylomastoid foramen, located between the mastoid tip and sty-loid process, is the site of passage of cranial nerve VII from the temporal bone to the extracranial compartment.

Axial high-resolution CT image(s) without contrast (▶ Fig. 8.29, ▶ Fig. 8.30, ▶ Fig. 8.31, ▶ Fig. 8.32). CT is excellent for the evaluation of detailed skull base bone anatomy including major foramina and fissures. Inferiorly, the PPF tapers into the greater palatine canal, ultimately leading to the greater and lesser pala-tine foramina. The greater palatine foramen transmits the greater palatine nerve and descending palatine vessels. The lesser palatine foramen transmits the lesser palatine nerves. Although commonly single, there can be two or rarely more than two lesser palatine foramina. More posteriorly in the posterior skull base, the hypoglossal canal transmits cranial nerve XII. The stylomastoid foramen, located between the mastoid tip and styloid process, is the site of passage of cranial nerve VII from the temporal bone to the extracranial compartment. The condyloid (or posterior condylar) canals transmit emissary veins and provide an anastomosis between the jugular bulb and the suboccipital venous plexus. These are among the largest emissary foramina in the skull and should not be misinterpreted as pathology.

Axial high-resolution CT image(s) without contrast (▶ Fig. 8.33, ▶ Fig. 8.34, ▶ Fig. 8.35, ▶ Fig. 8.36). CT is excellent

for the evaluation of detailed skull base bone anatomy including major foramina and fissures as well as other structures at the skull base. The greater palatine foramen transmits the greater palatine nerve and descending palatine vessels. The lesser pala-tine foramen transmits the lesser palatine nerves. Although commonly single, there can be two or rarely more than two lesser palatine foramina. There are important relationships of the skull base to adjacent spaces and cavities, including the nasopharynx. Seen here in the nasopharynx is the torus tubar-ius, the cartilaginous end of the Eustachian tube, and the fossa of Rosenmüller (or pharyngeal recess).

Axial high-resolution CT image(s) without contrast (▶ Fig. 8.37, ▶ Fig. 8.38, ▶ Fig. 8.39, ▶ Fig. 8.40). CT is excellent for the evaluation of detailed skull base bone anatomy including major foramina and fissures as well as other structures at the skull base.

## 8.2.2 Coronal Image Set
### Coronal Computed Tomography (No Contrast)

Coronal reformats from high-resolution CT images without con-trast (▶ Fig. 8.41, ▶ Fig. 8.42, ▶ Fig. 8.43, ▶ Fig. 8.44). The skull base and paranasal sinuses are formed by the fusion of multiple bones, as shown. The anterior skull base can be broadly described as constituting the floor of the anterior cranial fossa and the roof of the nose, ethmoid air cells, and orbits. These anatomic relationships are important and constitute different potential pathways of spread of pathology.

Coronal reformats from high-resolution CT images without contrast (▶ Fig. 8.45, ▶ Fig. 8.46, ▶ Fig. 8.47, ▶ Fig. 8.48). CT is

(*text continued on page 212*)

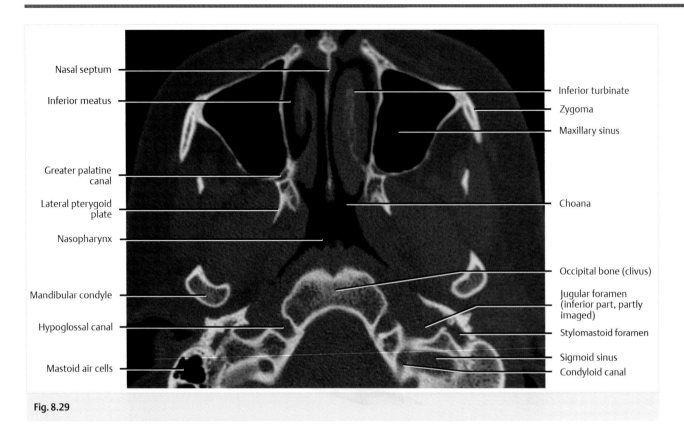

Nasal septum

Inferior meatus

Greater palatine canal

Lateral pterygoid plate

Nasopharynx

Mandibular condyle

Hypoglossal canal

Mastoid air cells

Inferior turbinate

Zygoma

Maxillary sinus

Choana

Occipital bone (clivus)

Jugular foramen (inferior part, partly imaged)

Stylomastoid foramen

Sigmoid sinus

Condyloid canal

**Fig. 8.29**

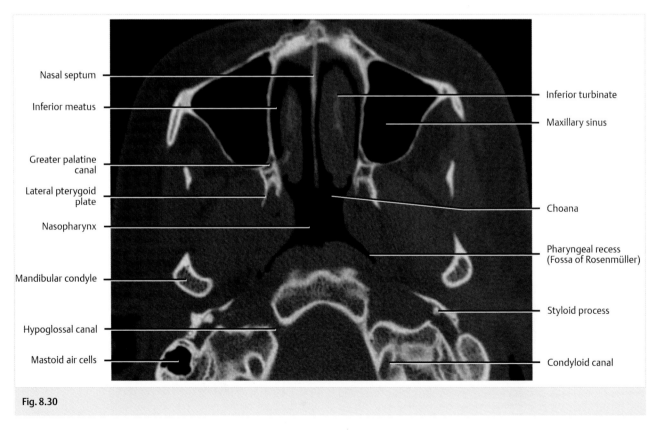

Nasal septum

Inferior meatus

Greater palatine canal

Lateral pterygoid plate

Nasopharynx

Mandibular condyle

Hypoglossal canal

Mastoid air cells

Inferior turbinate

Maxillary sinus

Choana

Pharyngeal recess (Fossa of Rosenmüller)

Styloid process

Condyloid canal

**Fig. 8.30**

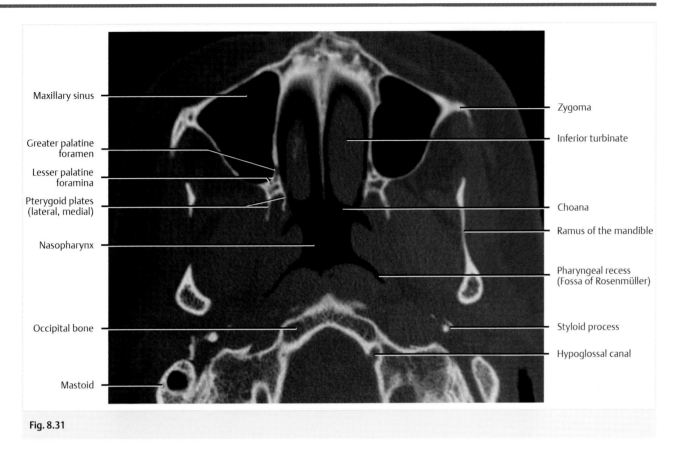

Maxillary sinus

Greater palatine foramen

Lesser palatine foramina

Pterygoid plates (lateral, medial)

Nasopharynx

Occipital bone

Mastoid

Zygoma

Inferior turbinate

Choana

Ramus of the mandible

Pharyngeal recess (Fossa of Rosenmüller)

Styloid process

Hypoglossal canal

Fig. 8.31

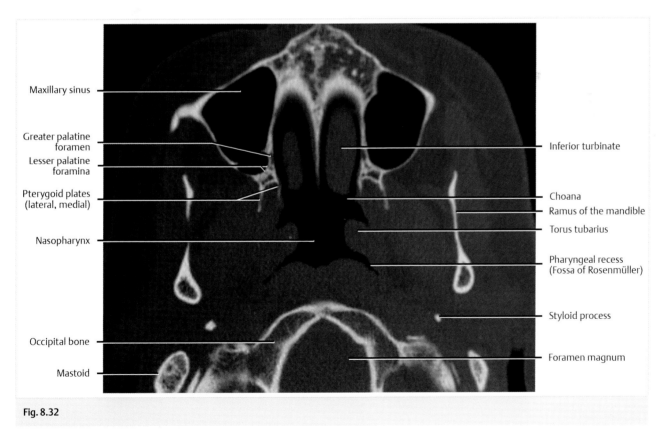

Maxillary sinus

Greater palatine foramen

Lesser palatine foramina

Pterygoid plates (lateral, medial)

Nasopharynx

Occipital bone

Mastoid

Inferior turbinate

Choana

Ramus of the mandible

Torus tubarius

Pharyngeal recess (Fossa of Rosenmüller)

Styloid process

Foramen magnum

Fig. 8.32

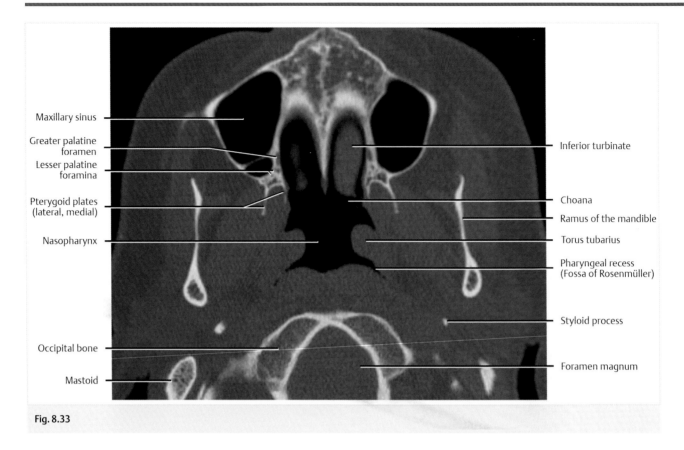

Maxillary sinus

Greater palatine foramen

Lesser palatine foramina

Pterygoid plates (lateral, medial)

Nasopharynx

Occipital bone

Mastoid

Inferior turbinate

Choana

Ramus of the mandible

Torus tubarius

Pharyngeal recess (Fossa of Rosenmüller)

Styloid process

Foramen magnum

**Fig. 8.33**

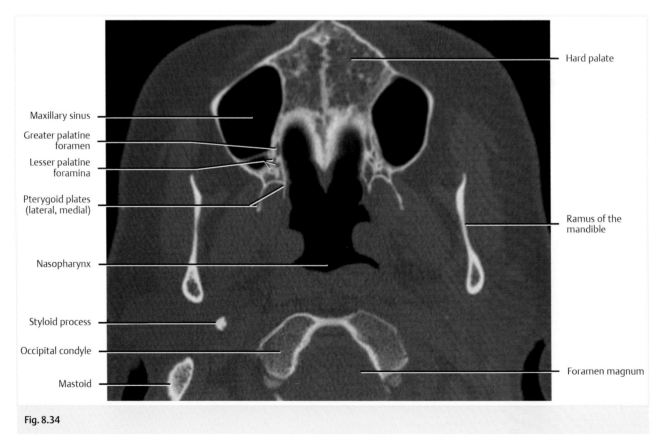

Hard palate

Maxillary sinus

Greater palatine foramen

Lesser palatine foramina

Pterygoid plates (lateral, medial)

Nasopharynx

Styloid process

Occipital condyle

Mastoid

Ramus of the mandible

Foramen magnum

**Fig. 8.34**

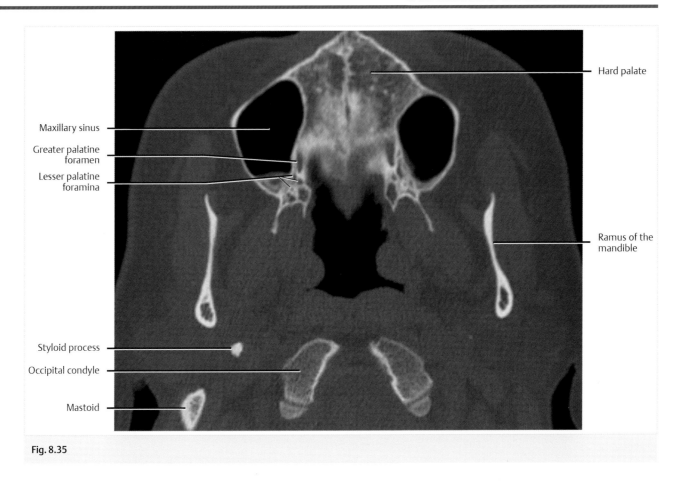

Hard palate

Maxillary sinus

Greater palatine foramen

Lesser palatine foramina

Ramus of the mandible

Styloid process

Occipital condyle

Mastoid

Fig. 8.35

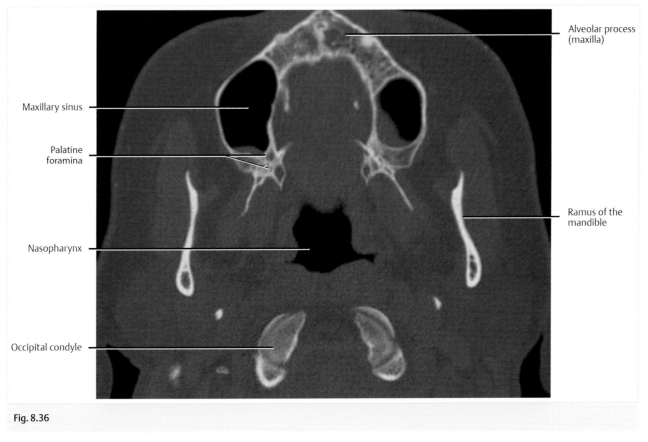

Alveolar process (maxilla)

Maxillary sinus

Palatine foramina

Ramus of the mandible

Nasopharynx

Occipital condyle

Fig. 8.36

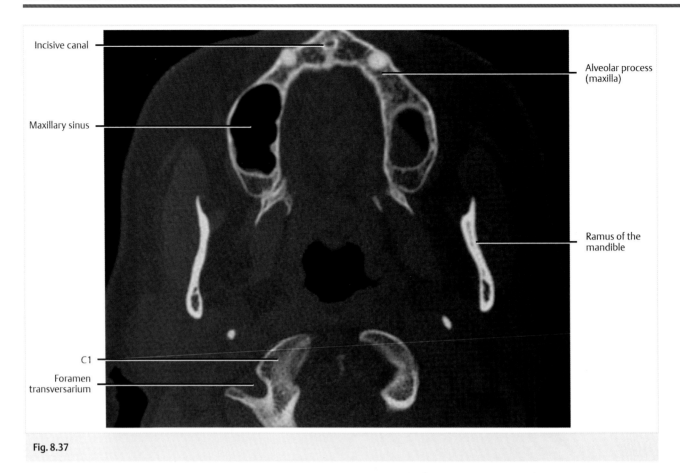

Incisive canal

Maxillary sinus

Alveolar process (maxilla)

Ramus of the mandible

C1

Foramen transversarium

**Fig. 8.37**

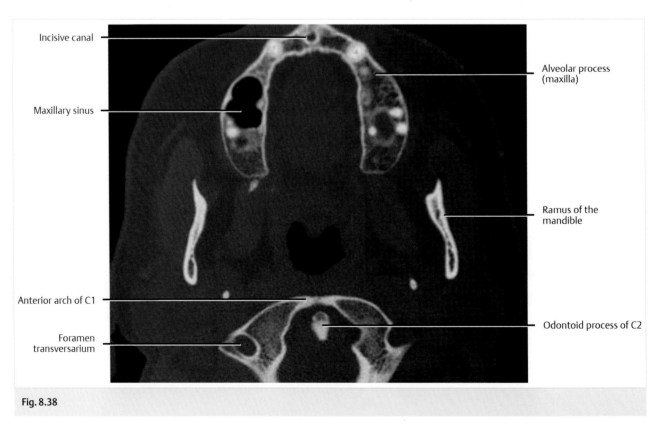

Incisive canal

Maxillary sinus

Alveolar process (maxilla)

Ramus of the mandible

Anterior arch of C1

Foramen transversarium

Odontoid process of C2

**Fig. 8.38**

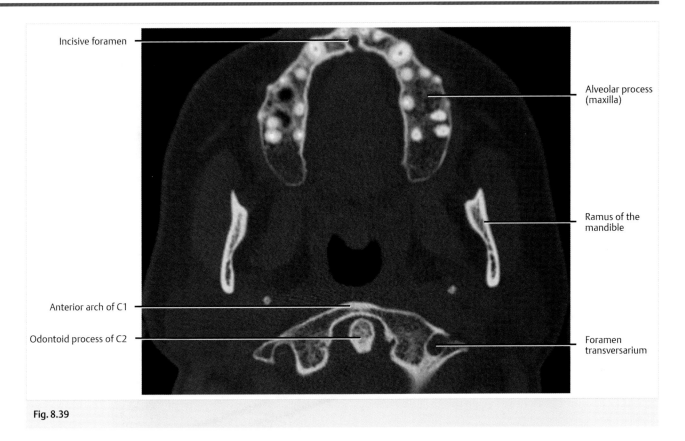

Incisive foramen

Alveolar process (maxilla)

Ramus of the mandible

Anterior arch of C1

Odontoid process of C2

Foramen transversarium

**Fig. 8.39**

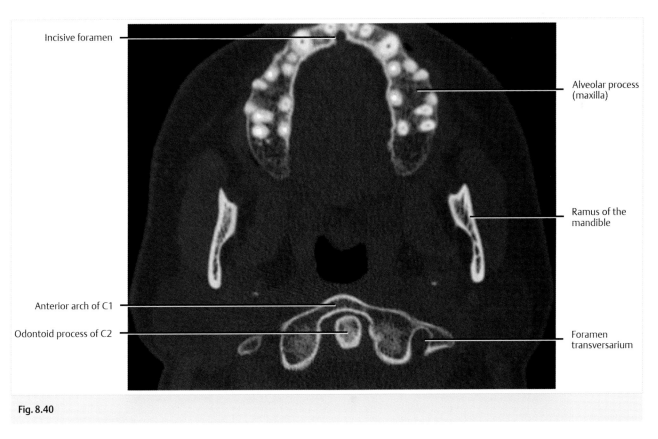

Incisive foramen

Alveolar process (maxilla)

Ramus of the mandible

Anterior arch of C1

Odontoid process of C2

Foramen transversarium

**Fig. 8.40**

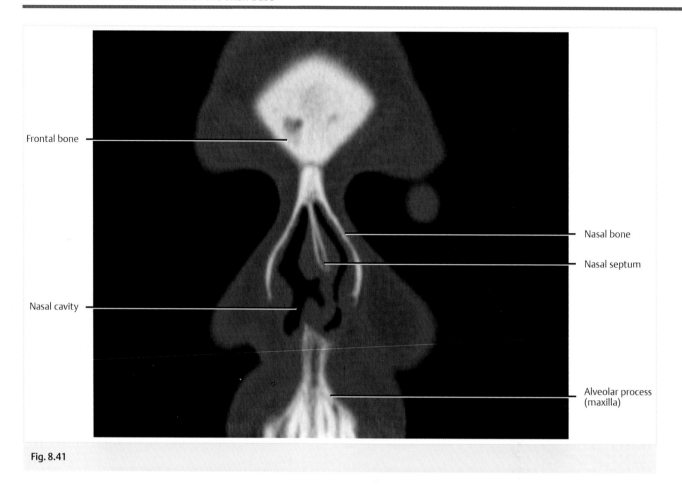

**Fig. 8.41**

Frontal bone

Nasal bone

Nasal septum

Nasal cavity

Alveolar process
(maxilla)

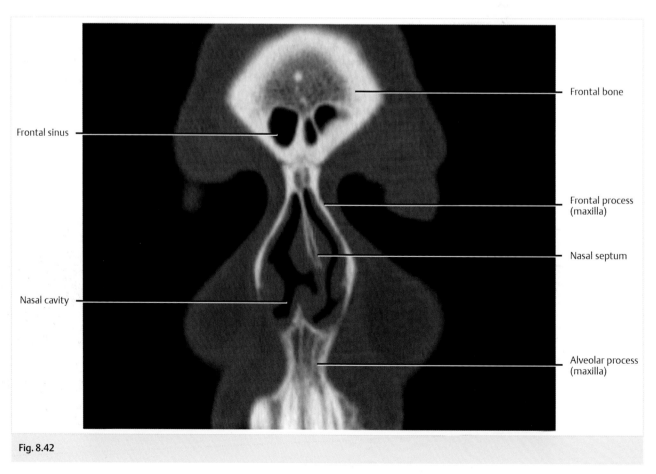

**Fig. 8.42**

Frontal sinus

Frontal bone

Frontal process
(maxilla)

Nasal septum

Nasal cavity

Alveolar process
(maxilla)

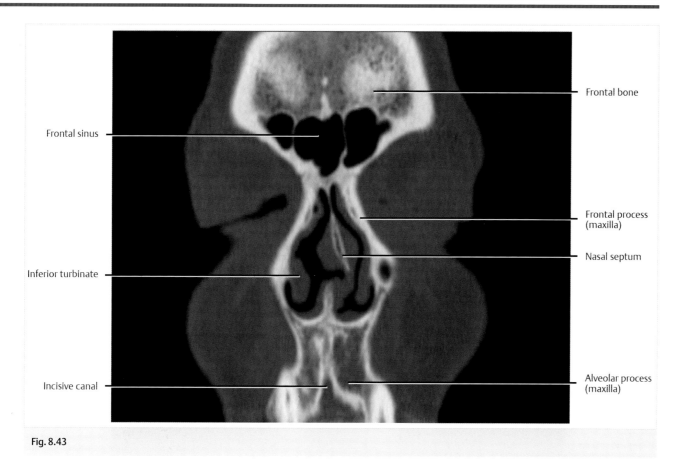

Frontal bone

Frontal sinus

Frontal process (maxilla)

Nasal septum

Inferior turbinate

Incisive canal

Alveolar process (maxilla)

Fig. 8.43

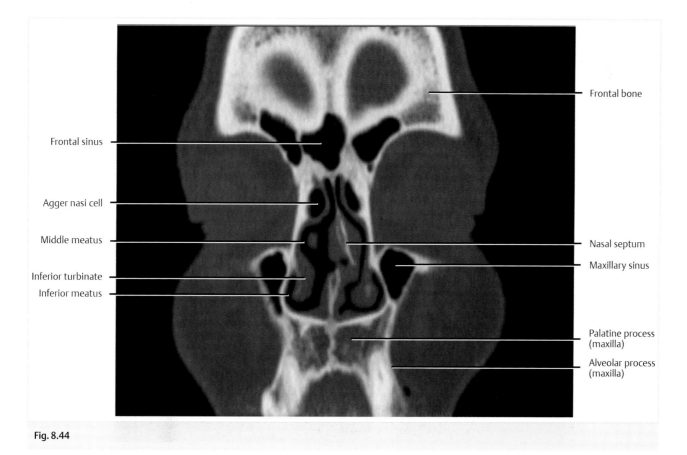

Frontal bone

Frontal sinus

Agger nasi cell

Middle meatus

Nasal septum

Maxillary sinus

Inferior turbinate

Inferior meatus

Palatine process (maxilla)

Alveolar process (maxilla)

Fig. 8.44

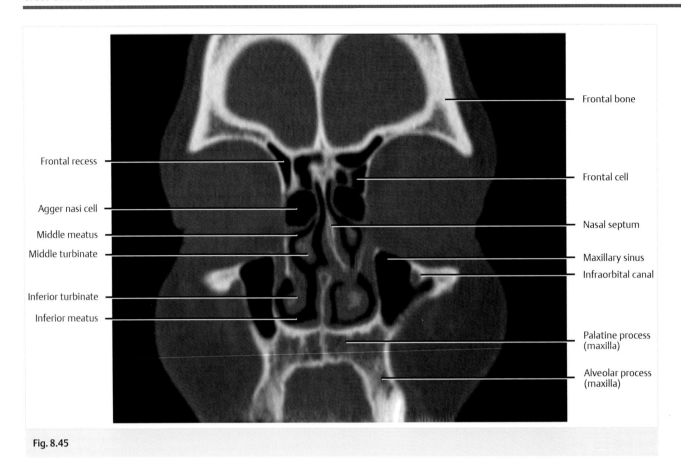

Frontal recess

Agger nasi cell

Middle meatus

Middle turbinate

Inferior turbinate

Inferior meatus

Frontal bone

Frontal cell

Nasal septum

Maxillary sinus

Infraorbital canal

Palatine process
(maxilla)

Alveolar process
(maxilla)

Fig. 8.45

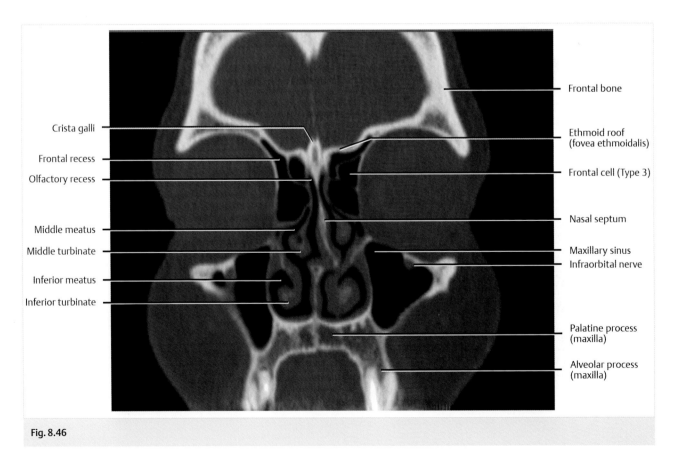

Crista galli

Frontal recess

Olfactory recess

Middle meatus

Middle turbinate

Inferior meatus

Inferior turbinate

Frontal bone

Ethmoid roof
(fovea ethmoidalis)

Frontal cell (Type 3)

Nasal septum

Maxillary sinus
Infraorbital nerve

Palatine process
(maxilla)

Alveolar process
(maxilla)

Fig. 8.46

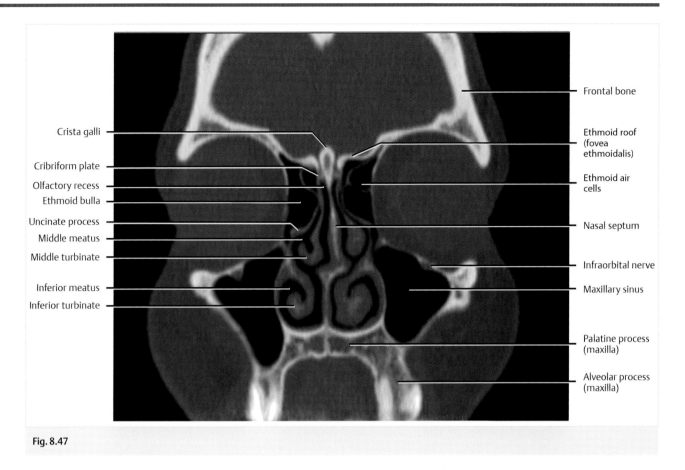

Crista galli

Cribriform plate

Olfactory recess

Ethmoid bulla

Uncinate process

Middle meatus

Middle turbinate

Inferior meatus

Inferior turbinate

Frontal bone

Ethmoid roof (fovea ethmoidalis)

Ethmoid air cells

Nasal septum

Infraorbital nerve

Maxillary sinus

Palatine process (maxilla)

Alveolar process (maxilla)

Fig. 8.47

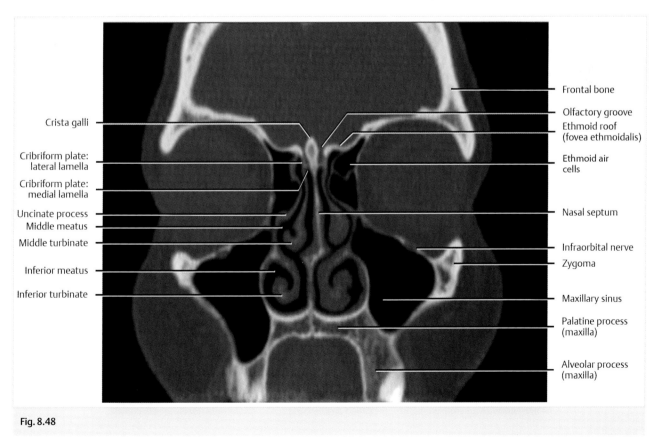

Crista galli

Cribriform plate: lateral lamella

Cribriform plate: medial lamella

Uncinate process

Middle meatus

Middle turbinate

Inferior meatus

Inferior turbinate

Frontal bone

Olfactory groove

Ethmoid roof (fovea ethmoidalis)

Ethmoid air cells

Nasal septum

Infraorbital nerve

Zygoma

Maxillary sinus

Palatine process (maxilla)

Alveolar process (maxilla)

Fig. 8.48

excellent for the evaluation of detailed skull base and paranasal sinus bony anatomy. The horizontal central part of the roof of the nasal cavity is formed by the cribriform plate. The cribriform plate has a medial lamella inferiorly and medially and a lateral lamella that is vertical or slanted. The lateral lamella of the cribriform plate is the thinnest structure in the skull base and as such represents a site of potential breach or injury during surgery. The fovea ethmoidalis forms the roof of the ethmoid labyrinth. The symmetry, slanting, and depth of the cribriform plate and fovea ethmoidalis are also important for surgical planning and well demonstrated on coronal CT images. Different anatomic variants of the paranasal sinuses, including Agger nasi cells and frontal cells, are well seen on coronal and sagittal reformats. The infraorbital canal transmits the infraorbital nerve, a branch of V2 (maxillary division of trigeminal nerve).

Coronal reformats from high-resolution CT images without contrast (▶ Fig. 8.49, ▶ Fig. 8.50, ▶ Fig. 8.51, ▶ Fig. 8.52). CT is excellent for the evaluation of detailed skull base and paranasal sinus bony anatomy. The horizontal central part of the roof of the nasal cavity is formed by the cribriform plate. The cribriform plate has a medial lamella inferiorly and medially and a lateral lamella that is vertical or slanted. The lateral lamella of the cribriform plate is the thinnest structure in the skull base and as such represents a site of potential breach or injury during surgery. The fovea ethmoidalis forms the roof of the ethmoid labyrinth. The symmetry, slanting, and depth of the cribriform plate and fovea ethmoidalis are also important for surgical planning and well demonstrated on coronal CT images. The olfactory fossa is also formed by the cribriform plate,

separated at the midline by the crista galli. Coronal reformats are also excellent for visualization of important paranasal sinus anatomy, such as structures of the ostiomeatal unit (OMU). The OMU refers to a functional unit of structures draining the frontal, anterior ethmoid, and maxillary sinuses, and includes the middle meatus, ethmoid bulla, uncinate process, hiatus semilunaris, infundibulum, and superomedial maxillary sinus/maxillary sinus ostium. The hiatus semilunaris is the area between uncinate process and ethmoid bulla that receives drainage from anterior ethmoid air cells and maxillary sinus (via the infundibulum).

Coronal reformats from high-resolution CT images without contrast (▶ Fig. 8.53, ▶ Fig. 8.54, ▶ Fig. 8.55, ▶ Fig. 8.56). CT is excellent for the evaluation of detailed skull base and paranasal sinus bony anatomy. The horizontal central part of the roof of the nasal cavity is formed by the cribriform plate and the fovea ethmoidalis forms the roof of the ethmoid labyrinth. The symmetry, slanting, and depth of the cribriform plate and fovea ethmoidalis are also important for surgical planning and well demonstrated on coronal CT images. Coronal reformats are also excellent for visualization of important nasal cavity and paranasal sinus anatomy, such as the nasal turbinates and meati.

Coronal reformats from high-resolution CT images without contrast (▶ Fig. 8.57, ▶ Fig. 8.58, ▶ Fig. 8.59, ▶ Fig. 8.60). CT is excellent for the evaluation of detailed skull base bone anatomy including major foramina and fissures. The PPF is an important elongated, vertically oriented, predominantly fat-filled region located lateral to the posterior aspect of the nasal cavity that has an important relationship to the skull base and paranasal sinuses. The PPF is an important site of anatomic convergence

(*text continued on page 218*)

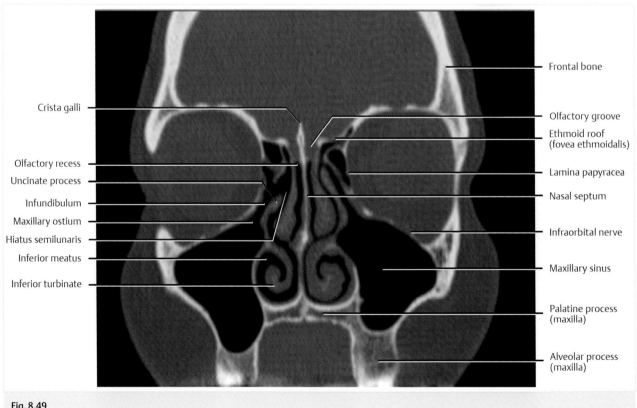

Fig. 8.49

Crista galli
Olfactory recess
Uncinate process
Infundibulum
Maxillary ostium
Hiatus semilunaris
Inferior meatus
Inferior turbinate

Frontal bone
Olfactory groove
Ethmoid roof (fovea ethmoidalis)
Lamina papyracea
Nasal septum
Infraorbital nerve
Maxillary sinus
Palatine process (maxilla)
Alveolar process (maxilla)

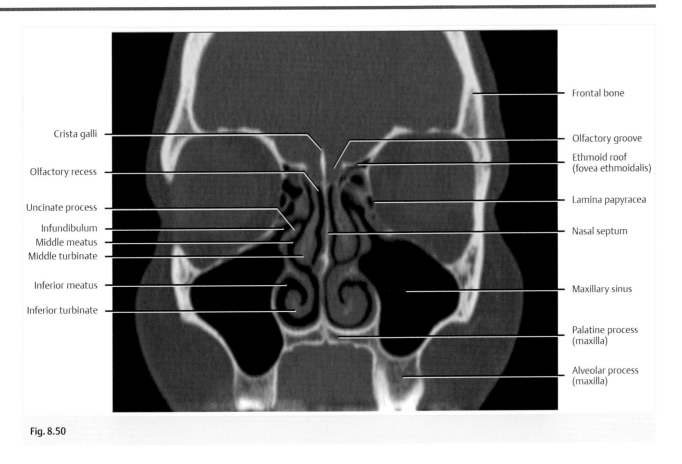

Crista galli

Olfactory recess

Uncinate process
Infundibulum
Middle meatus
Middle turbinate

Inferior meatus

Inferior turbinate

Frontal bone

Olfactory groove
Ethmoid roof
(fovea ethmoidalis)

Lamina papyracea

Nasal septum

Maxillary sinus

Palatine process
(maxilla)

Alveolar process
(maxilla)

Fig. 8.50

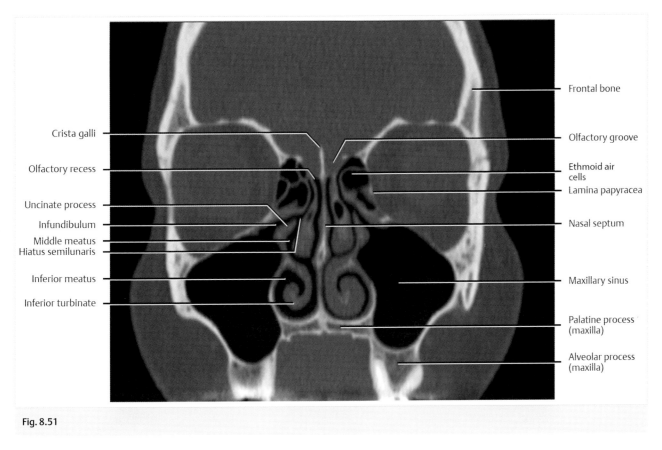

Crista galli

Olfactory recess

Uncinate process

Infundibulum

Middle meatus
Hiatus semilunaris

Inferior meatus

Inferior turbinate

Frontal bone

Olfactory groove

Ethmoid air
cells
Lamina papyracea

Nasal septum

Maxillary sinus

Palatine process
(maxilla)

Alveolar process
(maxilla)

Fig. 8.51

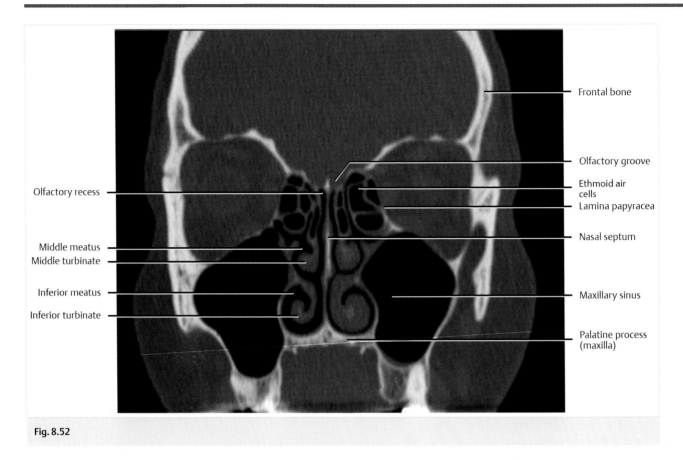

Frontal bone

Olfactory groove

Ethmoid air cells

Lamina papyracea

Nasal septum

Olfactory recess

Middle meatus

Middle turbinate

Inferior meatus

Inferior turbinate

Maxillary sinus

Palatine process (maxilla)

**Fig. 8.52**

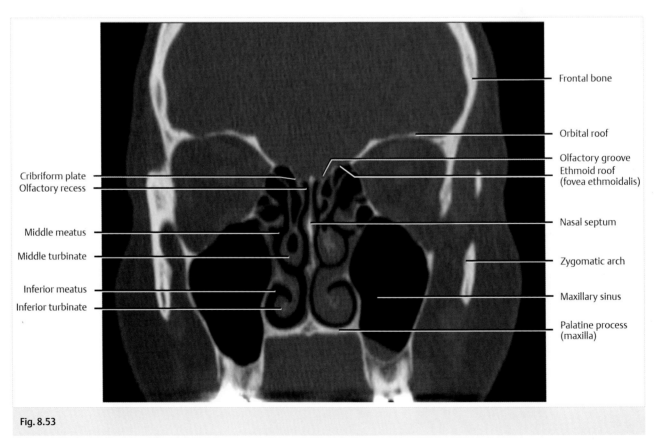

Frontal bone

Orbital roof

Olfactory groove

Ethmoid roof (fovea ethmoidalis)

Cribriform plate

Olfactory recess

Middle meatus

Middle turbinate

Inferior meatus

Inferior turbinate

Nasal septum

Zygomatic arch

Maxillary sinus

Palatine process (maxilla)

**Fig. 8.53**

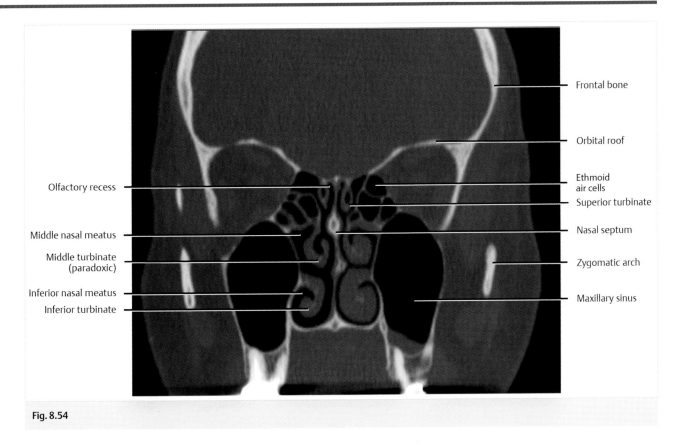

Frontal bone

Orbital roof

Olfactory recess

Ethmoid
air cells

Superior turbinate

Middle nasal meatus

Nasal septum

Middle turbinate
(paradoxic)

Zygomatic arch

Inferior nasal meatus

Maxillary sinus

Inferior turbinate

**Fig. 8.54**

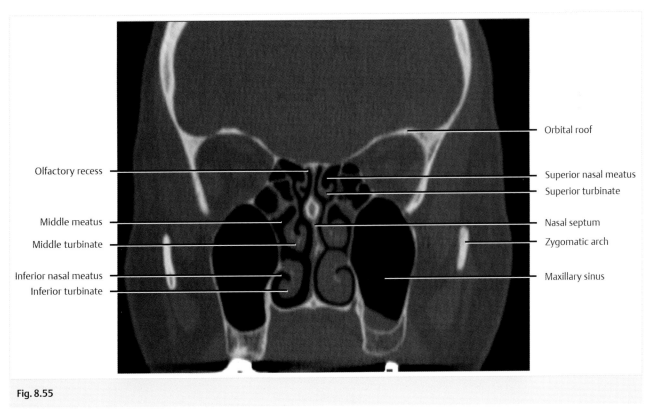

Orbital roof

Olfactory recess

Superior nasal meatus

Superior turbinate

Middle meatus

Nasal septum

Middle turbinate

Zygomatic arch

Inferior nasal meatus

Maxillary sinus

Inferior turbinate

**Fig. 8.55**

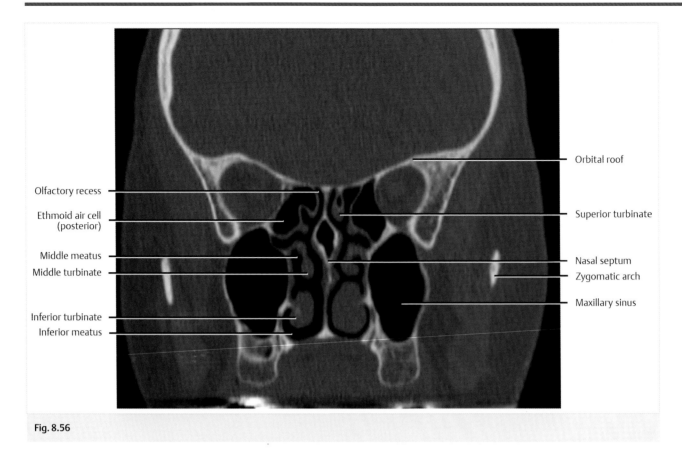

Orbital roof

Olfactory recess

Ethmoid air cell
(posterior)

Superior turbinate

Middle meatus
Middle turbinate

Nasal septum
Zygomatic arch

Maxillary sinus

Inferior turbinate
Inferior meatus

Fig. 8.56

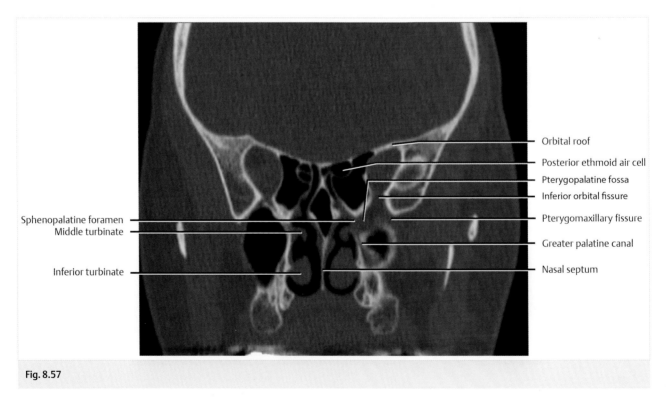

Orbital roof

Posterior ethmoid air cell

Pterygopalatine fossa

Inferior orbital fissure

Sphenopalatine foramen
Middle turbinate

Pterygomaxillary fissure

Greater palatine canal

Inferior turbinate

Nasal septum

Fig. 8.57

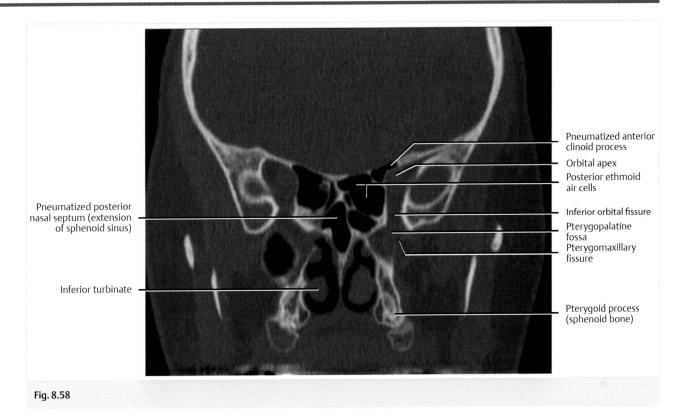

Pneumatized anterior clinoid process

Orbital apex

Posterior ethmoid air cells

Inferior orbital fissure

Pterygopalatine fossa

Pterygomaxillary fissure

Pterygoid process (sphenoid bone)

Pneumatized posterior nasal septum (extension of sphenoid sinus)

Inferior turbinate

**Fig. 8.58**

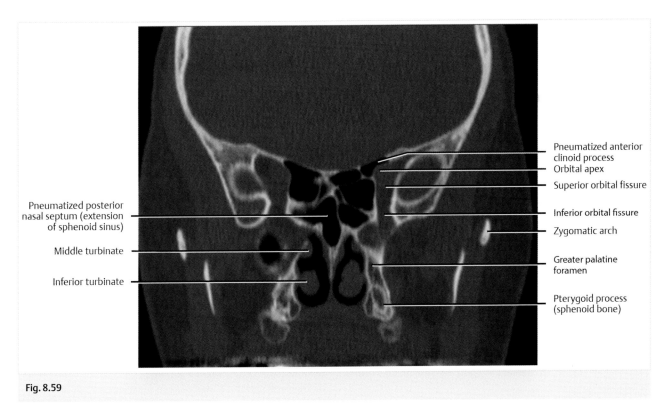

Pneumatized anterior clinoid process

Orbital apex

Superior orbital fissure

Inferior orbital fissure

Zygomatic arch

Greater palatine foramen

Pterygoid process (sphenoid bone)

Pneumatized posterior nasal septum (extension of sphenoid sinus)

Middle turbinate

Inferior turbinate

**Fig. 8.59**

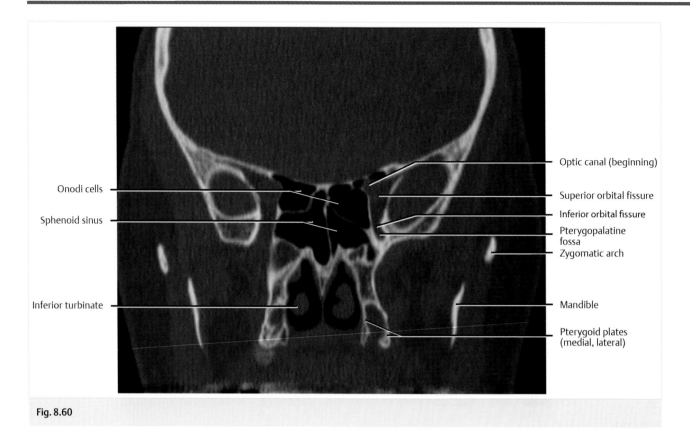

Onodi cells

Sphenoid sinus

Inferior turbinate

Optic canal (beginning)

Superior orbital fissure

Inferior orbital fissure

Pterygopalatine fossa

Zygomatic arch

Mandible

Pterygoid plates (medial, lateral)

**Fig. 8.60**

of multiple neural pathways, and familiarity with this area is critical, particularly for evaluation of tumors where there is potential for perineural spread of tumor. The PPF is well seen on axial images, but it is also important to be familiar with its appearance in other planes, such as the coronal plane, which in addition highlights the relation to adjacent spaces in a different way. The superior aspect of PPF is in continuity with the inferior orbital fissure, and, inferiorly, the PPF tapers into the greater palatine canal, ultimately leading to the greater and lesser palatine foramina. At the lateral boundary of the PPF, there is an opening referred to as the pterygomaxillary fissure, an elongated vertical communication with the infratemporal fossa. The coronal plane also demonstrates the relationship with and between other important foramina, fissures, and spaces well, including that of the superior and inferior orbital fissures, optic canal, and orbital apex. Anatomic variations of the paranasal sinuses such as Onodi cells are also well demonstrated in the coronal plane and important to recognize because there is potential for misidentification during endoscopic surgery that would put closely related critical structures, in particular the optic nerves, at risk for inadvertent surgical injury. The presence of a horizontal or near horizontal septation suggests the presence of an Onodi cell and should be sought on coronal reformats.

Coronal reformats from high-resolution CT images without contrast (► Fig. 8.61, ► Fig. 8.62, ► Fig. 8.63, ► Fig. 8.64). CT is excellent for the evaluation of detailed skull base bone anatomy including major foramina and fissures. Anatomic variations of the paranasal sinuses such as Onodi cells are also well demonstrated in the coronal plane and important to recognize because there is potential for misidentification during endoscopic sur-

gery that would put closely related critical structures, in particular the optic nerves, at risk for inadvertent surgical injury. The presence of a horizontal or near horizontal septation suggests the presence of an Onodi cell and should be sought on coronal reformats. Other important variations such as pneumatization of the anterior clinoid process also have an increased association with optic nerve exposure and dehiscence and are considered an indicator of optic nerve vulnerability during endoscopic sinus surgery. These relationships are well evaluated on coronal reformats. Among others, the foramen rotundum (containing the maxillary [V2] branch of the trigeminal nerve, artery of foramen rotundum, and emissary veins) and the Vidian (pterygoid) canal (containing the Vidian nerve) are well seen in the coronal plane.

Coronal reformats from high-resolution CT images without contrast (► Fig. 8.65, ► Fig. 8.66, ► Fig. 8.67, ► Fig. 8.68). CT is excellent for the evaluation of detailed skull base bone anatomy including major foramina and fissures. In the central skull base, the foramen ovale transmits the mandibular (V3) branch of the trigeminal nerve, lesser petrosal nerve, accessory meningeal branch of maxillary artery, and emissary vein, and provides a direct communication between the cranial cavity and the masticator space. Other, smaller foramina can also be seen reliably on high-resolution CT images from modern CT scanners.

Coronal reformats from high-resolution CT images without contrast (► Fig. 8.69, ► Fig. 8.70, ► Fig. 8.71, ► Fig. 8.72). CT is excellent for the evaluation of detailed skull base bone anatomy including different foramina and fissures. Among other structures, the carotid canal, foramen spinosum, and foramen lacerum are well seen here. There are important relationships of the skull base to adjacent spaces and cavities. Seen here in the

(*text continued on page 225*)

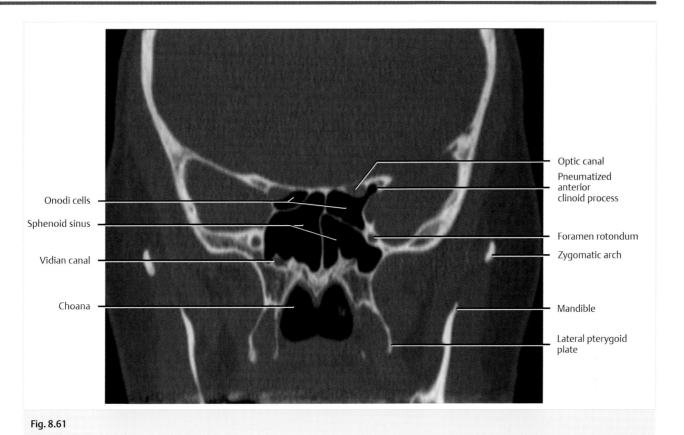

Onodi cells

Sphenoid sinus

Vidian canal

Choana

Optic canal

Pneumatized anterior clinoid process

Foramen rotondum

Zygomatic arch

Mandible

Lateral pterygoid plate

Fig. 8.61

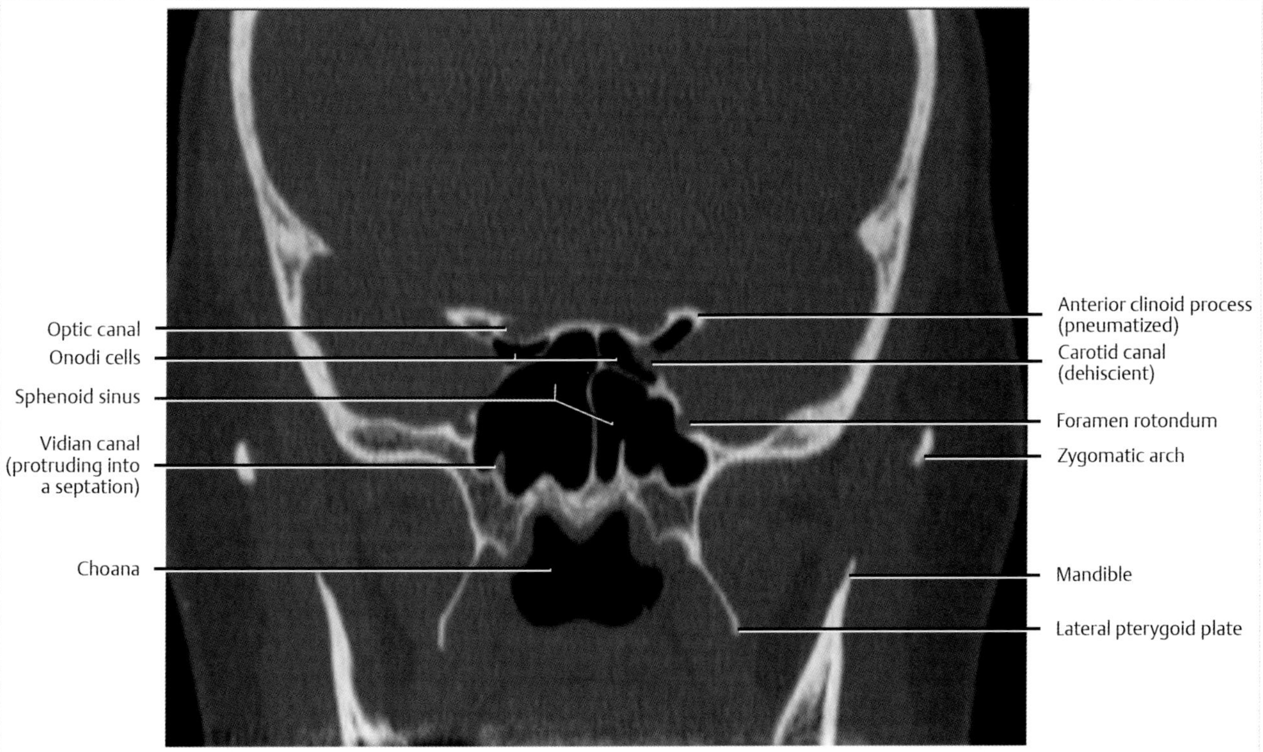

Optic canal

Onodi cells

Sphenoid sinus

Vidian canal (protruding into a septation)

Choana

Anterior clinoid process (pneumatized)

Carotid canal (dehiscent)

Foramen rotondum

Zygomatic arch

Mandible

Lateral pterygoid plate

Fig. 8.62

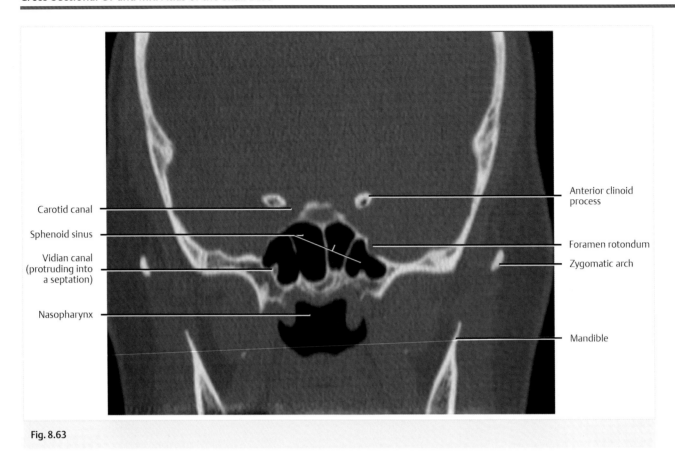

Carotid canal

Sphenoid sinus

Vidian canal
(protruding into
a septation)

Nasopharynx

Anterior clinoid
process

Foramen rotondum

Zygomatic arch

Mandible

Fig. 8.63

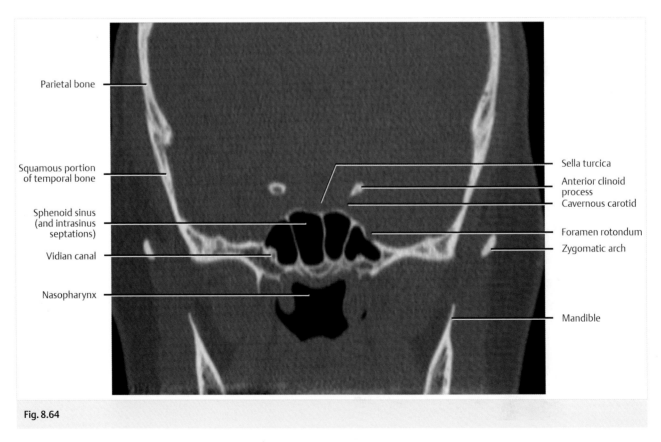

Parietal bone

Squamous portion
of temporal bone

Sphenoid sinus
(and intrasinus
septations)

Vidian canal

Nasopharynx

Sella turcica

Anterior clinoid
process

Cavernous carotid

Foramen rotondum

Zygomatic arch

Mandible

Fig. 8.64

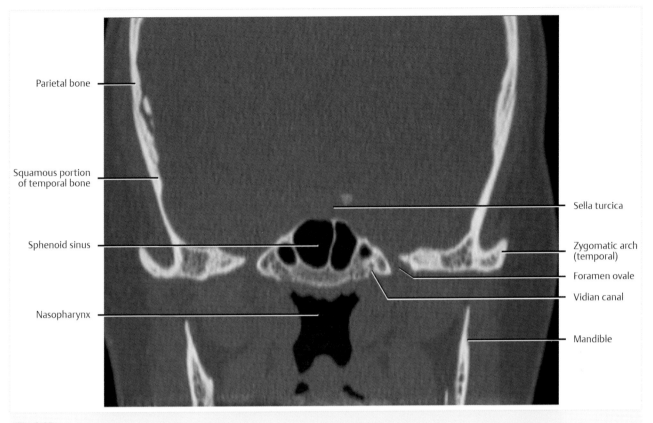

Fig. 8.65

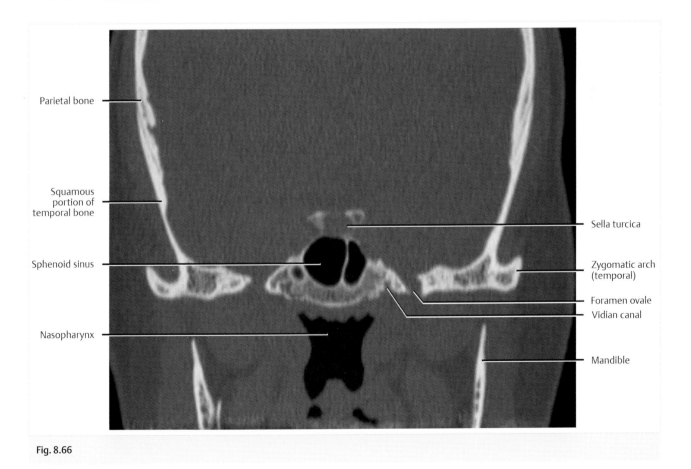

Fig. 8.66

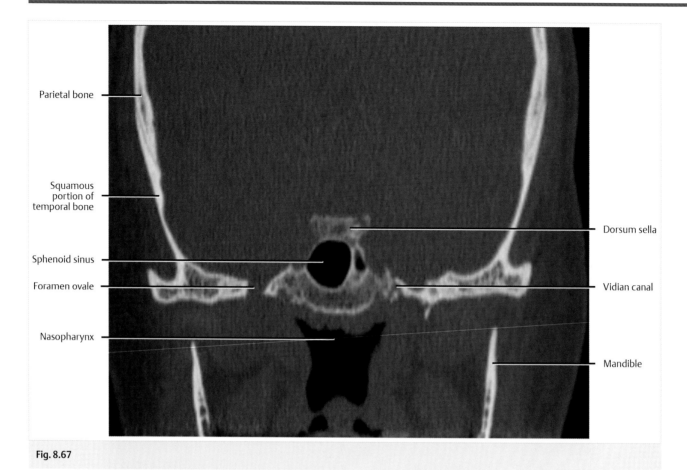

Parietal bone

Squamous portion of temporal bone

Sphenoid sinus

Foramen ovale

Nasopharynx

Dorsum sella

Vidian canal

Mandible

**Fig. 8.67**

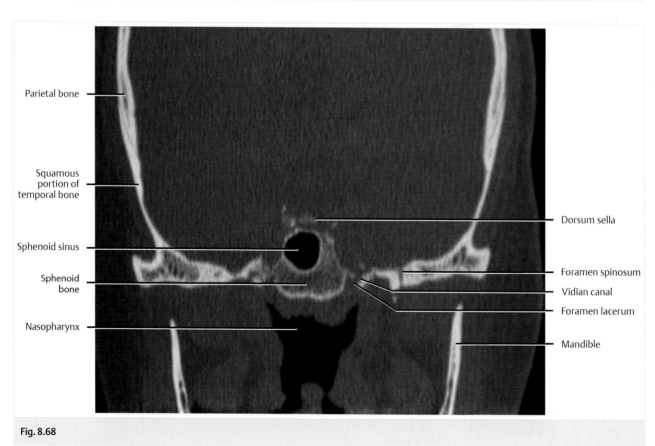

Parietal bone

Squamous portion of temporal bone

Sphenoid sinus

Sphenoid bone

Nasopharynx

Dorsum sella

Foramen spinosum

Vidian canal

Foramen lacerum

Mandible

**Fig. 8.68**

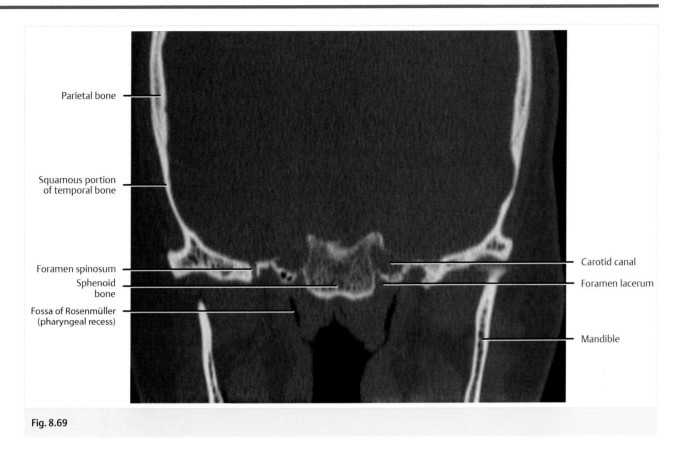

Parietal bone

Squamous portion
of temporal bone

Foramen spinosum

Sphenoid
bone

Fossa of Rosenmüller
(pharyngeal recess)

Carotid canal

Foramen lacerum

Mandible

**Fig. 8.69**

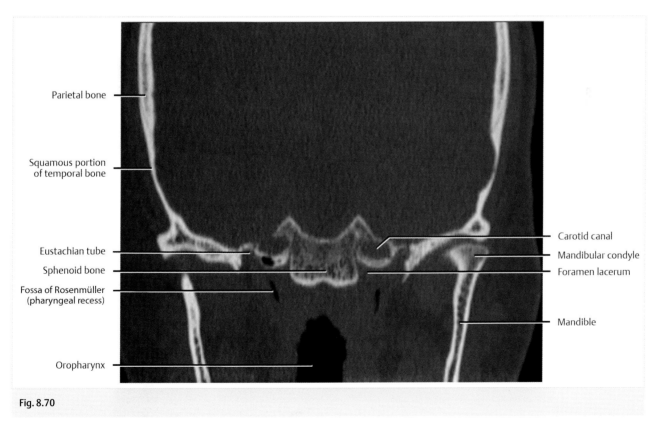

Parietal bone

Squamous portion
of temporal bone

Eustachian tube

Sphenoid bone

Fossa of Rosenmüller
(pharyngeal recess)

Oropharynx

Carotid canal

Mandibular condyle

Foramen lacerum

Mandible

**Fig. 8.70**

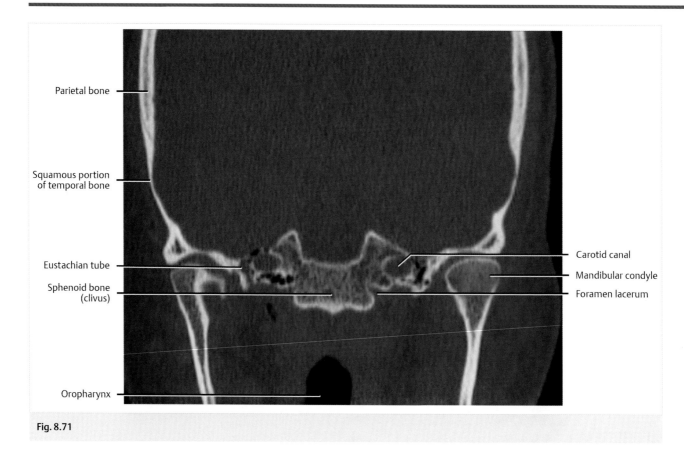

Parietal bone

Squamous portion of temporal bone

Eustachian tube

Sphenoid bone (clivus)

Oropharynx

Carotid canal

Mandibular condyle

Foramen lacerum

Fig. 8.71

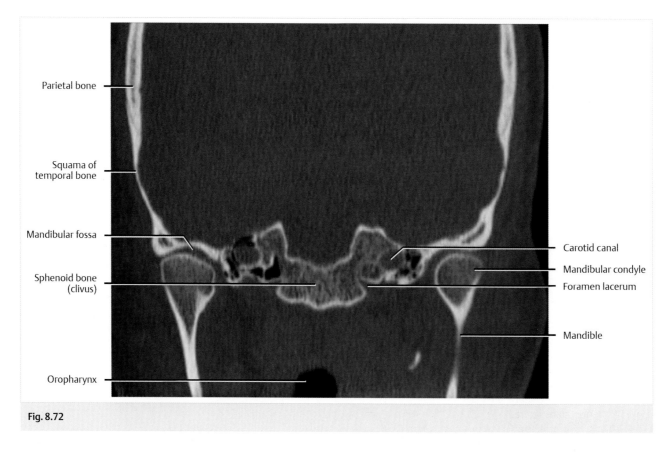

Parietal bone

Squama of temporal bone

Mandibular fossa

Sphenoid bone (clivus)

Oropharynx

Carotid canal

Mandibular condyle

Foramen lacerum

Mandible

Fig. 8.72

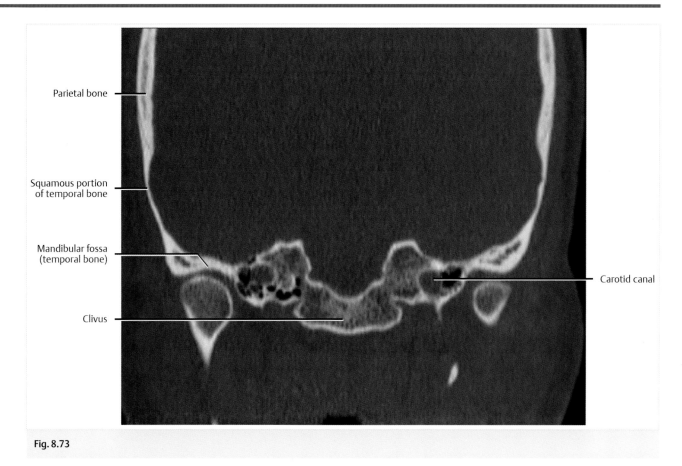

Parietal bone

Squamous portion of temporal bone

Mandibular fossa (temporal bone)

Clivus

Carotid canal

**Fig. 8.73**

nasopharynx is the fossa of Rosenmüller (or lateral pharyngeal recess).

Coronal reformats from high-resolution CT images without contrast (▶ Fig. 8.73, ▶ Fig. 8.74, ▶ Fig. 8.75, ▶ Fig. 8.76). CT is excellent for the evaluation of detailed skull base bone anatomy including major foramina and fissures. In the posterior skull base, the jugular foramen has two parts, the pars nervosa and pars vascularis. The pars nervosa is the more medial and anteriorly located part, and transmits cranial nerve IX, Jacobson nerve, and inferior petrosal sinus. The larger pars vascularis is more posterior and laterally located and transmits cranial nerves X and XI, Arnold nerve, jugular bulb, and posterior meningeal artery. The internal auditory canal contains cranial nerves VII and VIII, and the stylomastoid foramen, located between the mastoid tip and styloid process, also transmits cranial nerve VII from the temporal bone to the extracranial compartment. The hypoglossal canal transmits cranial nerve XII.

Coronal reformats from high-resolution CT images without contrast (▶ Fig. 8.77, ▶ Fig. 8.78, ▶ Fig. 8.79, ▶ Fig. 8.80). CT is excellent for the evaluation of detailed skull base bone anatomy including major foramina and fissures. In the posterior skull base, the jugular foramen has two parts, the pars nervosa and pars vascularis. The pars nervosa is the more medial and anteriorly located part, and transmits cranial nerve IX, Jacobson nerve, and inferior petrosal sinus. The larger pars vascularis is more posterior and laterally located and transmits cranial nerves X and XI, Arnold nerve, jugular bulb, and posterior meningeal artery. The condyloid (or posterior condylar) canals transmit emissary veins and provide an anastomosis between

the jugular bulb and suboccipital venous plexus. These are among the largest emissary foramina in the skull and should not be misinterpreted as pathology.

Coronal reformats from high-resolution CT images without contrast (▶ Fig. 8.81, ▶ Fig. 8.82, ▶ Fig. 8.83). CT is excellent for the evaluation of detailed skull base bone anatomy including major foramina and fissures as well as other structures at the skull base.

## 8.2.3 Sagittal Image Set

### Sagittal Computed Tomography (No Contrast)

Sagittal reformats from high-resolution CT images without contrast (▶ Fig. 8.84, ▶ Fig. 8.85, ▶ Fig. 8.86, ▶ Fig. 8.87). CT is excellent for the evaluation of detailed skull base bone anatomy including major foramina and fissures as well as other structures at the skull base.

Sagittal reformats from high-resolution CT images without contrast (▶ Fig. 8.88, ▶ Fig. 8.89, ▶ Fig. 8.90, ▶ Fig. 8.91). CT is excellent for the evaluation of detailed skull base and paranasal sinus bony anatomy. Among others, these images show the carotid canal, internal auditory canal, jugular foramen, foramen spinosum, and stylomastoid foramen.

Sagittal reformats from high-resolution CT images without contrast (▶ Fig. 8.92, ▶ Fig. 8.93, ▶ Fig. 8.94, ▶ Fig. 8.95). CT is excellent for the evaluation of detailed skull base and paranasal sinus bony anatomy. The ability to create high-resolution

(*text continued on page 234*)

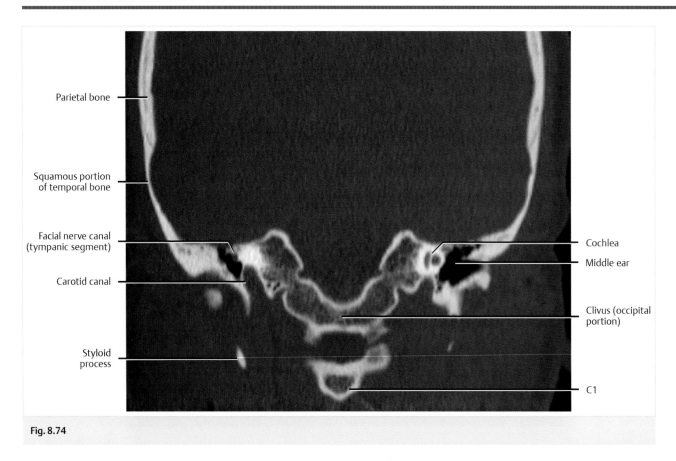

Parietal bone

Squamous portion
of temporal bone

Facial nerve canal
(tympanic segment)

Carotid canal

Styloid
process

Cochlea

Middle ear

Clivus (occipital
portion)

C1

**Fig. 8.74**

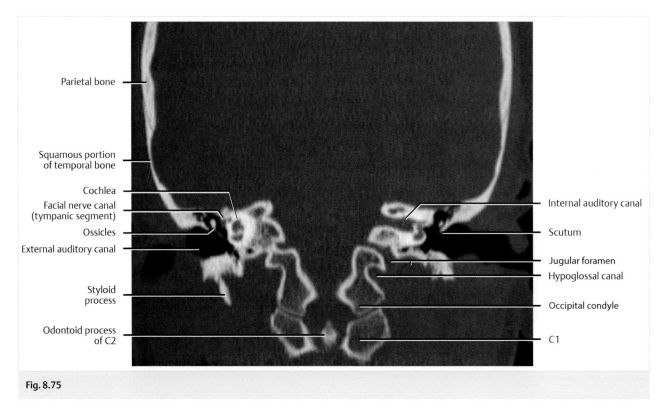

Parietal bone

Squamous portion
of temporal bone

Cochlea

Facial nerve canal
(tympanic segment)

Ossicles

External auditory canal

Styloid
process

Odontoid process
of C2

Internal auditory canal

Scutum

Jugular foramen

Hypoglossal canal

Occipital condyle

C1

**Fig. 8.75**

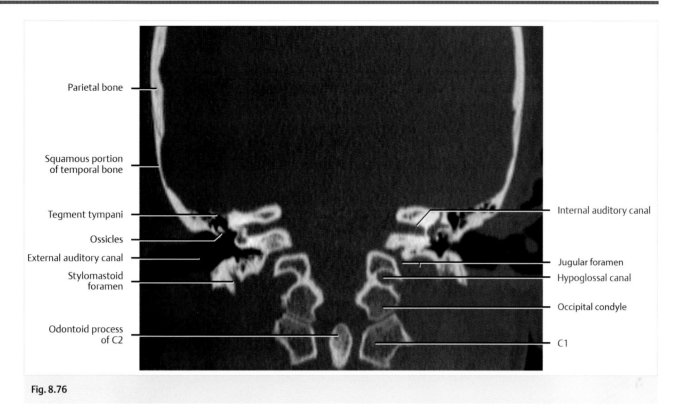

Parietal bone

Squamous portion of temporal bone

Tegment tympani

Ossicles

External auditory canal

Stylomastoid foramen

Odontoid process of C2

Internal auditory canal

Jugular foramen

Hypoglossal canal

Occipital condyle

C1

Fig. 8.76

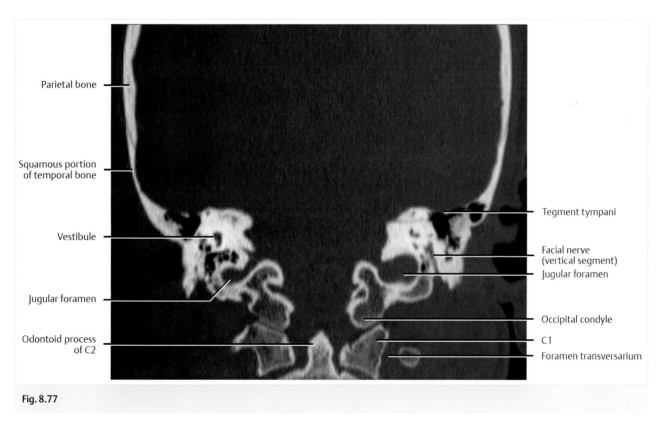

Parietal bone

Squamous portion of temporal bone

Vestibule

Jugular foramen

Odontoid process of C2

Tegment tympani

Facial nerve (vertical segment)

Jugular foramen

Occipital condyle

C1

Foramen transversarium

Fig. 8.77

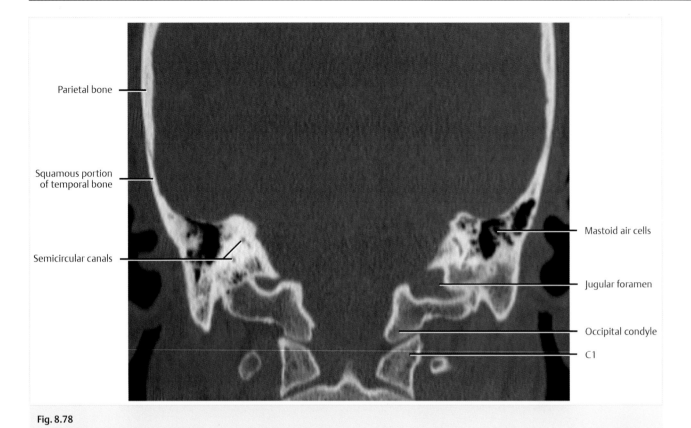

Parietal bone

Squamous portion of temporal bone

Semicircular canals

Mastoid air cells

Jugular foramen

Occipital condyle

C1

Fig. 8.78

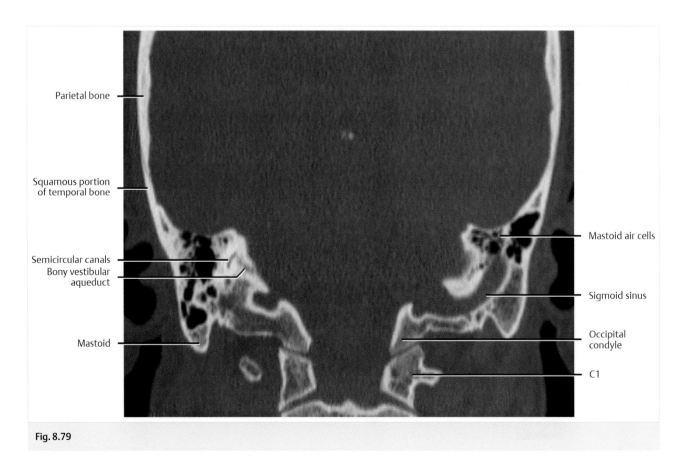

Parietal bone

Squamous portion of temporal bone

Semicircular canals
Bony vestibular aqueduct

Mastoid

Mastoid air cells

Sigmoid sinus

Occipital condyle

C1

Fig. 8.79

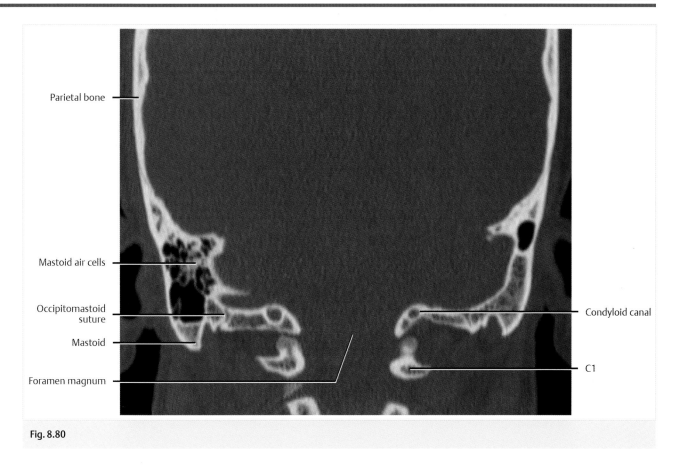

Parietal bone

Mastoid air cells

Occipitomastoid suture

Mastoid

Foramen magnum

Condyloid canal

C1

Fig. 8.80

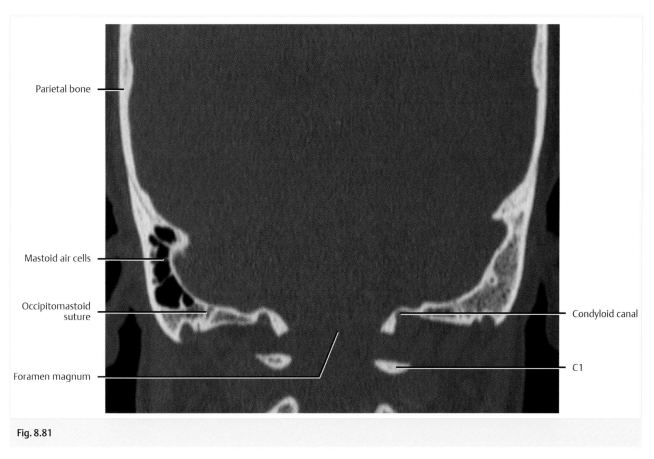

Parietal bone

Mastoid air cells

Occipitomastoid suture

Foramen magnum

Condyloid canal

C1

Fig. 8.81

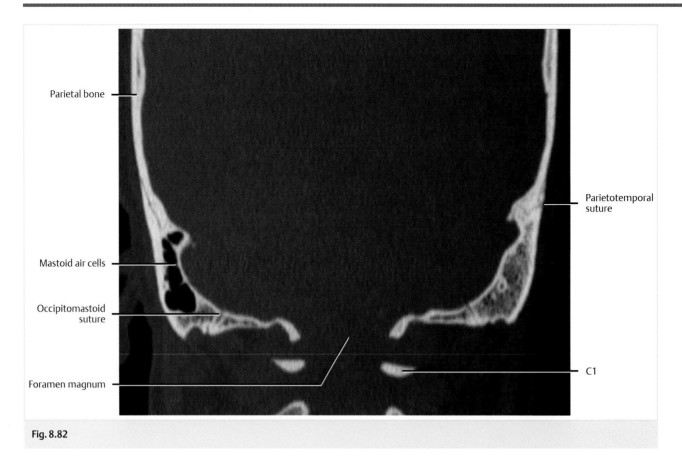

Parietal bone

Mastoid air cells

Occipitomastoid suture

Foramen magnum

Parietotemporal suture

C1

**Fig. 8.82**

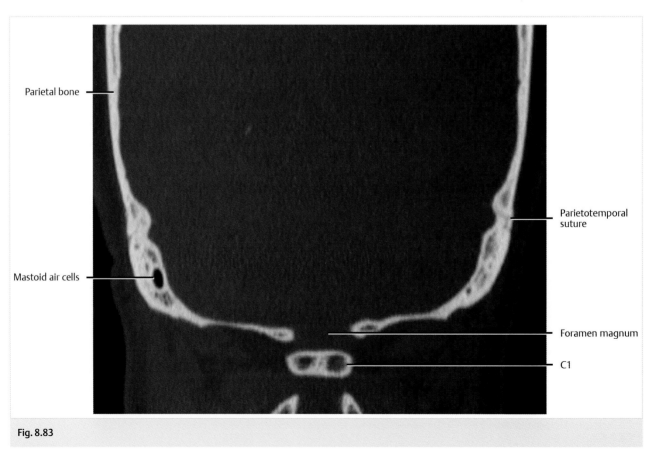

Parietal bone

Mastoid air cells

Parietotemporal suture

Foramen magnum

C1

**Fig. 8.83**

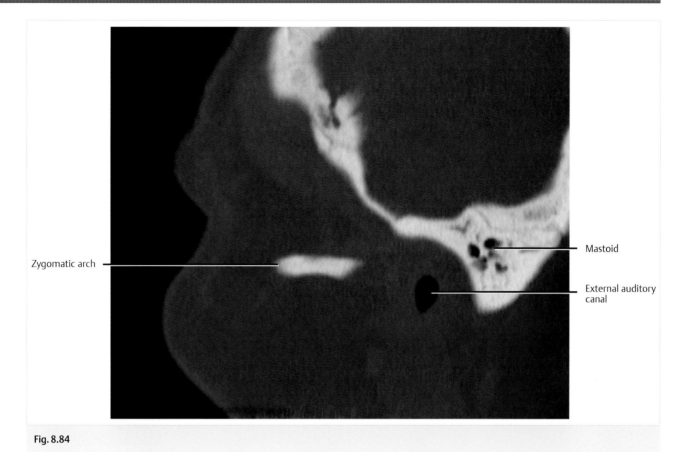

Zygomatic arch

Mastoid

External auditory canal

**Fig. 8.84**

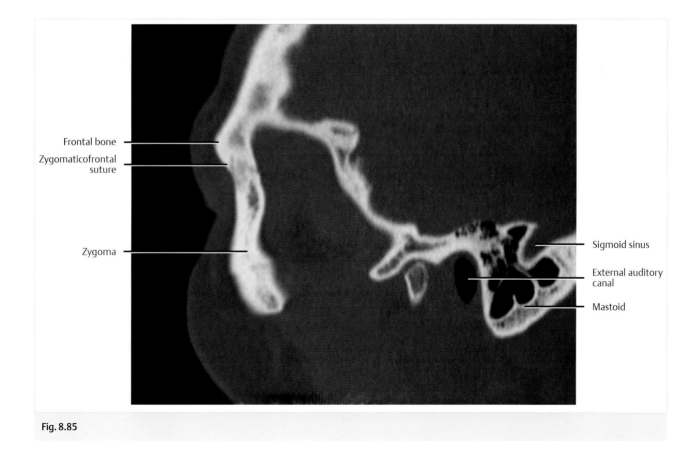

Frontal bone

Zygomaticofrontal suture

Zygoma

Sigmoid sinus

External auditory canal

Mastoid

**Fig. 8.85**

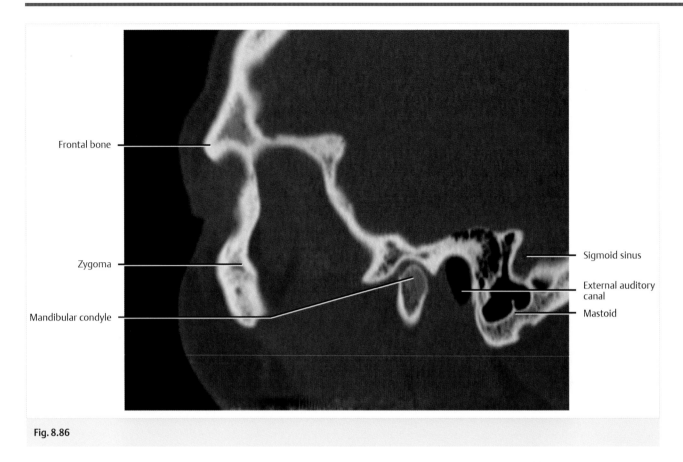

Frontal bone

Zygoma

Mandibular condyle

Sigmoid sinus

External auditory canal

Mastoid

Fig. 8.86

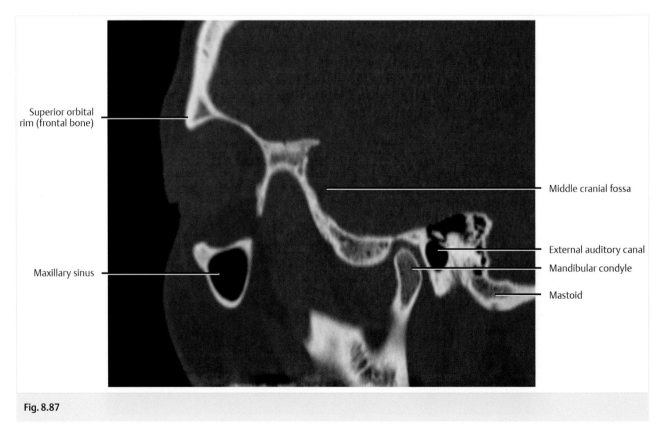

Superior orbital rim (frontal bone)

Maxillary sinus

Middle cranial fossa

External auditory canal

Mandibular condyle

Mastoid

Fig. 8.87

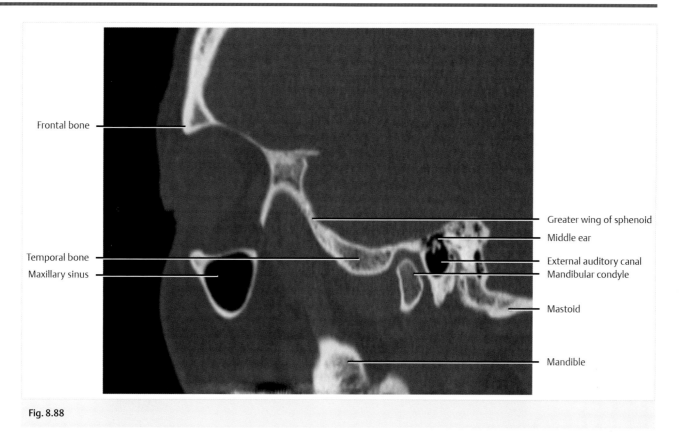

Frontal bone

Greater wing of sphenoid
Middle ear
Temporal bone
Maxillary sinus
External auditory canal
Mandibular condyle

Mastoid

Mandible

**Fig. 8.88**

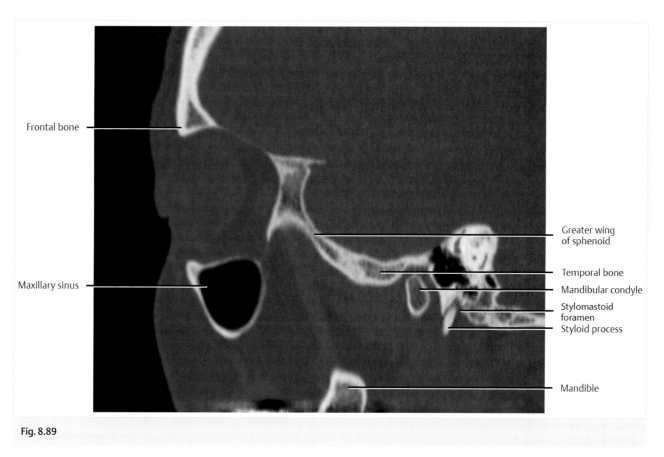

Frontal bone

Greater wing
of sphenoid

Temporal bone

Maxillary sinus
Mandibular condyle

Stylomastoid
foramen
Styloid process

Mandible

**Fig. 8.89**

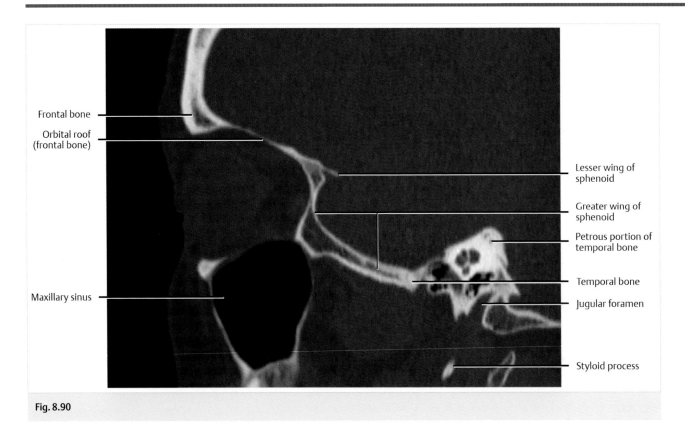

Frontal bone

Orbital roof
(frontal bone)

Maxillary sinus

Lesser wing of
sphenoid

Greater wing of
sphenoid

Petrous portion of
temporal bone

Temporal bone

Jugular foramen

Styloid process

Fig. 8.90

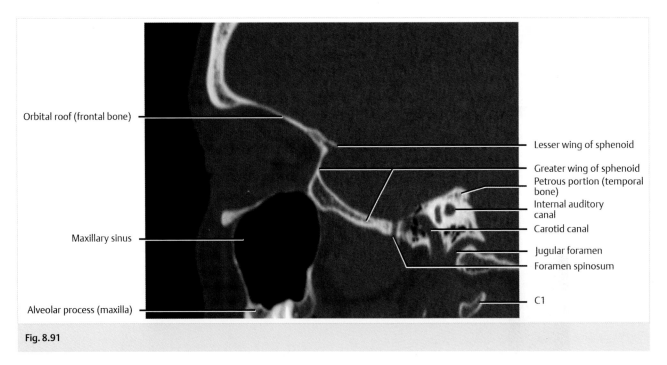

Orbital roof (frontal bone)

Maxillary sinus

Alveolar process (maxilla)

Lesser wing of sphenoid

Greater wing of sphenoid
Petrous portion (temporal bone)
Internal auditory canal

Carotid canal

Jugular foramen
Foramen spinosum

C1

Fig. 8.91

reformats in different planes is important and provides an appreciation of a variety of important structures and their relationships from different perspectives. The superior orbital fissure is a cleft between the lesser and greater wings of the sphenoid through which cranial nerves (III, IV, V1, VI) and the superior ophthalmic vein traverse into the orbit. The inferior orbital fissure transmits the zygomatic branch of V2 (maxillary division of trigeminal nerve) and the inferior ophthalmic vein. The inferior orbital fissure is also in continuity with the superior aspect of the PPF, an important site of anatomic convergence of multiple neural pathways. The PPF is an important elongated, vertically oriented, predominantly fat-filled region located lateral to the posterior aspect of the nasal cavity that has an important relationship to the skull base and paranasal

(*text continued on page 236*)

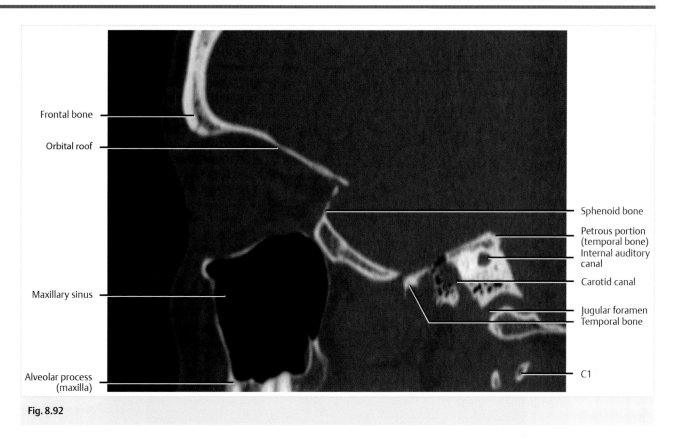

Frontal bone

Orbital roof

Maxillary sinus

Alveolar process
(maxilla)

Sphenoid bone

Petrous portion
(temporal bone)

Internal auditory
canal

Carotid canal

Jugular foramen
Temporal bone

C1

**Fig. 8.92**

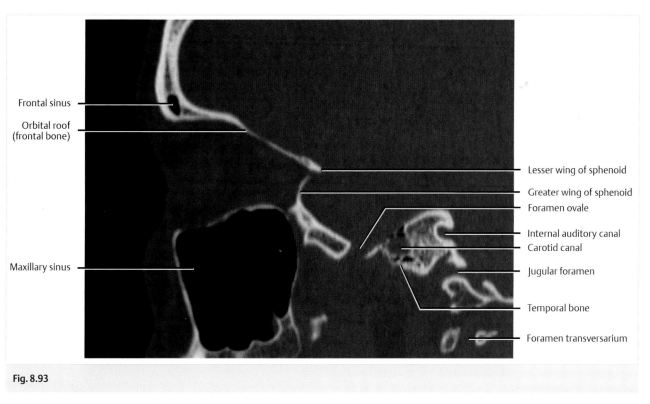

Frontal sinus

Orbital roof
(frontal bone)

Maxillary sinus

Lesser wing of sphenoid

Greater wing of sphenoid

Foramen ovale

Internal auditory canal

Carotid canal

Jugular foramen

Temporal bone

Foramen transversarium

**Fig. 8.93**

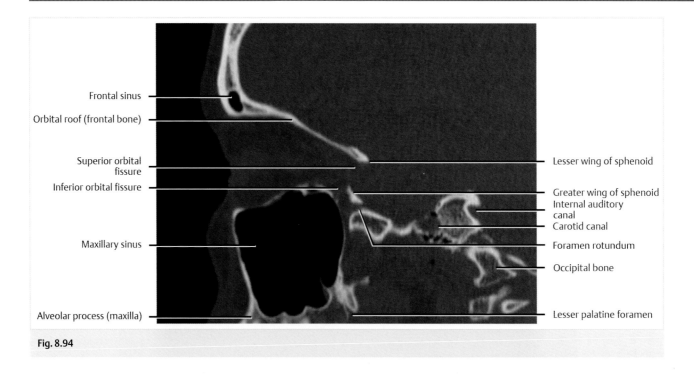

Frontal sinus

Orbital roof (frontal bone)

Superior orbital fissure

Inferior orbital fissure

Maxillary sinus

Alveolar process (maxilla)

Lesser wing of sphenoid

Greater wing of sphenoid
Internal auditory canal

Carotid canal

Foramen rotundum

Occipital bone

Lesser palatine foramen

**Fig. 8.94**

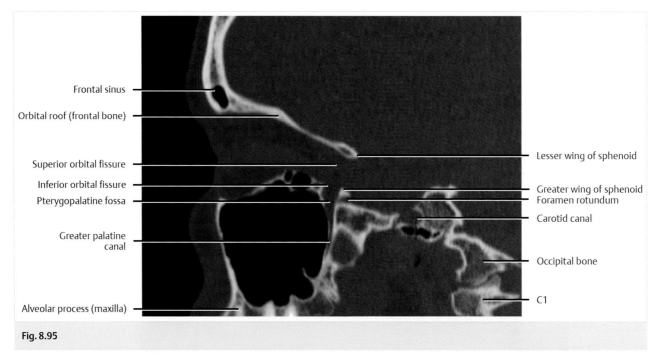

Frontal sinus

Orbital roof (frontal bone)

Superior orbital fissure

Inferior orbital fissure

Pterygopalatine fossa

Greater palatine canal

Alveolar process (maxilla)

Lesser wing of sphenoid

Greater wing of sphenoid
Foramen rotundum

Carotid canal

Occipital bone

C1

**Fig. 8.95**

sinuses. Inferiorly, the PPF tapers into the greater palatine canal, ultimately leading to the greater and lesser palatine foramina. Posteriorly, the foramen rotundum provides a communication between the PPF and the middle cranial fossa, transmitting the maxillary (V2) branch of the trigeminal nerve, artery of foramen rotundum, and emissary veins. More posteriorly in the central skull base, the foramen ovale transmits the mandibular (V3) branch of the trigeminal nerve, lesser petrosal nerve, accessory meningeal branch of maxillary artery, and emissary vein, and provides a direct communication between the cranial cavity and the masticator space.

Sagittal reformats from high-resolution CT images without contrast (► Fig. 8.96, ► Fig. 8.97, ► Fig. 8.98, ► Fig. 8.99). CT is excellent for the evaluation of detailed skull base and paranasal sinus bony anatomy. The ability to create high-resolution reformats in different planes is important and provides an appreciation of a variety of important structures and their relationships from different perspectives. The optic nerve and ophthalmic artery pass through the optic canal where variations such as dehiscence and/or pneumatization of the anterior clinoid process have an increased association with optic nerve exposure and considered an indicator of optic nerve vulnerability during

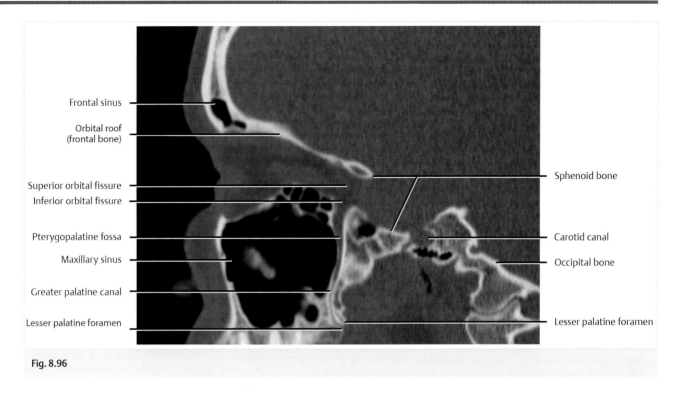

Frontal sinus

Orbital roof
(frontal bone)

Superior orbital fissure

Inferior orbital fissure

Pterygopalatine fossa

Maxillary sinus

Greater palatine canal

Lesser palatine foramen

Sphenoid bone

Carotid canal

Occipital bone

Lesser palatine foramen

**Fig. 8.96**

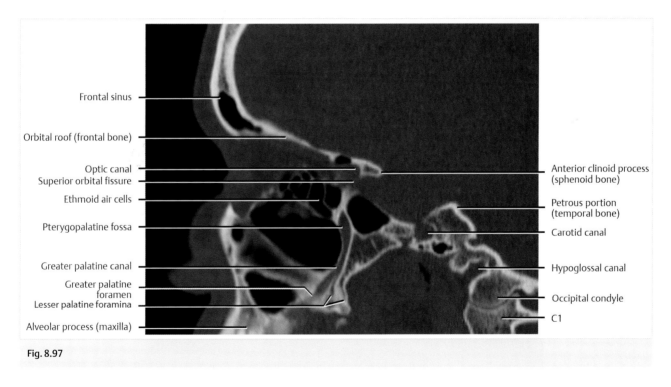

Frontal sinus

Orbital roof (frontal bone)

Optic canal

Superior orbital fissure

Ethmoid air cells

Pterygopalatine fossa

Greater palatine canal

Greater palatine
foramen

Lesser palatine foramina

Alveolar process (maxilla)

Anterior clinoid process
(sphenoid bone)

Petrous portion
(temporal bone)

Carotid canal

Hypoglossal canal

Occipital condyle

C1

**Fig. 8.97**

endoscopic sinus surgery. The superior orbital fissure is a cleft between the lesser and greater wings of the sphenoid through which cranial nerves (III, IV, V1, VI) and the superior ophthalmic vein traverse into the orbit. The inferior orbital fissure transmits the zygomatic branch of V2 (maxillary division of trigeminal nerve) and the inferior ophthalmic vein. The inferior orbital fissure is also in continuity with the superior aspect of the PPF, an important site of anatomic convergence of multiple

neural pathways. The PPF is an important elongated, vertically oriented, predominantly fat-filled region located lateral to the posterior aspect of the nasal cavity that has an important relationship to the skull base and paranasal sinuses. Inferiorly, the PPF tapers into the greater palatine canal, ultimately leading to the greater and lesser palatine foramina. The greater palatine foramen transmits the greater palatine nerve and descending palatine vessels. The lesser palatine foramen transmits the

(*text continued on page 239*)

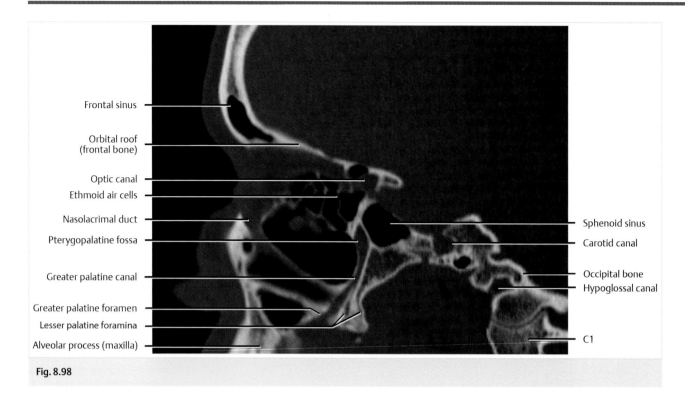

Frontal sinus

Orbital roof
(frontal bone)

Optic canal

Ethmoid air cells

Nasolacrimal duct

Pterygopalatine fossa

Greater palatine canal

Greater palatine foramen

Lesser palatine foramina

Alveolar process (maxilla)

Sphenoid sinus

Carotid canal

Occipital bone

Hypoglossal canal

C1

**Fig. 8.98**

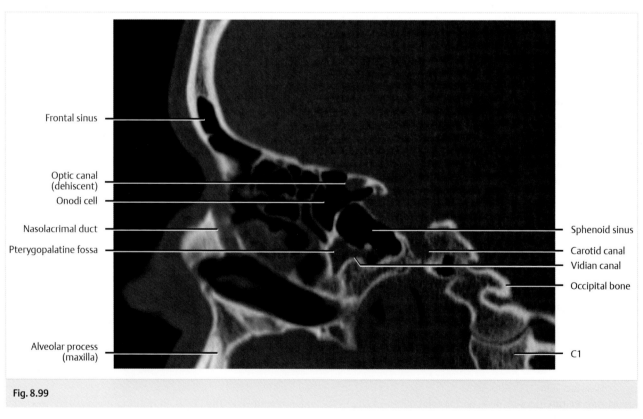

Frontal sinus

Optic canal
(dehiscent)

Onodi cell

Nasolacrimal duct

Pterygopalatine fossa

Alveolar process
(maxilla)

Sphenoid sinus

Carotid canal

Vidian canal

Occipital bone

C1

**Fig. 8.99**

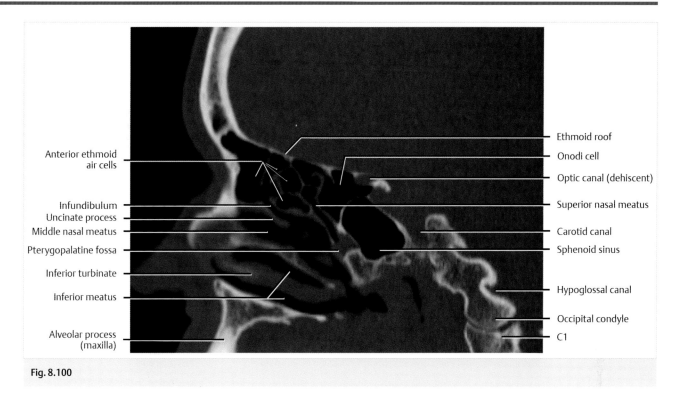

Anterior ethmoid air cells

Infundibulum
Uncinate process
Middle nasal meatus
Pterygopalatine fossa

Inferior turbinate

Inferior meatus

Alveolar process (maxilla)

Ethmoid roof
Onodi cell
Optic canal (dehiscent)
Superior nasal meatus

Carotid canal
Sphenoid sinus

Hypoglossal canal

Occipital condyle
C1

**Fig. 8.100**

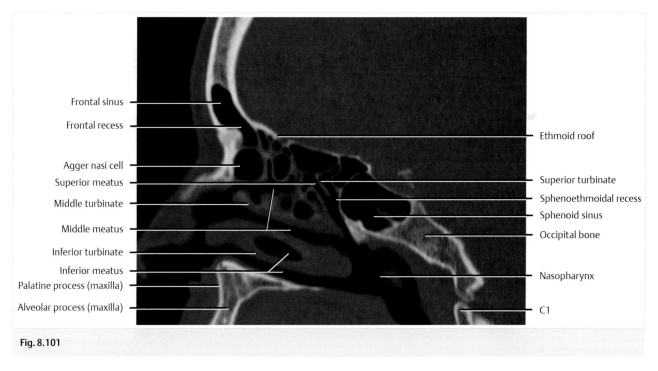

Frontal sinus

Frontal recess

Agger nasi cell
Superior meatus

Middle turbinate

Middle meatus

Inferior turbinate
Inferior meatus
Palatine process (maxilla)

Alveolar process (maxilla)

Ethmoid roof

Superior turbinate
Sphenoethmoidal recess
Sphenoid sinus
Occipital bone

Nasopharynx

C1

**Fig. 8.101**

lesser palatine nerves. Although commonly single, there can be two or rarely more than two lesser palatine foramina. Posteriorly, the foramen rotundum provides a communication between the PPF and the middle cranial fossa, transmitting the maxillary (V2) branch of the trigeminal nerve, artery of foramen rotundum, and emissary veins. More posteriorly in the central skull base, the foramen ovale transmits the mandibular (V3) branch of the trigeminal nerve, lesser petrosal nerve, accessory meningeal branch of maxillary artery, and emissary vein, and provides a direct communication between the cranial cavity and the masticator space. In the posterior skull base, the hypoglossal canal transmits cranial nerve XII.

Sagittal reformats from high-resolution CT images without contrast (▶ Fig. 8.100, ▶ Fig. 8.101, ▶ Fig. 8.102, ▶ Fig. 8.103). CT is excellent for the evaluation of detailed skull base and paranasal sinus bony anatomy. This includes visualization of important paranasal sinus anatomy, such as the complex anatomy of the middle turbinate and structures of the OMU. The OMU

(*text continued on page 241*)

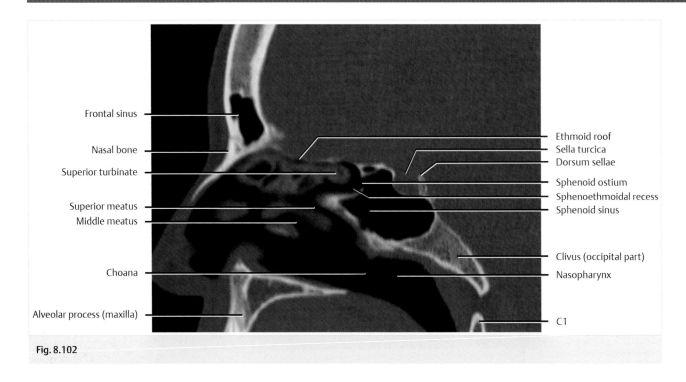

Frontal sinus

Nasal bone

Superior turbinate

Superior meatus

Middle meatus

Choana

Alveolar process (maxilla)

Ethmoid roof

Sella turcica

Dorsum sellae

Sphenoid ostium

Sphenoethmoidal recess

Sphenoid sinus

Clivus (occipital part)

Nasopharynx

C1

**Fig. 8.102**

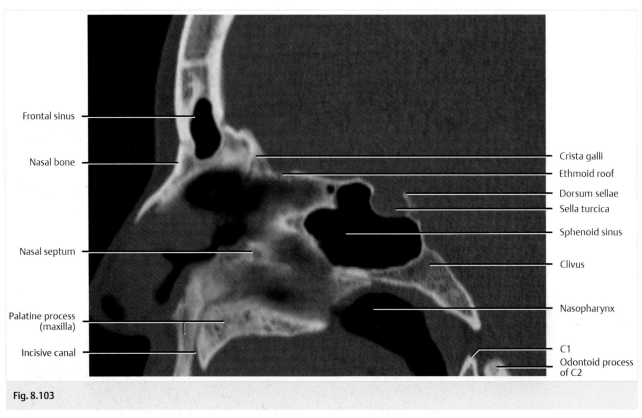

Frontal sinus

Nasal bone

Nasal septum

Palatine process (maxilla)

Incisive canal

Crista galli

Ethmoid roof

Dorsum sellae

Sella turcica

Sphenoid sinus

Clivus

Nasopharynx

C1

Odontoid process of C2

**Fig. 8.103**

refs to a functional unit of structures draining the frontal, anterior ethmoid, and maxillary sinuses, and includes the middle meatus, ethmoid bulla, uncinate process, hiatus semilunaris, infundibulum, and superomedial maxillary sinus/maxillary sinus ostium.

## 8.3 Magnetic Resonance Imaging: Anatomy of the Sella, Cavernous Sinus, and Posterior Fossa

### 8.3.1 Anatomy of the Sella

#### Coronal T2-Weighted Magnetic Resonance Imaging

The sella is a concave midline depression in the central skull base (basisphenoid) and contains the pituitary gland or hypophysis (▶ Fig. 8.104, ▶ Fig. 8.105, ▶ Fig. 8.106, ▶ Fig. 8.107). The pituitary gland consists of the larger adenohypophysis (anteriorly) and the smaller neurohypophysis posteriorly, with a small pars intermedia in between. The pituitary stalk or

infundibulum is the midline structure that extends from the median eminence of hypothalamus to the pituitary gland. There are multiple important relations of the sella and pituitary gland including the optic pathways/chiasm superiorly, cavernous sinuses laterally, and the sphenoid bone and sphenoid sinus inferiorly.

#### Sagittal T2-Weighted Magnetic Resonance Imaging

The sella is a concave midline depression in the central skull base (basisphenoid) and contains the pituitary gland or hypophysis (▶ Fig. 8.108, ▶ Fig. 8.109). The pituitary gland consists of the larger adenohypophysis (anteriorly) and the smaller neurohypophysis posteriorly, with a small pars intermedia in between. The pituitary stalk or infundibulum is the midline structure that extends from the median eminence of hypothalamus to the pituitary gland. There are multiple important relations of the sella and pituitary gland including the optic pathways/chiasm superiorly, cavernous sinuses laterally, and the sphenoid bone and sphenoid sinus inferiorly.

(*text continued on page 244*)

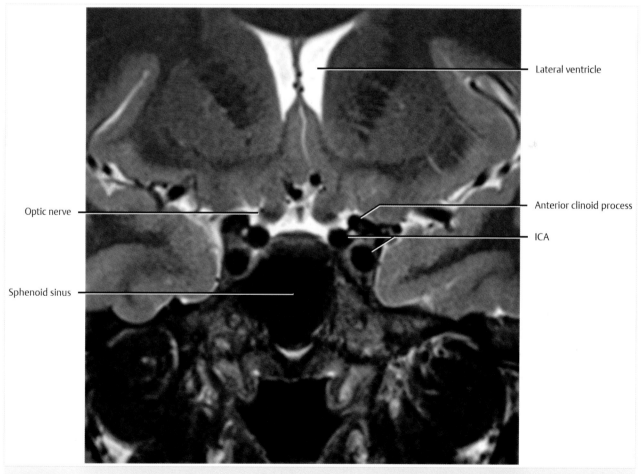

Fig. 8.104

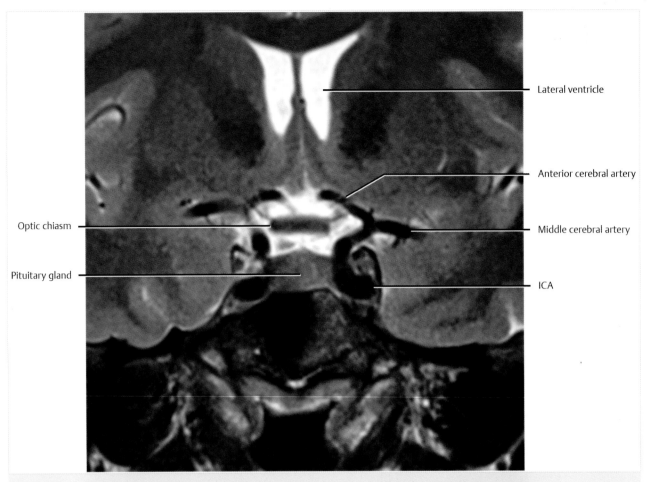

Lateral ventricle

Anterior cerebral artery

Optic chiasm

Middle cerebral artery

Pituitary gland

ICA

Fig. 8.105

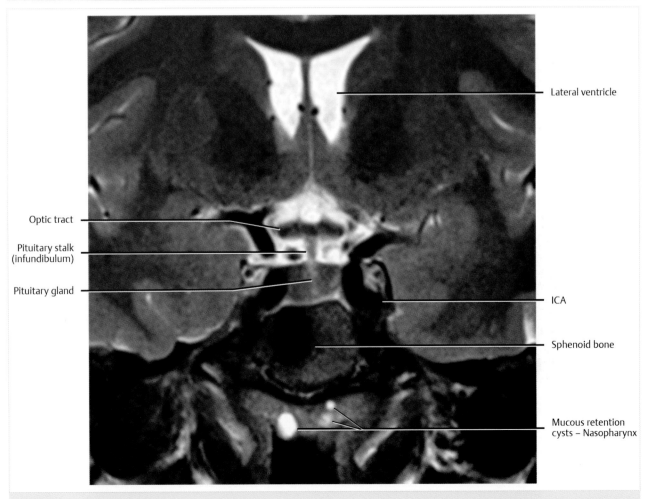

Lateral ventricle

Optic tract

Pituitary stalk
(infundibulum)

Pituitary gland

ICA

Sphenoid bone

Mucous retention
cysts – Nasopharynx

Fig. 8.106

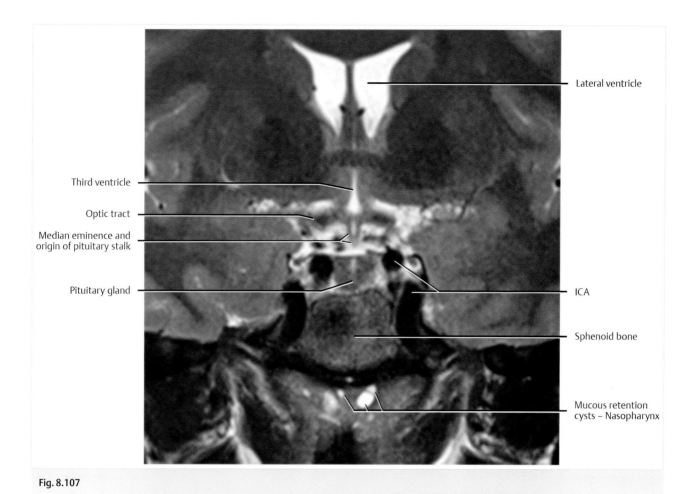

Lateral ventricle

Third ventricle

Optic tract

Median eminence and origin of pituitary stalk

Pituitary gland

ICA

Sphenoid bone

Mucous retention cysts – Nasopharynx

**Fig. 8.107**

Corpus callosum

Lateral ventricle

Third ventricle

Chiasmatic and infundibular recess, third ventricle

Optic chiasm

Pituitary stalk (infundibulum)

Pituitary gland

Sphenoid sinus

Mamillary body

Median eminence

**Fig. 8.108**

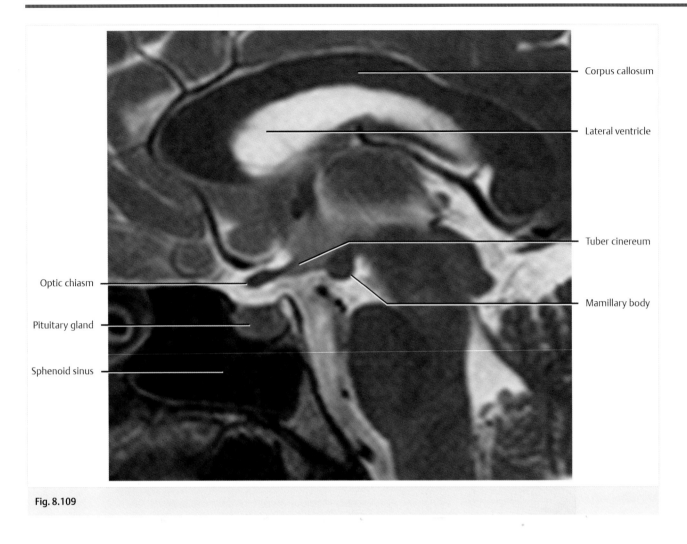

Corpus callosum

Lateral ventricle

Tuber cinereum

Optic chiasm

Mamillary body

Pituitary gland

Sphenoid sinus

**Fig. 8.109**

## Sagittal T1-Weighted C–/C + Magnetic Resonance Imaging

The sella is a concave midline depression in the central skull base (basisphenoid) and contains the pituitary gland or hypophysis (▶ Fig. 8.110, ▶ Fig. 8.111). The pituitary gland consists of the larger adenohypophysis (anteriorly) and the smaller neurohypophysis posteriorly, with a small pars intermedia in between. The pituitary stalk or infundibulum is the midline structure that extends from the median eminence of hypothalamus to the pituitary gland. On T1-weighted images performed without contrast, the neurohypophysis typically has high signal secondary to its content that includes vasopressin and oxytocin. After administration of contrast, the pituitary gland demonstrates strong enhancement. There are multiple important relations of the sella and pituitary gland including the optic pathways/chiasm superiorly, cavernous sinuses laterally, and the sphenoid bone and sphenoid sinus inferiorly.

## Coronal T1-Weighted C–/C + Magnetic Resonance Imaging

The sella is a concave midline depression in the central skull base (basisphenoid) and contains the pituitary gland or hypophysis (▶ Fig. 8.112, ▶ Fig. 8.113). The pituitary gland consists of the larger adenohypophysis (anteriorly) and the smaller neurohypophysis posteriorly, with a small pars intermedia in between. The pituitary stalk or infundibulum is the midline structure that extends from the median eminence of hypothalamus to the pituitary gland. There are multiple important relations of the sella and pituitary gland including the optic pathways/chiasm superiorly, cavernous sinuses laterally, and the sphenoid bone and sphenoid sinus inferiorly.

(*text continued on page 247*)

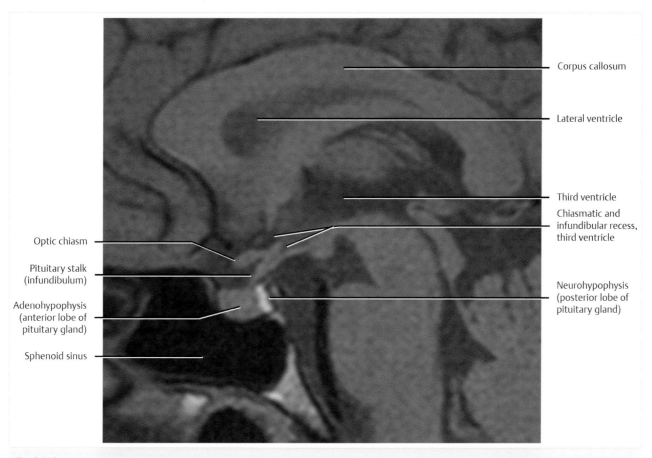

Corpus callosum

Lateral ventricle

Third ventricle

Chiasmatic and
infundibular recess,
third ventricle

Optic chiasm

Pituitary stalk
(infundibulum)

Adenohypophysis
(anterior lobe of
pituitary gland)

Neurohypophysis
(posterior lobe of
pituitary gland)

Sphenoid sinus

Fig. 8.110

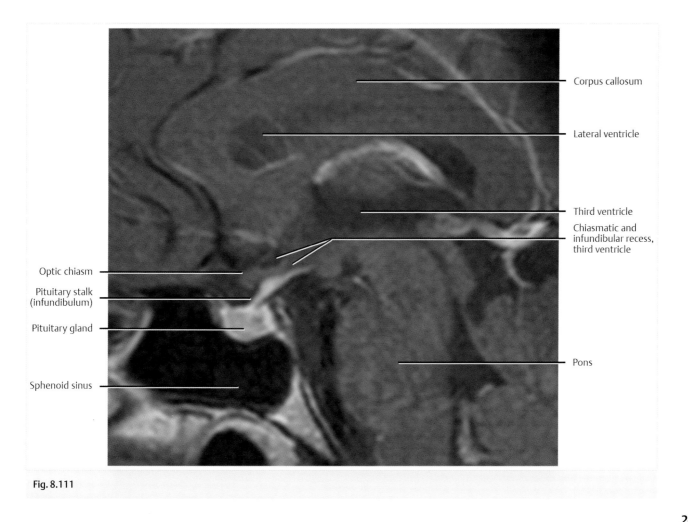

Corpus callosum

Lateral ventricle

Third ventricle

Chiasmatic and
infundibular recess,
third ventricle

Optic chiasm

Pituitary stalk
(infundibulum)

Pituitary gland

Pons

Sphenoid sinus

Fig. 8.111

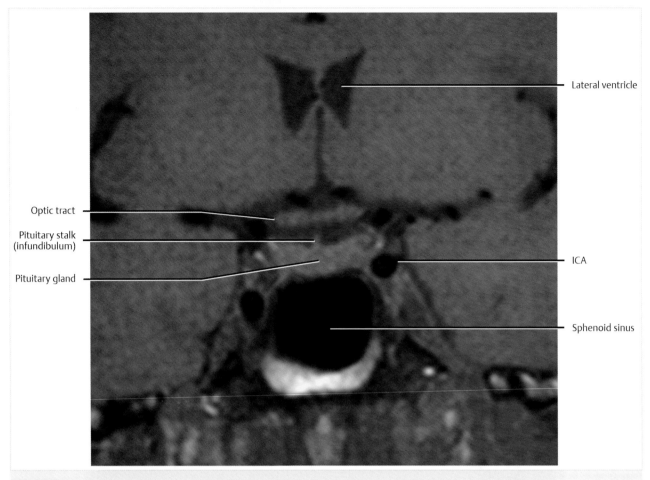

Optic tract

Pituitary stalk (infundibulum)

Pituitary gland

Lateral ventricle

ICA

Sphenoid sinus

Fig. 8.112

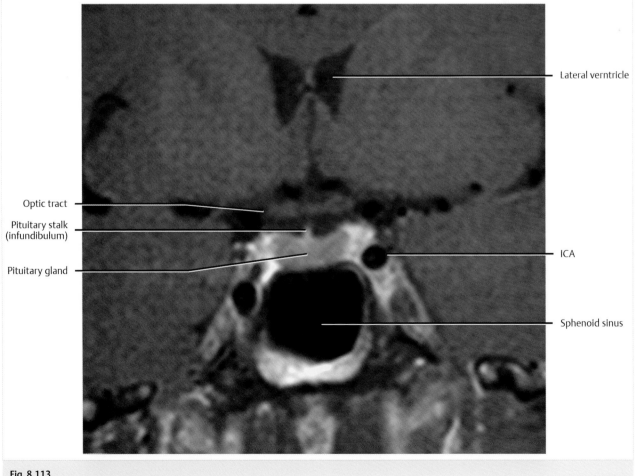

Optic tract

Pituitary stalk (infundibulum)

Pituitary gland

Lateral verntricle

ICA

Sphenoid sinus

Fig. 8.113

## 8.3.2 Cavernous Sinus

### Coronal T1-Weighted C + Magnetic Resonance Imaging

The cavernous sinuses are the paired dural-lined venous sinuses on each side of the sella where the cavernous segment of the internal carotid artery and accompanying sympathetic plexus are also located (▶ Fig. 8.114, ▶ Fig. 8.115). In addition to the vascular component, the cavernous sinuses contain multiple cranial nerves that may be visible on high-resolution MR images. These include cranial nerves III, IV, V1 (ophthalmic division of trigeminal nerve), and V2 (maxillary division of trigeminal nerve), located along the lateral cavernous sinus wall from superior to inferior, respectively. Cranial nerve VI lies more medially within the cavernous sinus proper rather than along its lateral wall. Cranial nerve V3 (mandibular division of trigeminal) does not travel within the cavernous sinus. It extends from Meckel's cave into foramen ovale inferiorly.

## 8.3.3 Posterior Fossa

### Axial SPACE Magnetic Resonance Imaging

Multiple important structures including the cranial nerves, vessels, cisterns, foramina, and their relationships can be seen with a high level of detail on high-resolution MR images through the posterior fossa (▶ Fig. 8.116, ▶ Fig. 8.117, ▶ Fig. 8.118, ▶ Fig. 8.119, ▶ Fig. 8.120, ▶ Fig. 8.121, ▶ Fig. 8.122, ▶ Fig. 8.123, ▶ Fig. 8.124, ▶ Fig. 8.125, ▶ Fig. 8.126, ▶ Fig. 8.127, ▶ Fig. 8.128, ▶ Fig. 8.129, ▶ Fig. 8.130, ▶ Fig. 8.131, ▶ Fig. 8.132, ▶ Fig. 8.133).

### Axial T2 Three-Dimensional Magnetic Resonance Imaging

Multiple important structures including cranial nerves, vessels, cisterns, foramina, and their relationships can be seen with a high level of detail on high-resolution MR images through the posterior fossa (▶ Fig. 8.134, ▶ Fig. 8.135).

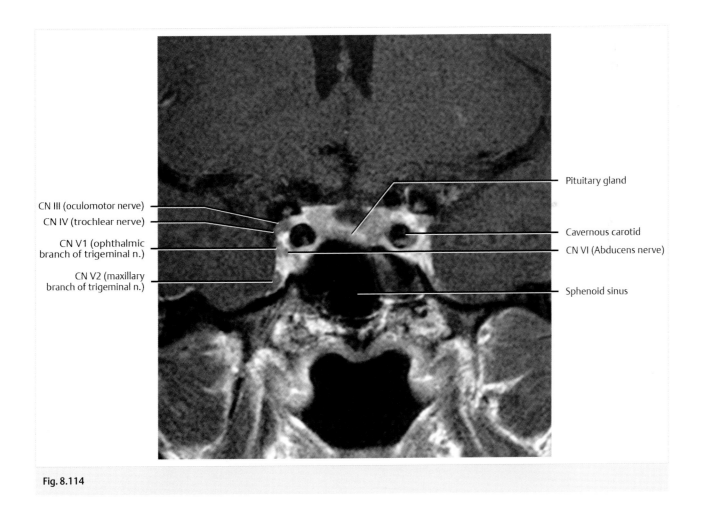

CN III (oculomotor nerve)
CN IV (trochlear nerve)
CN V1 (ophthalmic branch of trigeminal n.)
CN V2 (maxillary branch of trigeminal n.)

Pituitary gland
Cavernous carotid
CN VI (Abducens nerve)
Sphenoid sinus

Fig. 8.114

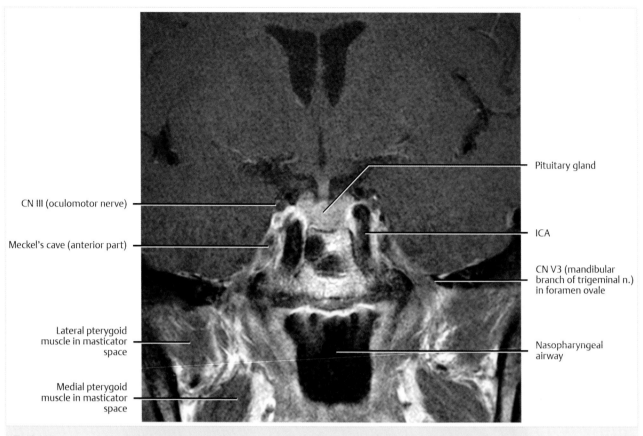

CN III (oculomotor nerve)

Meckel's cave (anterior part)

Lateral pterygoid muscle in masticator space

Medial pterygoid muscle in masticator space

Pituitary gland

ICA

CN V3 (mandibular branch of trigeminal n.) in foramen ovale

Nasopharyngeal airway

Fig. 8.115

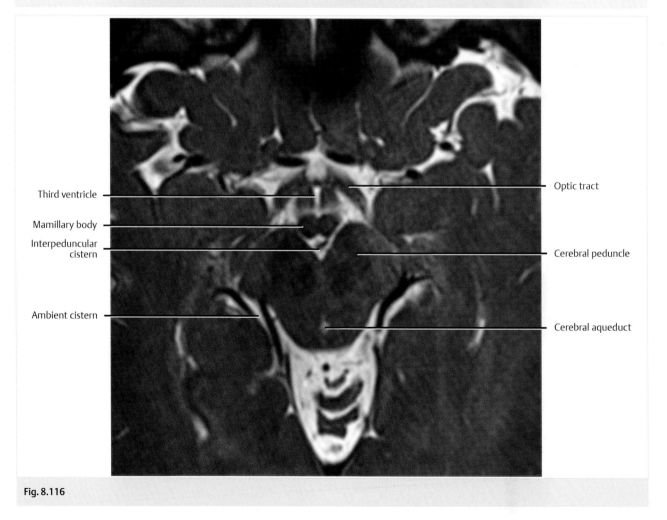

Third ventricle

Mamillary body

Interpeduncular cistern

Ambient cistern

Optic tract

Cerebral peduncle

Cerebral aqueduct

Fig. 8.116

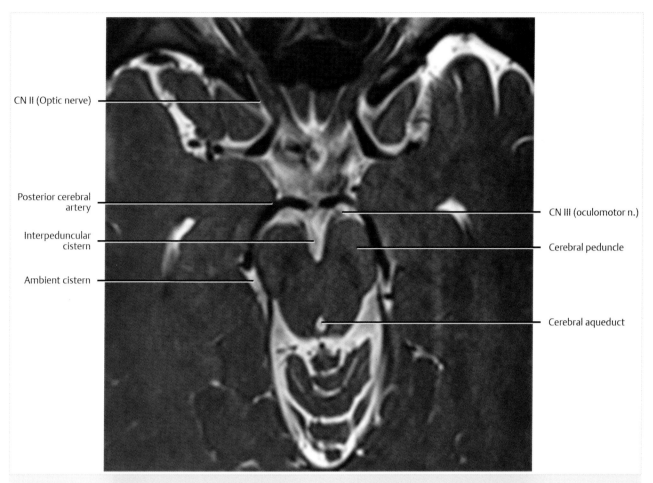

CN II (Optic nerve)

Posterior cerebral artery

Interpeduncular cistern

Ambient cistern

CN III (oculomotor n.)

Cerebral peduncle

Cerebral aqueduct

**Fig. 8.117**

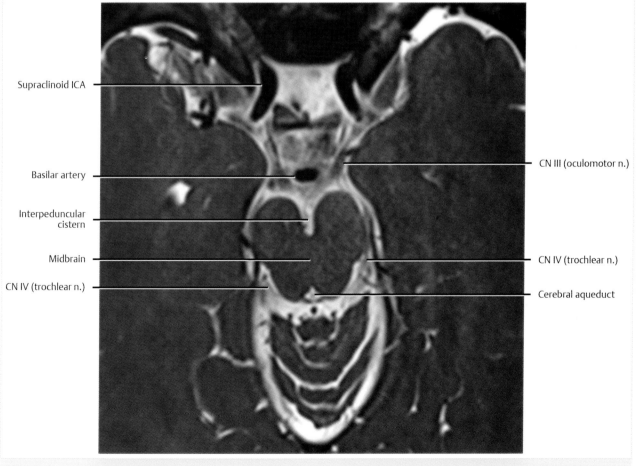

Supraclinoid ICA

Basilar artery

Interpeduncular cistern

Midbrain

CN IV (trochlear n.)

CN III (oculomotor n.)

CN IV (trochlear n.)

Cerebral aqueduct

**Fig. 8.118**

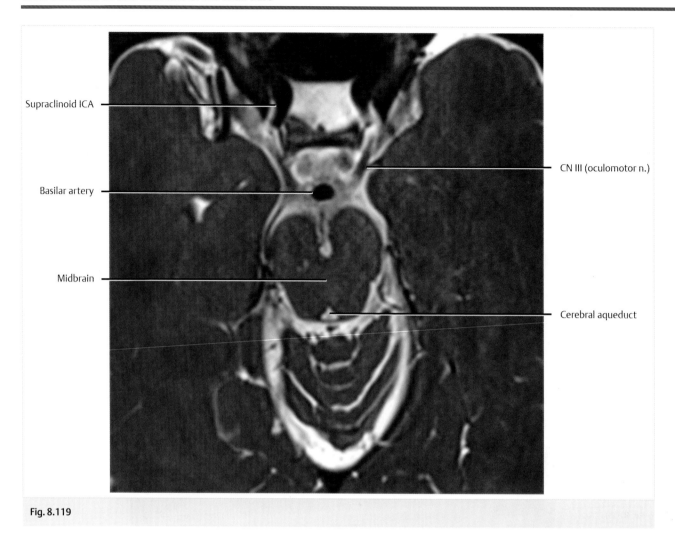

Supraclinoid ICA

Basilar artery

Midbrain

CN III (oculomotor n.)

Cerebral aqueduct

Fig. 8.119

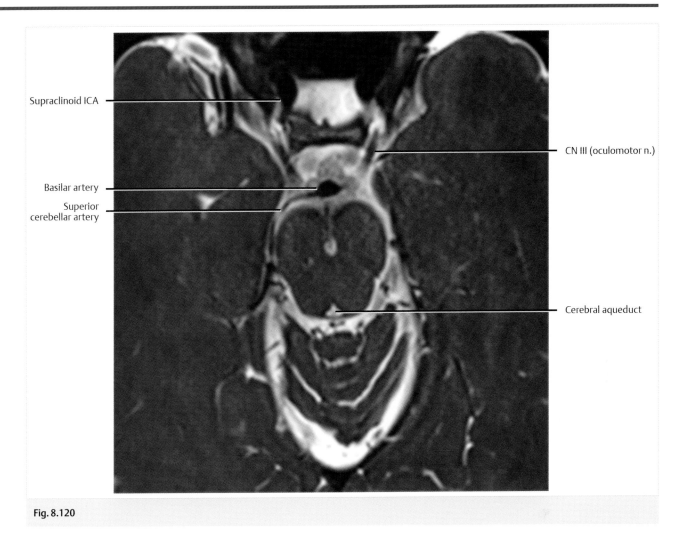

Supraclinoid ICA

CN III (oculomotor n.)

Basilar artery

Superior
cerebellar artery

Cerebral aqueduct

Fig. 8.120

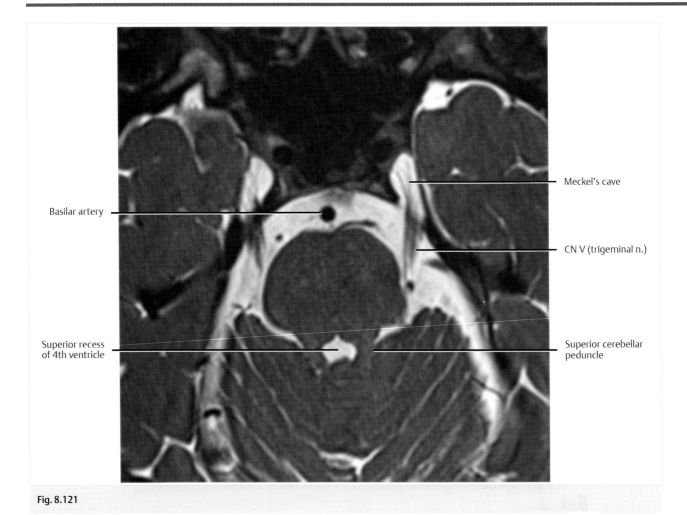

Basilar artery

Meckel's cave

CN V (trigeminal n.)

Superior recess
of 4th ventricle

Superior cerebellar
peduncle

**Fig. 8.121**

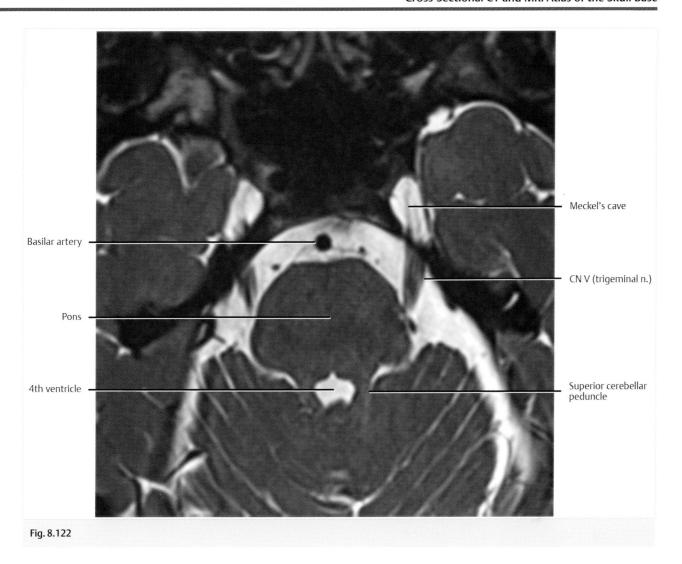

Basilar artery

Pons

4th ventricle

Meckel's cave

CN V (trigeminal n.)

Superior cerebellar peduncle

**Fig. 8.122**

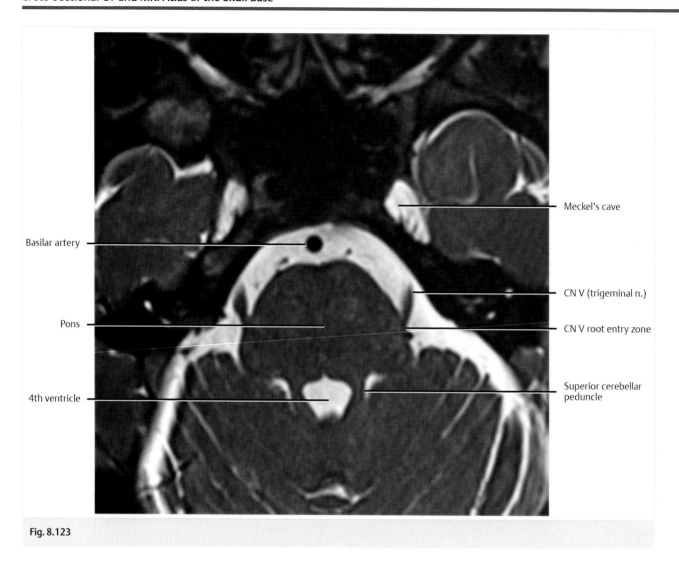

Basilar artery

Pons

4th ventricle

Meckel's cave

CN V (trigeminal n.)

CN V root entry zone

Superior cerebellar peduncle

Fig. 8.123

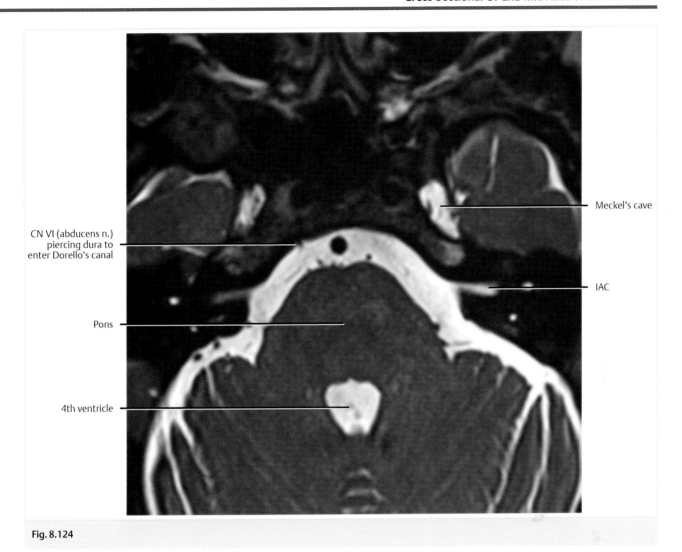

CN VI (abducens n.) piercing dura to enter Dorello's canal

Meckel's cave

IAC

Pons

4th ventricle

**Fig. 8.124**

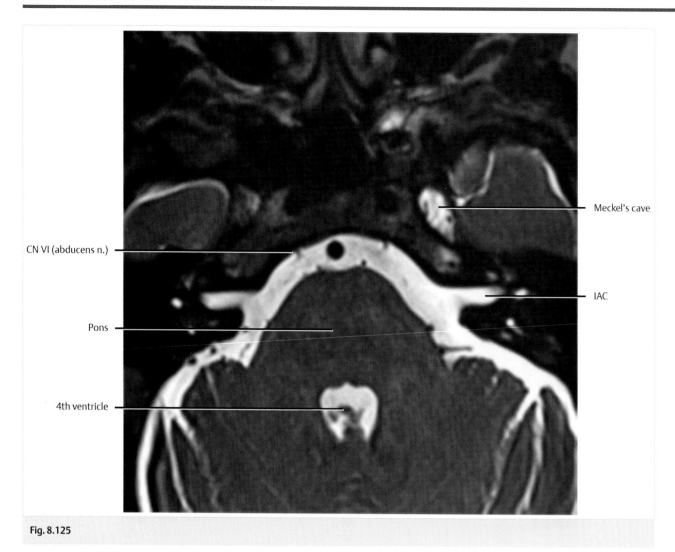

**Fig. 8.125**

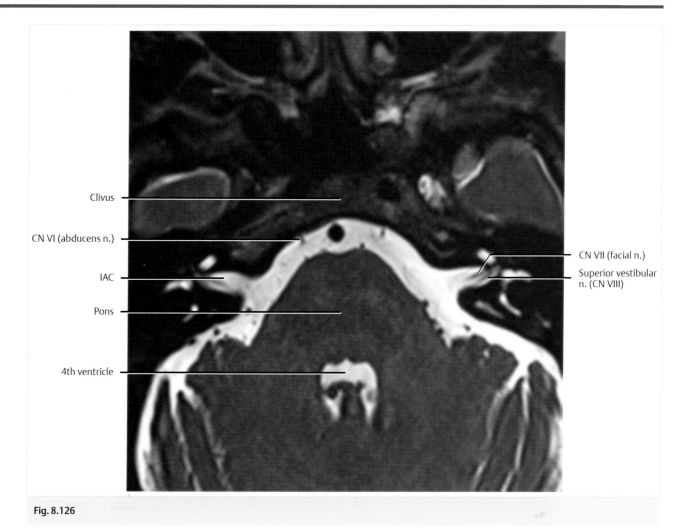

Clivus

CN VI (abducens n.)

IAC

Pons

4th ventricle

CN VII (facial n.)

Superior vestibular n. (CN VIII)

Fig. 8.126

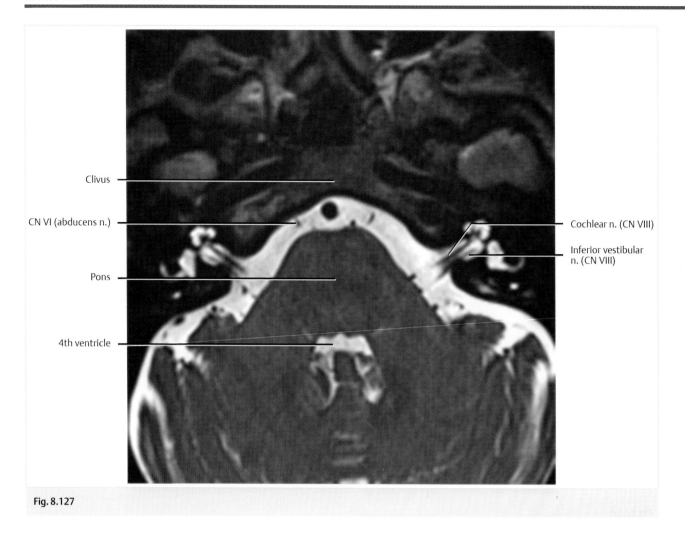

Clivus

CN VI (abducens n.)

Pons

4th ventricle

Cochlear n. (CN VIII)

Inferior vestibular
n. (CN VIII)

**Fig. 8.127**

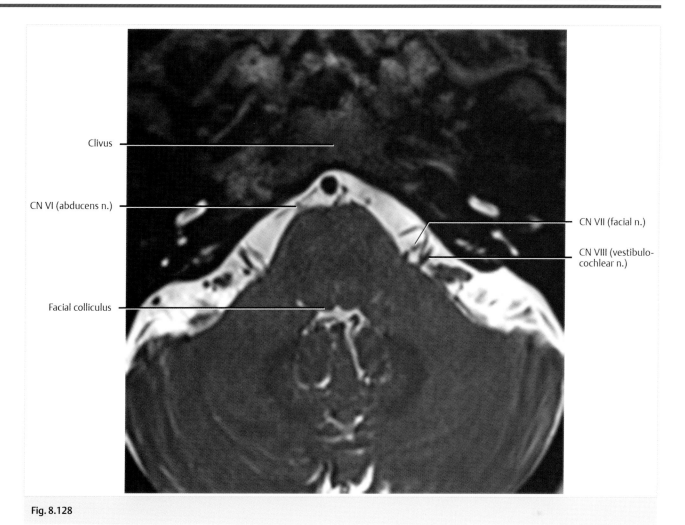

Clivus

CN VI (abducens n.)

Facial colliculus

CN VII (facial n.)

CN VIII (vestibulo-cochlear n.)

**Fig. 8.128**

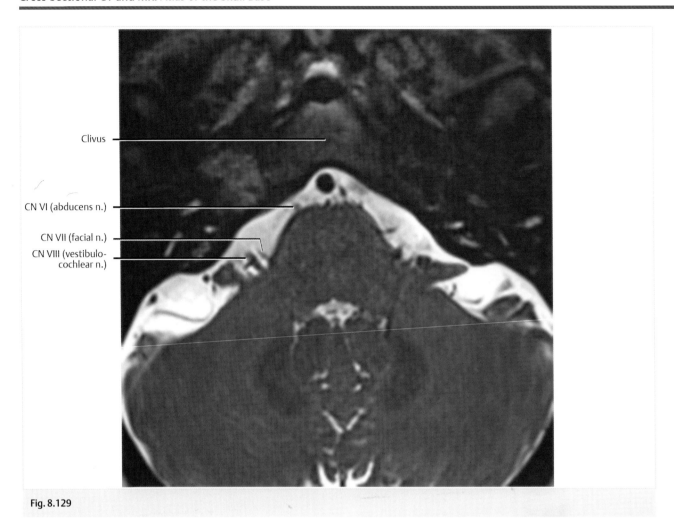

Clivus

CN VI (abducens n.)

CN VII (facial n.)

CN VIII (vestibulo-
cochlear n.)

Fig. 8.129

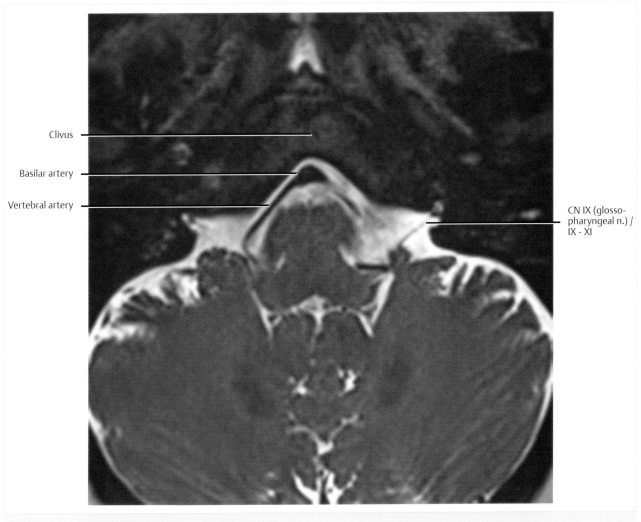

Clivus

Basilar artery

Vertebral artery

CN IX (glosso-pharyngeal n.) / IX - XI

Fig. 8.130

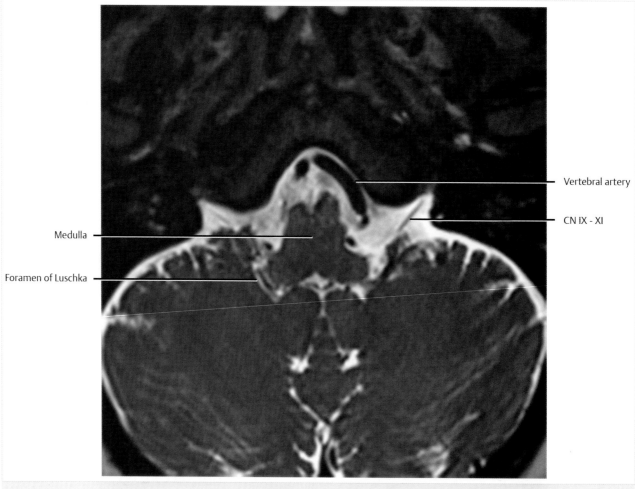

Vertebral artery

CN IX - XI

Medulla

Foramen of Luschka

Fig. 8.131

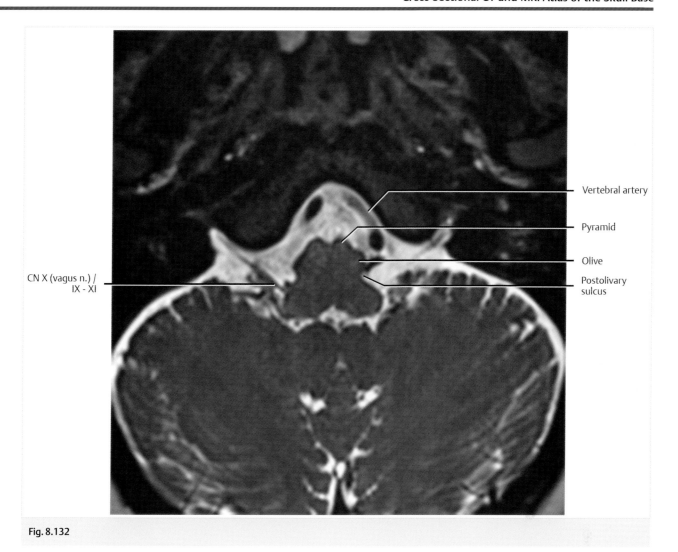

Vertebral artery

Pyramid

Olive

Postolivary sulcus

CN X (vagus n.) /
IX - XI

Fig. 8.132

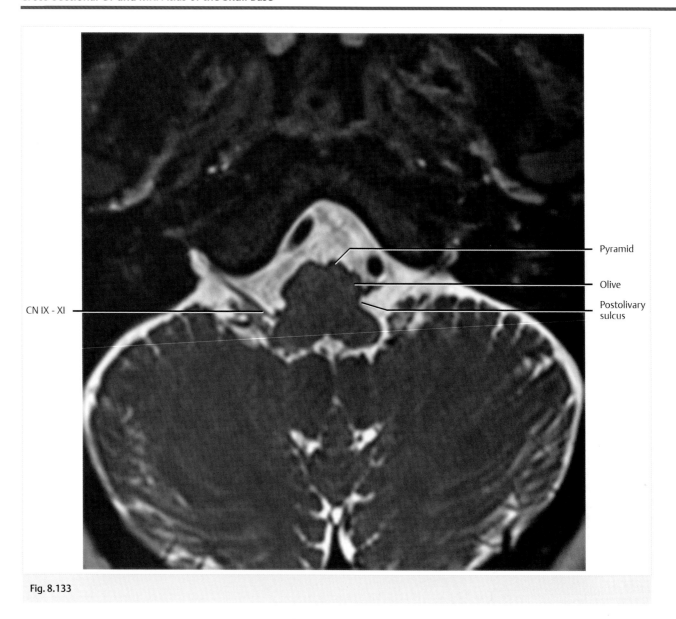

CN IX - XI

Pyramid

Olive

Postolivary
sulcus

Fig. 8.133

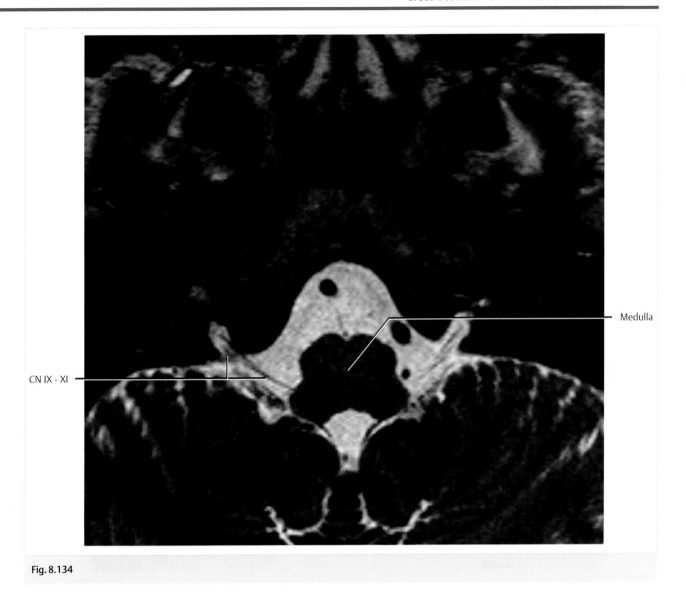

Fig. 8.134

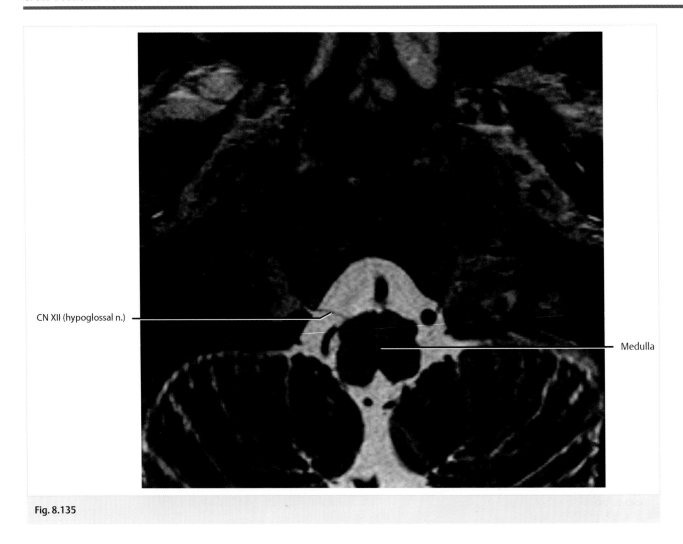

CN XII (hypoglossal n.)

Medulla

Fig. 8.135

# Index

Note: Page numbers set **bold** or *italic* indicate headings or figures, respectively.